Dictionary of Ophthalmic Optics

Dictionary of Ophthalmic Optics

Arthur H. Keeney, M.D., D.SC.
Professor of Ophthalmology,
University of Louisville School of Medicine;
Attending Staff, Department of Ophthalmology,
University of Louisville Hospital, Louisville

Robert E. Hagman, A.B.O.M., F.N.A.O.
Chairman, Ohio State Optical Company,
Columbus, Ohio

Cosmo J. Fratello, M.SC. VOCH. TECH. ED., F.N.A.O.
Professor and Department Head, Emeritus,
Ophthalmic Dispensing Curriculum,
Erie Community College–North Campus, Buffalo

NATIONAL ACADEMY OF OPTICIANRY, INC.

Foreword by
Floyd H. Holmgrain, Jr., ED.D.
Executive Director
National Academy of Opticianry, Inc.
Bowie, Maryland

BUTTERWORTH–HEINEMANN

Boston London Oxford Singapore Sydney Toronto Wellington

Every effort has been made to ensure that the drug dosage schedules within this text are accurate and conform to standards accepted at time of publication. However, as treatment recommendations vary in the light of continuing research and clinical experience, the reader is advised to verify drug dosage schedules herein with information found on product information sheets. This is especially true in cases of new or infrequently used drugs.

Recognizing the importance of preserving what has been written, Butterworth–Heinemann prints its books on acid-free paper whenever possible.

Library of Congress Cataloging-in-Publication Data
Keeney, Arthur H. (Arthur Hail)
Dictionary of ophthalmic optics / Arthur H. Keeney, Cosmo J. Fratello, Robert E. Hagman : foreword by Floyd H. Holmgrain, Jr.
p. cm.
Includes bibliographical references.
ISBN 0-7506-9592-7 (alk. paper)
1. Ophthalmic lenses—Dictionaries. 2. Physiological optics—Dictionaries. I. Fratello, Cosmo J. II. Hagman, Robert E.
[DNLM: 1. Optics—dictionaries. 2. Optometry—dictionaries. 3. Lenses—dictionaries. WW 13 K26d 1994]
RE976.K43 1995
617.7'5'03--dc20
DNLM/DLC
for Library of Congress 94-38287
CIP

British Library Cataloguing-in-Publication Data
A catalogue record for this book is available from the British Library.

Butterworth–Heinemann
313 Washington Street
Newton, MA 02158

10 9 8 7 6 5 4 3 2
Printed in the United States of America

Contents

Contributing Authors

Raymond Dennis, A.A.S., B.S., M.A.
Associate Professor and Coordinator
Ophthalmic Design and Dispensing
Middlesex Community Technical College
Middletown, Connecticut

Cosmo J. Fratello, M.SC. VOCH. TECH. ED., F.N.A.O.
Professor and Department Head, Emeritus
Ophthalmic Dispensing Curriculum
Erie Community College–North Campus
Buffalo

Robert E. Hagman, A.B.O.M., F.N.A.O.
Chairman, Ohio State Optical Company
Columbus, Ohio

Arthur H. Keeney, M.D., D.SC.
Professor of Ophthalmology
University of Louisville School of Medicine;
Attending Staff, Department of Ophthalmology
University of Louisville Hospital
Louisville

René "Skip" Rivard, F.C.L.S.A. (H.)
Ophthalmic Design and Dispensing
Middlesex Community Technical College
Middletown, Connecticut

Foreword

Over 80,000,000 pairs of eyeglasses and contact lenses are sold each year in the United States. Today's complex eye care and eyewear system involves many interrelated disciplines, including ophthalmology, optometry, opticianry, photobiology, and polymer chemistry. With an increasing number of specialties involved, the need for standardization of understanding among these disciplines becomes essential.

The National Academy of Opticianry recognized the need for an industrywide standard of optical terms. In 1988, Academy president K. Richard Davenport appointed a committee to develop a dictionary of optical terms and related functions that could be used by all eye care professionals. Continued advances in eye health care demand complete, widely understood definitions.

This dictionary is not just for the practicing professional; it is aimed to be of interest to and instructive for students in opticianry, optometry, and ophthalmology training programs. It should also be helpful to contact lens technicians, ophthalmic laboratory technicians, third-party administrators, and others who provide eye care to the public.

The authors of this dictionary, Robert E. Hagman, Committee Chairman; Arthur H. Keeney, M.D.; and Cosmo J. Fratello, as well as contributing authors Raymond Dennis and René "Skip" Rivard, are to be highly commended for preparing a text so comprehensive, standardized, and authoritative.

The National Academy of Opticianry is indebted to past presidents Cindy L. Clancy and J. Norman Clay, current president William B. Mueller, and the Academy Directors for providing initial funding and support staff time to generate this project. Special thanks also go to George C. Chase, Ph.D., for his technical assistance, and to Robin Feik and Joy Pierce for their suggestions and initial clerical input.

Floyd H. Holmgrain, Jr., Ed.D.
Executive Director
National Academy of Opticianry, Inc.
Bowie, Maryland

Preface

The science of optics, with a history of more than 2,000 years, has suffered from differences in vocabulary and word interpretation. This is particularly true for Chinese optics. Mo Zi (Mo-tsu, or Mo-i), c. 479–381 B.C., devised the straight-line projection of light, the focal center of spheres, the camera obscura, and many other basics of geometric optics. His work, known as Mohist optics, has been nearly unknown to the Western world. The same is true for fourteenth century Zhao Youqin whose work involved catoptrics and early dioptrics.[1]

The ancient Mesopotamians (1800 to 1000 B.C.) evolved a tabulating system based on units of 60; this system is still used for measuring degrees, minutes, and seconds of arc in astronomy and in the alignment of cylinders in spectacle lenses.

Pythagoras (c. 560–480 B.C.), though a boon to geometry and acoustics, stifled visual optics for nearly 900 years because of his erroneous hypothesis that light went out from the eyes to "see" the world. An extraordinarily inventive engineer in the first century A.D., Hero of Alexandria, produced the book *On the Dioptra* with clear discussions of ray tracing, reflections, and mirrors. Unfortunately, it also included Pythagoras' hypothesis regarding emission of light from the eyes. In addition, Pythagoras' theory was adopted by one of the great astronomers of antiquity, Claudius Ptolemy (c. 90–160 A.D.), in his volume *Optica*, which shows an understanding of dioptrics.

Although Pythagoras' misconception lingered well into the early 1600s from Galen of Pergamon (c. 130–200 A.D.) and his continuing influence, it is from Greek scholars that the foundations of optics arise. The great mathematician, Euclid of Athens (c. 330–280 B.C.), gave much to geometry and codified mathematics. Much of optics has evolved from geometry, hence the term "geometric optics." The brilliant, but sometimes overlooked, Greek scholars of optics, Aristotle (382–322 B.C.) and Epicurus (342?–270 B.C.), both clearly displayed their genuine evidence that light travels in straight lines from its source to the eye.

After the fall of the Roman Empire (c. 450 A.D.), western European scientific thought entered the Dark Ages which lasted into the thirteenth century. During the Dark Ages European scholars turned to Arabia and Islamic Spain to access the organization and systemization of the Greek knowledge base. Several Arabic scholars clarified and added to the Greek accomplishments. Al-Hazen (Ibn Al-Haitham) of Cairo (c. 965–1040 A.D.) created the *Opticae Thesaurus* (*Book of Optics*) discarding the misleading theories of light emitting from the eye; he adopted the view of the Greek scholars Epicurus and Aristotle that rays of light travel from objects to the eye. Al-Hazen also had insights into dioptrics, and he refined catoprics. Ibn Rushd (Averroes) (1126–1198 A.D.) correctly identified that photoreceptors of the eye are located in the retina, not in the lens. Greek insight, amended by a few Arab scholars, provided a framework for the launching of Renaissance knowledge.

Roger Bacon (1220–1292)—no relative of the often politically correct Sir Francis Bacon—was one of the major scholars and experimentalists to research Arabic material for information on optics. He constructed magnifying glasses, suggested the use of spectacles, and predicted the design details of a telescope. His foundation of experimentation and mathematics provided for rapid growth in optics but his explanation of presbyopia was in error. The advent of crude reading glasses and spectacles between the end of the thirteenth and early fourteenth centuries extended a scholar's useful visual life and contributed to the wonders of the Renaissance.

The exchange of scientific thought across Europe during the Renaissance was facilitated by using nomenclature with word stems from Greek and Latin scholarly writings. Science, however, is a heavily quantitative discipline; the units of measurement were a confused substratum. Further development of science and optics necessitated improvement in units of measurement to avoid ill-defined results in the laboratory and international confusion in the literature. Development of common terminology for units, physical forces, weights, degrees of time and temperature, and other measurements in the 1600s greatly accelerated quantitative optical science. Thus, opticians gained stature long before major evolutions in ocular disease and ophthalmology occurred.

The fundamental achievements of the seventeenth and early eighteenth centuries laid the groundwork for extensive development of optical and ophthalmic instrumentation in the nineteenth century. Documentation of these achievements fills the sixteen volumes of Frederick C. Blodi's (1982–1992) translation of Julius Hirschberg's *History of Ophthalmology* (written 1889 to 1911). The developments of this period, however, preceded an even larger growth in the field of optics in the twentieth century.

In this century, the professions of physicist, optician, and physician have branched widely into several types of opticians, the ophthalmologist, the optometrist, the photobiologist, the ocularist, the orthoptist, the contact lens specialist, the design engineer, the polymer chemist, the radiation physicist, the ocular bacteriologists, and numerous other specialists.

The continuing evolution has brought us high precision in measuring nanometers, diopters, wavelengths, ultrasonic echoes, and light intensities in both radiometric and photometric units. All quantifications in this volume move toward the Système Internationale des Unités (S.I.), the logical and steady expansion of the metric system, whose origins date back nearly 200 years.

The authors and sources undergirding the definitions in this volume rely preponderantly on English language construction and formalities, and less frequently informalities, of its expression. Precision is espoused even though at times a less familiar wording or construction results. Consider for example, the difference between *distant*, the adjective, and *distance*, the noun. *Distance* has been used, very loosely and improperly, as the adjective describing an interocular measurement such as "*distance* interocular distance" rather than the correct "*distant* interocular distance" or "*far* interocular distance." Also, common practice is to call a prescription for infinite viewing a "*distance* Rx" rather than the correct "*distant* Rx" or "Rx for *distant* viewing."

This dictionary seeks to bring together differing disciplines and differing levels of technological precision in nomenclature. Shop jargon and abbreviated expressions will always be part of personal interchange, but accomplishing growth of science and scientific interchange is dependent upon clarity of definition. The authors of this dictionary use some shop nomenclature, but overall, tighter constructions and word sequences are used to achieve precision. We hope these will be improvements in specificity. Thus, a *pupillometer* is defined as measuring the size of the pupil, not the distance between the pupils. Similarly, a *keratometer* is an anterior corneal surface measuring instrument, which is sometimes improperly called an ophthalmometer.

Dictionaries are living and unending creations. The authors of this volume hope to achieve a scientific and unifying effect within parameters such as Sir Stewart Duke-Elder used in describing optical functions as "approximations close enough to reality to be justified, inaccuracies, small enough to be ignored."[2]

The science of optics relating to vision, visual appliances, and the eyes themselves come under many headings and include geometric optics, physical optics, statistical optics, linear optics, fiber optics, laser optics, non-linear optics, even cosmetic optics. Much of the applied field is based on fundamentals of Euclidean optics, Cartesian optics, elaborated by the French scientist René Descartes in the early seventeenth century; Gaussian optics as simplified by the brilliant German mathematician Karl Gauss in the early nineteenth century; Maxwellian optics, uncovering three-dimensional electromagnetic wave forms by James Maxwell in the latter nineteenth century; and today's laser optics with exotic elements in lasers and spectacle frames, in addition to the rapidly changing science of optical polymers.

Scientific opticianry has a long, distinguished history that considerably antedates scientific ophthalmology. In the present century, scientific optometry has also contributed to the advancement and understanding of physical optics. These functions are most significantly involved in the human need to enhance vision for daily work as well as in the astronomic explorations of space and the microscopic exploration of subcellular structures.

Without question, all who today practice the scientific and technical care of patients' vision are greatly enhanced by the work of giants who have gone before us in previous years. This dictionary reflects such current indebtedness, and the authors specifically express their appreciation to those many individuals who have contributed to present-day advances. The authors have not only relied on their relatively extensive personal experience in ophthalmic optics, but have also labored to note those earlier scholars and the dates of their contributions.

Frequently, the authors have imposed on others for consultation by telephone and letter to clarify terms or specific meanings. For several aspects of contact lens nomenclature the authors thank René Rivard and Ray Dennis for their contributions. Many new friendships have been generated over the nearly six years in preparation and verification of details in these definitions. We are particularly indebted to those students of optical science who have left carefully documented notes and publications in their respective fields. The authors also express their thanks to the National Academy of Opticianry for the agency's assistance with this *Dictionary*.

The authors anticipate that there will be additions and corrections, and welcome such suggestions at any time. We hope the quality of this work will justify future and even enlarged editions.

A.H.K.
R.E.H.
C.J.F.

References

1. Institute of the History of Natural Sciences. *Ancient China's Technology and Science.* Jin Qiupeng, Optics, Chinese Academy of Sciences, Beijing: Beijing Foreign Language Press, 1983:166-175.
2. Duke-Elder S. *System of Ophthalmology,* Vol. V. St. Louis: C. V. Mosby, 1970:27.

How to Use This Dictionary

Organization

The organization of this dictionary, in common with most English language dictionaries, relies on entry words or key words (**bold**) in phrases or descriptors.

Guide words appear at the top of each page; the first word defined on the left page appears as the left running head and the last word on the right page appears as the right running head.

Entries

Entries that are modified by an adjective are listed by both the adjective and the noun. The listing under the adjective, however, contains only a cross-reference to the noun under which it has been defined. For example,

center line, geometric See *line, geometric center.*

line, geometric center A horizontal line, passing through the intersection of diagonal lines joining opposite corners of a box, that circumscribes the lens shape; previously called normal mounting line. See Figure 22; see also *bisector, horizontal lens (HLB).*

Phonetics

Phonetic spelling is indicated for entry terms with complex, difficult, or obscure phonetic values, but not for commonly known words.

Subentries

Multiple meanings have been added to entry words where applicable. These subentries, however, are listed arbitrarily: the order does not denote either historical priority or presumed importance.

Definitions which are generally obsolete, superseded, or used very rarely will appear at times only for clarification or to reduce confusion. Effort has been made to avoid rare or archaic terms or definitions except when such notation adds to the understanding of the entry word.

Cross-Referencing

Generous use of cross-referencing appears for eponyms, acronyms (mnemonics), synonyms, or initialized shortening of complex, multiple word entries. Entry words are followed by instructions to see the full definition under the complete spelling of the entry term. Thus, the initials J.C.A.H.P.O., which do not form an easily pronounceable acronym (as does RADAR, radio detection and ranging), are cross-referenced to the full entry, Joint Commission on Allied Health Personnel in Ophthalmology.

Opposite terms or antonyms have been added where they enhance the definition of an entry word. Suggestions to compare (cf.) entries have been added to increase understanding.

Plurals

In general, the singular form is used for entry nouns. Plurals of nouns are not indicated when formed by a standard suffix such as -s or -es. When there is an irregular or variant spelling, as the singular *iris* and the plural *irides,* the plural form is spelled out fully. Combining forms are indicated by a following hyphen for prefixes and a preceding hyphen for suffixes or terminal combining forms.

Historical Acknowledgments

Although this is not a biographical dictionary, eponyms are liberally indicated, particularly when they are commonly used as adjectival modifiers for an entry noun. To enhance the understanding of eponyms, where possible, the full name is given followed in parentheses by dates of birth and death, plus an indication of the field of endeavor and principal location of the individual.

Similarly, a strong effort has been made to acknowledge a discoverer or inventor of a structure, process, device, etc., where known. Sometimes, only a single name has survived in common usage or the actual year of birth or death may be unknown. At other times, an early but perhaps not well-documented discoverer is isolated from one who has been credited with a carefully documented or organized discovery.

A further option has been weighed by the authors when an individual's name is closely associated with popularization of a product which was devised or primitively described elsewhere; for example, Edward Jackson broadly popularized a retinoscope in North America. Although he did not invent it, both retinoscopy and the Jackson cross cylinders are associated with his name as a championing individual.

List of Figures

Dictionary of Ophthalmic Optics

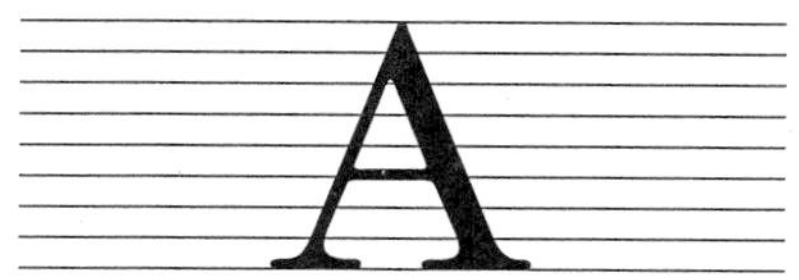

A **1.** The horizontal distance in millimeters between vertical tangents to the apex of the rim groove of a lens opening on the temporal and nasal sides of a spectacle frame (see Figure 19).
2. Horizontal distance in millimeters between vertical tangents to the apex of the bevel on the temporal and nasal edges of a spectacle lens (see Figure 20).
3. Abbreviation for the numerical aperture in a dioptric system. See *aperture.*

Å Symbol for Ångström unit or Ångström; q.v.

a-, an- Prefix meaning not.

A-scan Ultrasound, the linear mode (contrasted to two-dimensional B-scan ultrasound) of echography of the globe, commonly used for measurement of the axial length of the eye. Trade names: Storz, Compuscan LT; Mentor O. & O., Inc., Bio-Pen XL.

A.A.A.H.C Abbreviation for Accreditation Association for Ambulatory Health Care; q.v.

A.A.C.O. Abbreviation for American Association of Certified Orthoptists; q.v.

A.A.O. Abbreviation for:
1. American Academy of Ophthalmology; q.v.
2. American Academy of Optometry; q.v.
3. American Association of Ophthalmology; q.v.
4. American Association of Orthodontists.

A.B.M.S. Abbreviation for American Board of Medical Specialties; q.v.

A.B.O. Abbreviation for:
1. American Board of Ophthalmology; q.v.
2. American Board of Opticianry; q.v.

3. American Board of Otolaryngology (sometimes abbreviated A.B.Ot.); q.v.

A.B.O.C. Abbreviation for American Board of Opticianry Certified; q.v.

A.B.O.M. Abbreviation for American Board of Opticianry, Master; q.v.

A.C.G.I.H. Abbreviation for American Conference of Governmental Industrial Hygienists; q.v.

A.C.O.E.M. Abbreviation for American College of Occupational and Environmental Medicine; q.v.

A.C.S.M. Abbreviation for American College of Sports Medicine; q.v.

A.N.S.I. Abbreviation for American National Standards Institute; q.v.

A.O.A. Abbreviation for:
1. Alpha Omega Alpha; q.v.
2. American Optometric Association; q.v.
3. American Osteopathic Association; q.v.
4. American Orthopaedic Association.

A.O.C. Abbreviation for American Orthoptic Council; q.v.

A.O.S. Abbreviation for:
1. American Ophthalmological Society; q.v.
2. American Otological Society.

A.R.C. In visual physiology, abbreviation for:
1. Anomalous Retinal Correspondence as occurs in adaptation to longstanding strabismus; also
2. Abrasion Resistance Coating (coating, scratch resistant; q.v.)
3. Aids Related Complex,
4. American Red Cross.

A.R.V.O. Abbreviation for Association for Research in Vision and Ophthalmology; q.v.; originally, Association for Research in Ophthalmology.

A.S.O. Abbreviation for American Society of Ocularists; q.v.

A.S.O.A. Abbreviation for American Society of Ophthalmic Administrators; q.v.

A.S.O.R.N. Abbreviation for American Society of Ophthalmic Registered Nurses; q.v.

A.S.P. Abbreviation for American Society for Photobiology; q.v.

A.S.T.M. Abbreviation for American Society for Testing and Materials; q.v.

A.T.P.O. Abbreviation for Association of Technical Personnel in Ophthalmology; q.v.

A.U.P.O. Abbreviation for Association of University Professors of Ophthalmology; q.v.

A.W.S. Abbreviation for American Welding Society; q.v.

ab- Prefix meaning away from, or off.

abaxial (ab-ak'se-al) Situated out of, or directed away from an axis.

Abbé number See *number, Abbé.*

Abbé value See *number, Abbé.*

abduct (ab-dukt') In ocular physiology, to turn the eye laterally (outward) from the primary gaze position; away from the median plane.

abductor In ocular anatomy, an extraocular muscle responsible for turning the eye away from the median plane or outward; principally, the lateral rectus muscle.

aberration A deviation from the normal or correct; in optics, the creation of a blurred or distorted image due to physical properties of the optical elements. Five aberrations are classically considered as "Seidel aberrations," 1) longitudinal spherical; 2) coma; 3) astigmatic; 4) Petzval curvature; 5) distortion. Named for German scientist L.P. Seidel (1821–1896) who identified these imperfections that represent the largest and most conspicuous defects in an uncorrected lens system.

aberration, astigmatic (as"tig-mat'ik) Undesirable, unequal refraction of an optical system in which an object point is imaged as line foci.

aberration, chromatic (kro-mat'ik) Unequal refraction of different wavelengths of light; commonly producing colored fringes about an image; particularly encountered with strong plus lenses, and lenses of high refractive index material; (differential refraction; chromatic dispersion; color blur); divided into longitudinal (on axis) and lateral (off axis or oblique).

aberration, coma A defect in imaging objects off the optical axis in which there is a bright central area and a tail of lesser brightness.

aberration, curvature of field An optical defect in which a flat object is imaged as a curved surface (Petzval curvature). See also *curvature of field.*

aberration, lens The failure of a refracting surface or lens to bring all rays from an object point toward a desired image point. This can result in image blur. See *error*; *peripheral power*. Aberration also results in curvature in the image of a straight line. See *distortion*. Aberration may be inherent in the design of a lens or may result from errors in processing. See *warpage*; *wave*.

aberration, spherical An optical defect caused by peripheral and paraxial rays focusing at different points along the optical axis of a lens; longitudinal spherical aberrations.

ablepharon (ah-blef'ah-ron) Congenital absence of the eyelids. See *cryptophthalmos*.

abrasion A scraped spot or area.

abrasion, corneal A scraping or scratching of the corneal epithelium, causing the loss of superficial tissue.

abscess A localized, circumscribed collection of pus.

absorption

1. In radiation physics, the ability of a material to transform radiant energy (e.g., light), to a different form of energy (usually heat); the negative log of transmittance; absorptivity.
2. In spectacle optics, the reduction of transmission of radiant energy (e.g., light), through a transparent medium.

absorptive lens See *lens, absorptive*.

acanthamoeba (ah-kan"tha-mē'bah) A genus of parasites that cause an extremely serious corneal and ocular infection, usually very painful, associated with contact lens wear. Classified as a free-living ameboid protozoa, usually found in fresh water or moist soil; opportunistically may cause chronic or acute fatal infection.

accommodation The dioptric adjustment of the crystalline lens of the eye to attain maximal sharpness of retinal imagery for an object of regard; change in shape of the lens when focusing at different distances had been described in 1792 by Thomas Young (1773–1892), English physicist and physician, while he was a medical student; a term introduced in 1841 by C. August Burrow (1809–1874), German physician and ophthalmologist.

accommodation, amplitude of The difference, expressed in diopters, between the farthest point and the nearest point of accommodation with respect to the spectacle plane, the entrance pupil, or some other reference point of the eye. Varies from a maximum of about 18 diopters in infancy to almost zero at 60 years of age. (cf. *accommodation, range of*.)

accommodation, negative The adjustment of the crystalline lens from near to far regard; occurs by relaxation of the ciliary muscles and decreasing the curvature of the crystalline lens.

accommodation, positive The adjustment of the crystalline lens from far to near regard; occurs by contraction of the ciliary muscles and increasing the curvature of the crystalline lens.

accommodation, range of The linear distance from the farthest point of clear vision to the nearest point of focus or clear vision attainable by the human eye; usually expressed in centimeters or inches from far point to near point. (cf. *accommodation, amplitude of.*)

accommodative convergence See *convergence, accommodative.*

accommodative esotropia See *esotropia, accommodative.*

accommodometer A mechanical–optical device for measuring the limits of accommodation. (cf. *optometer, Prince's rule.*)

achromat (ak'rō-mat) A lens corrected for chromatic aberration (achromatic lens).

achromate (ak'rō-māt) A totally color-blind individual; a patient with hereditary, total color blindness (all colors appear as neutral gray with varying darkness), usually associated with nystagmus, photophobia, and poor visual acuity (rod monochromaticity); when accompanied by relatively normal visual acuity is referred to as cone monochromaticity.

achromatic lens See *lens, achromatic.*

achromatopsia (ah-kro"mah-top'se-ah) Absence of ability to see colors; due to absence or severe deficiency of cone cells; may be complete (rod chromatism) with poor visual acuity, photophobia and nystagmus, incomplete (cone chromatism) with only modest reduction of acuity and with little or no nystagmus and photophobia, or progressive with concurrent decrease in vision (monochromatism, achromatism).

acronym (ak'ro-nim) A word formed from the first letter of a series of words; usually written without periods following the letters (e.g., laser, **l**ight **a**mplification by **s**timulated **e**mission of **r**adiation—LASER).

acrylic Synthetic, chain-linked polymers of acrylic acid, (2-propenoic acid) or methacrylic acid; used in the manufacture of hard contact lenses and some spectacle frames since the 1930s.

actinic (ak-tin'ik) Pertaining to the chemical and biological effect of ultraviolet radiation; generally considered within the UVB and UVC wavelengths.

actinic keratitis See *keratitis, actinic.*

acuity

1. From the Latin, sharpness.

2. Clarity or clearness, especially of vision.

acuity, binocular visual The resultant resolving power (acuity) obtained with both eyes open; usually slightly better than with either eye alone. In patients with latent nystagmus (nystagmus appearing only when one eye is covered), it is much better than acuity with one eye alone.

acuity, central visual The resolving power of the dioptric system of the eye; a measurement of sharpness of sight at the fovea centralis of the retina.

acuity, vernier Central visual acuity as measured by ability to detect offset between contiguous line segments; generally is of higher capability than is resolving acuity; aligning power. See *vernier.*

acuity, visual Resolving power or form discrimination dependent upon the sharpness of the retinal image, the sensitivity of the neural elements and the interpretation facility of the brain.

ad- Prefix meaning toward.

adaptation, visual Adjustments of the visual system to the brightness (luminosity) of environmental light conditions and the viewed objects; includes light adaptation and dark adaptation; this function is served by changes in retinal sensitivity and pupillary area; concept elaborated and term introduced in 1865 by Hermann Aubert (1826–1892), optical physiologist of Rostock, Germany.

addition (spectacle add) In spectacle optics, the difference in vertex power (on the lens surface containing the add) between the reading or intermediate portion of a multifocal lens and its distance portion. For progressive lenses, this difference is determined at the locations specified by its manufacturer. An addition (add) is commonly equivalent to a positive sphere superimposed on a distance prescription to permit the wearer to focus near objects more easily.

addition power See *addition.*

adduct (ad-dukt') In ocular physiology, to turn the eye nasally (inward) from the primary gaze position; toward the median plane.

adductor In ocular anatomy, an extraocular muscle responsible for turning the eye toward the median plane or inward; principally, the medial rectus muscle.

adnexa oculi (ad-nek'sah ok'yu-lī) Associated structures or adjunct parts related to the eye, including the lacrimal apparatus, eyelids, orbital fascia, adipose tissue, lacrimal gland, nerves, blood vessels, and eyebrows.

Adopted Names Council (A.N.C.) See *United States Adopted Names Council* (U.S.A.N.).

Advisory Group for Aerospace Research Development (AGARD) A treaty organization composed of North Atlantic nation members; facilitates exchange and advancement of scientific and technical relevance to the North Atlantic Military Committee. Has issued several reports on visual problems, aids, and eye protection, particularly for the aviator.

Aerospace Medical Association (A.M.A.) Established in 1929 as Aeromedical Association; 4,500 members interested in medical aspects of air and space travel. Office: Alexandria, Virginia 22314-3524.

aesthesiometer See *esthesiometer.*

afferent Conveying from the periphery to the center, centripetal, as optic nerve fibers carrying visual impulses from the eye to the brain.

Ag Chemical symbol for the metallic element silver; q.v.

against motion See *motion, against.*

against the rule astigmatism See *astigmatism, against the rule.*

AGARD Acronym for Advisory Group for Aerospace Research Development; q.v.

agonist

1. A prime mover; opposite of antagonist; q.v.
2. A muscle that acts in the primary or desired direction, though opposed in action by another muscle, the antagonist; in ocular anatomy this is an attribute of the extraocular muscles.
3. A drug that stimulates physiologic or normal activity.

aids, low-vision Optical or non-optical appliances and devices designed to assist the partially sighted patient; may include magnification, illumination, telescopic devices, or any combination of these.

Al Chemical symbol for the metallic element aluminum; q.v.

albedo (al-bē'dō)

1. Reflective power.
2. The fraction of incident light that is reflected from a surface.
3. Whiteness; sometimes expressed as Bond albedo for George Phillips Bond (1825–1865), director of Harvard College Observatory and specialist in brightness measures of stars; initially described and published in Latin (albedo, L for whiteness) in 1760 by Johann Heinrich Lambert (1728–1777), German mathematician, for whom the unit of brightness, the Lambert, is named.

albinism, ocular (al'bi-nizm) A type of hereditary deficiency of pigment in the eyes marked by pale irides, nystagmus, photophobia, decreased vision; the hair and skin may be normal. Divided into two basic types, tyrosine-negative and tyrosine-positive depending on absence or presence of the amino acid tyrosine, which may be determined from analysis of a hair bulb.

alexia A neurological (brain) deficit in which the previously acquired ability to read has been lost.

alginate (al'ji-nāt) A viscous impression material made from a salt of alginic acid originally extracted from marine kelp. Used to make impression molds of the orbit after enucleation, or of the cornea for the purpose of fitting scleral contact lenses. Moldite powder, developed in 1942 by New York optician Theodore E. Obrig (1895–1967).

aligner, axis Any device used for placing a cylinder axis at its proper angle. Normally a focimeter, a protractor, or protractor-type instrument. Loosely, may refer to an axis-aligning plier.

alignment, apical A contact lens design which is contoured to the apex of the cornea with only a light pooling of fluorescein between the lens and the cornea.

alignment fitting In contact lenses, a fitting technique such that the CPC (base curve) is designed to fit parallel to the flattest meridian of the cornea.

alignment reference marking See *marking, alignment reference.*

allergic conjunctivitis See *conjunctivitis, allergic.*

allergic reaction See *reaction, allergic.*

allergy A state of hypersensitivity induced by exposure to a particular antigen, resulting in harmful immunologic reaction on subsequent exposure.

alloy A substance that is a mixture, as by fusion, of two or more substances, usually metals, but may include other substances.

alloy, low melting point See *indium.*

allyl diglycol carbonate (al'il dī-glī'kol kar'bon-āt) See *CR-39.*

alopecia (al"o-pe'she-a) Loss of hair; may be congenital, drug induced or disease-related; may occur in localized areas, as the eyebrows, over the entire scalp, or the entire body.

alpha, ***A*****,** α
1. The beginning of anything.
2. First letter of the Greek alphabet.
3. First in order of importance.

Alpha Omega Alpha (A.O.A.) An honor society of medical students, founded in 1902; now has chapters in 122 medical schools. Office: Menlo Park, California 94025-3480.

alpine skiing goggles See *goggles, alpine skiing.*

alternating strabismus See *strabismus, alternating.*

alternating vision See *vision, alternating.*

aluminum A lightweight (specific gravity about 2.7) relatively strong metallic chemical element, highly resistant to oxidation, used in ophthalmic frame construction; can be anodized to yield a variety of colors; also, when coated with silicon monoxide, useful as a broad band reflective coating for visible and infrared light; chemical symbol Al, atomic number 13. The most abundant metallic element in the earth's crust. Metallic aluminum was first isolated in 1825 by Danish physicist Hans Christian Oersted (1777–1851).

amaurosis fugax (am"aw-rō'sis fyoo'jax) Short attacks of partial blindness; usually due to circulatory insufficiency and suggestive of a potential vascular accident.

amblyopia (am"ble-ō'pe-ah) Decreased vision in an eye without detectable anatomic damage to the eye or visual pathway and uncorrectable by usual optical devices; commonly is related to unequal refractive status of the two eyes, monocular strabismus, or disease of an eye from the early months or years of life.

amblyopia ex anopsia (ex an-op'se-ah) "Lazy eye." Decreased vision due to lack of use; visual pathway fails to mature; usually associated with strabismus or anisometropia early in life; term being superceded by more physiologic classification of amblyopia.

amblyoscope (am'ble-o-skōp") Orthoptic instrument for analysis of sensory impairment to vision and for training to reduce such impairment (synoptophore, haploscope, troposcope); developed in 1901 by London ophthalmologist Claud Worth (1869–1936).

American Academy of Ophthalmology (A.A.O.) A voluntary, professional association of eye physicians and surgeons; established in 1896 as American Academy of Ophthalmology and Otolaryngology; approximately 17,000 members from the United States, Canada, and foreign nations. Publishes monthly journal, *Ophthalmology*, (formerly, *Transactions of American Academy of Ophthalmology and Otolaryngology*). Office: P.O. Box 7424, San Francisco, California 94120-7424.

American Academy of Optometry (A.A.O.) A voluntary professional organization established in 1922 for the scientific development of optometry. Publishes monthly journal, *Optometry and Visual Science* (formerly, *Journal of Physiologic Optics and Optometry,* and, earlier, *Journal of American Academy of Optometry*). Office: 4330 East West Hwy., Bethesda, Maryland 20814.

American Association for Pediatric Ophthalmology and Strabismus (A.A.P.O.S.) A voluntary professional association of ophthalmologists; since 1963, publishes bimonthly *Journal of Pediatric Ophthalmology and Strabismus.*

American Association of Certified Orthoptists (A.A.C.O.) Established in 1940 by technical personnel certified by the American Orthoptic Council; approximately 350 members. Since 1951, annually publishes *American Orthoptic Journal.* Office: Houston, Texas 77030-1693.

American Association of Ophthalmology Voluntary professional association of eye physicians established in 1965 from previous National Medical Foundation for Eyecare (est. 1956); merged in 1981 with American Academy of Ophthalmology.

American Board of Medical Specialties (A.B.M.S.) The governing authority for the organization and operation of the current 23 specialty boards in American medicine; created in 1933 as Advisory Board for Medical Specialties, a federation of individual specialty boards. Reorganized in 1970 as a new and independent corporation. Office: Evanston, Illinois 60201.

American Board of Ophthalmology (A.B.O.) A voluntary examining and certifying agency for physicians specializing in eye diseases, their correction, and related medical, optical, surgical and rehabilitation care; governed by the American Board of Medical Specialties; established in 1916 as the American Board for Ophthalmic Examinations, the first of current 23 examining Boards; name changed in 1933 to American Board of Ophthalmology. Office: Bala-Cynwyd, Pennsylvania 19004.

American Board of Opticianry (A.B.O.) A voluntary certifying agency established in 1947 to develop credentialing examinations at two levels and requirements for voluntary certification and recertification of opticians. The two levels are American Board of Opticianry Certified, A.B.O.C., and American Board of Opticianry Master, A.B.O.M.; approximately 23,000 certified at first level and 300 at second level. Office: 10341 Democracy Lane, P.O. Box 10110, Fairfax, Virginia 22030.

American Board of Otolaryngology (A.B.Ot.) The voluntary certifying agency established in 1924 for physicians involved with ear, nose, and throat disease.

American College of Occupational Medicine (A.C.O.M.) See *American College of Occupational and Environmental Medicine.*

American College of Occupational and Environmental Medicine (A.C.O.E.M.) Established in 1915 as American Occupational Medical Association; renamed in 1991. Publishes monthly *Journal of Occupational and Environmental Medicine.* Office: Arlington Heights, Illinois 60005.

American College of Sports Medicine (A.C.S.M.) Established 1954; 12,000 members in voluntary professional association; bimonthly publication, *Medicine and Science in Sports and Exercise.* Office: Indianapolis, Indiana 46206-1440.

American Conference of Governmental Industrial Hygienists (A.C.G.I.H.) Voluntary, professional association of scientists, concerned with manufacturing and commercial toxicology; establishes threshold limit values (TLV) for laser energy, various radiations, including ultraviolet light; established in 1938; 3,800 members. Office: Cincinnati, Ohio 45211-4438.

American Foundation for the Blind, Inc. (A.F.B.) National research, information, and consultation agency founded in 1921. Serves as a national clearinghouse for information about blindness. Office: 15 West 16th St., New York, New York 10016.

American National Standards Institute (A.N.S.I.) The coordinator of the voluntary standards system in the United States, established in 1918 as American Standards Association, from 1966 to 1969 name changed to United States of America Standards Institute (U.S.A.S.I.); current name adopted 1969. Provides a correlation with standards of other nations, the International Organization for Standardization (I.S.O.) and the International Electrotechnical Commission (I.E.C.).

A.N.S.I. is the primary entry point from the United States into the international standardization efforts of I.S.O. and I.E.C.. The use of

American National Standards is voluntary; its existence does not preclude anyone, from manufacturing, marketing, purchasing, or using products, processes, or procedures not conforming to the standards, unless otherwise required by law or government regulation. A.N.S.I. issues Z80 and Z87 standards for spectacles, safety eye wear, intraocular implants and low-vision aids. Also issues standard Z136, Safe Use of Lasers and Z49, Safety in Welding and Cutting.

American Ophthalmological Society (A.O.S.) Established in 1864 as the first specialized medical society in the U.S.; a limited and elective membership of 225 senior ophthalmologists in North America; issues annual *Transactions of the A.O.S.*

American Optometric Association (A.O.A.) A national organization of approximately 27,000 optometrists; established in 1898. Its prime purpose is to unite optometrists into a nationally representative group for the improvement of the optometric profession. Publishes monthly *Journal of American Optometric Association.* The American Optometric Association, Paraoptometric Section, is the association of optometric assistants, technicians, office managers, and receptionists. Office: 243 N. Lindbergh Blvd., St. Louis, Missouri 63141.

American Orthoptic Council (A.O.C.) Governing and standardizing body for orthoptists (q.v.) in the United States; 19 members comprised of ophthalmologists and orthoptists; established in 1935. Office: Madison, Wisconsin 53711.

American Osteopathic Association (A.O.A.) Voluntary professional organization established in 1887; 23,800 osteopathic physician members. Office: 212 E. Ohio St., Chicago, Illinois 30914.

American Society for Photobiology (A.S.P.) A voluntary professional group of scientists concerned with the effects of light on living organisms; established in 1972 as successor to the U.S. National Committee for Photobiology; publishes monthly journal *Photochemistry and Photobiology.* Office: Augusta, Georgia 30914.

American Society for Testing and Materials (A.S.T.M.) A voluntary, standard-setting agency established in Philadelphia in 1898 to define various simple and complex materials, and to formalize methods for evaluating and judging those materials and products made from them. Issues F8 standards for sports eye protection. Office: 1916 Race St., Philadelphia, Pennsylvania 19103.

American Society of Cataract and Refractive Surgery (A.S.C.R.S.) A voluntary association of ophthalmic surgeons established in 1974; 4,500 members; publishes bimonthly *Journal of Cataract and Refractive Surgery.* Office: Fairfax, Virginia 22030.

American Society of Ocularists (A.S.O.) A voluntary association of ocularists (q.v.) established in 1955 for improvement of patient care by prosthetics; 185 members; since 1970, publishes annual *Journal of American Society of Ocularists,* formerly *Today's Ocularist.*

American Society of Ophthalmic Registered Nurses (A.S.O.R.N.) A voluntary, professional organization of registered nurses caring for eye patients; established 1976; 1,800 members. Office: San Francisco, California 94119.

American Society of Ophthalmic Administrators (A.S.O.A.) A voluntary group of controllers or fiscal management officers charged with the financial or business management of ophthalmic offices, clinics, hospitals, research institutes, and the like.

American Welding Society (A.W.S.) Association established in 1919; 38,000 members; publishes with A.N.S.I. recommended standards for selecting protective lens shades (A6.2) and using electron beams (F2.1). Office: Miami, Florida 33126.

ametropia (am″e-tro′pe-ah) A general term for any error of refraction in the eye.

amplitude of accommodation See *accommodation, amplitude of.*

amplitude of convergence See *convergence, amplitude of.*

Amsler's grid See *grid, Amsler's.*

anaglyphs (an′a-glif) A stereoscopic pair of computer-generated "random dot" plates or drawings of the same subject printed in complementary colors; when looked at through a pair of corresponding color filters, give the impression of three-dimensional representation with no monocular cues.

analgesic (an″al-jē′zik) A medicine that relieves pain.

anatomical Of or pertaining to the form and structure of an organism.

anatomy The study of the form and structure of an organism.

anemia A condition in which there is a deficiency in the number of red blood cells or in the quantity of hemoglobin.

anesthetic, topical An agent applied as a drop to a membrane or the surface of the eye which produces insensitivity to pain or touch; a local anesthetic (e.g., cocaine).

angiography, fluorescein An ophthalmic diagnostic procedure to evaluate blood flow dynamics within the retina; uses a sterile intravenous injection of 10% or 25% fluorescein sodium solution, and subsequent serial fundus photography demonstrating details of

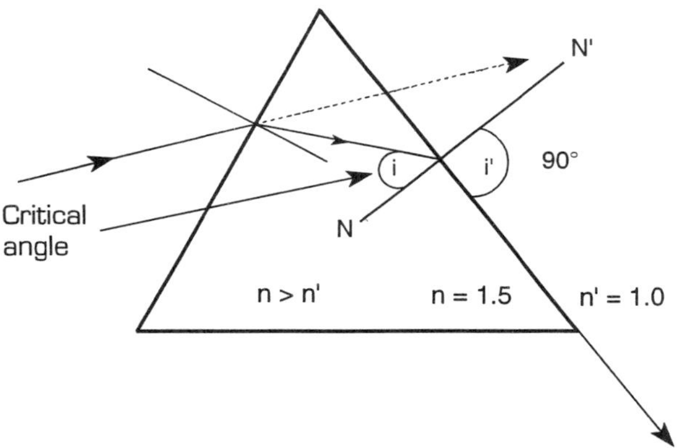

Figure 1 Critical (i.e., incident) angle. Angle i = 41.8° for glass, n = 1.5.

blood flow, leakage, pigment changes, areas of hemorrhage, and the like. Technique introduced in 1961 by H.R. Novotny (b. 1932) and D.L. Alvis (b. 1935), when medical students in Indianapolis, Indiana.

angle The relationship made by two straight lines meeting at a common point or vertex; the arc enclosed by two such straight lines; commonly measured in degrees.

angle alpha The angle formed by the intersection of the optic axis and the visual axis at the first nodal point of an eye.

angle, anterior chamber In ocular anatomy, the angle in the periphery of the front (i.e., aqueous) chamber of the eye created by the posterior surface of the cornea (endothelium) and the anterior surface of the iris.

angle, critical In geometric optics, where n > n', the maximum angle of incidence which results in an angle of refraction of 90°, that is, the emerging (refracted) ray just grazes the surface of the interface; rays at greater angles of incidence will be totally reflected within the first medium; also called limiting angle (Figure 1).

angle, cross See *angle, temple fold.*

angle, frame pantoscopic (down angle) (pan″tō̄-skop′ik) The angular value in degrees determined by measuring from a perpendicular through the spectacle lens plane at the temple hinge, intersecting the center line of the temple in the open position (straight line from

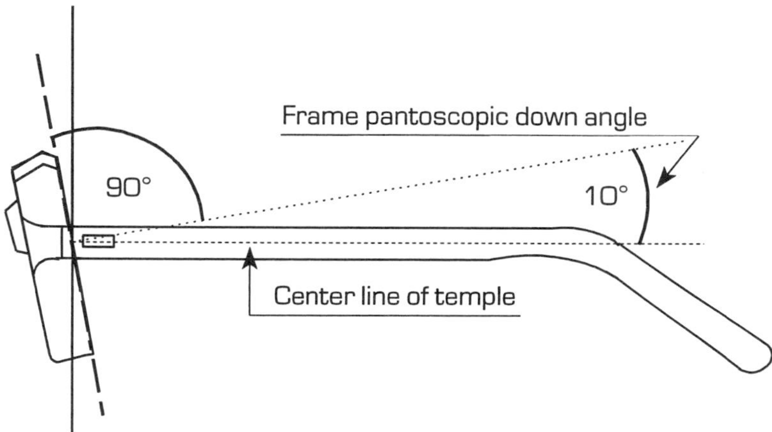

Figure 2 Frame pantoscopic angle (down angle).

the median hinge barrel through a point at the center of the ear bend) (Figure 2).

angle, frontal, of the nasal bones The angle by which each side of the nose deviates from the vertical. The nose usually widens as it approaches the tip (cf. *angle, splay*).

angle gamma The angle formed at the center of rotation of an eye between its optic axis and fixation axis; a theoretical consideration without significant clinical value because the center of rotation changes with movement of the globe.

angle, groove The included angle formed by the V-shape in the rim groove of a spectacle front.

angle kappa The angle between the visual axis and the pupillary axis of the eye; commonly estimated by reflection of light from the surface of the cornea; expressed as positive or negative—when the pupillary axis is temporal to the fixation axis, termed positive, and may simulate exotropia; when the pupillary axis appears nasal to the fixation axis, termed negative, and may simulate esotropia. The size of the angle is usually estimated visually as the patient fixes on a small penlight; the examiner notes how far this appears to be nasal or temporal from the apparent pupillary center.

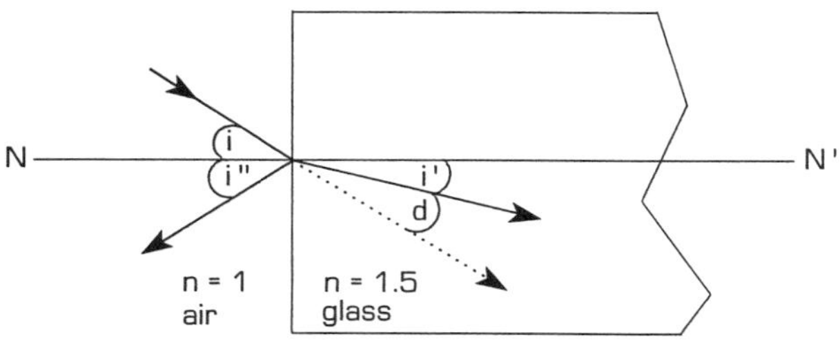

Figure 3 Angles of: Incidence = i; Reflection = i"; Refraction = i'; and Deviation = d.

angle, lens bevel The included angle at the apex on the periphery of an edged ophthalmic lens.

angle, minimum separable The smallest angle of separation at which the eye recognizes two points, lines, or objects as being set apart, usually 1 minute of arc; resolving power of the human eye; the basis of Snellen visual acuity measurement; originally described in 1669 by Robert Hooke (1635–1703), experimenter of the Royal Society of England.

angle, nasal splay See *angle, splay*.

angle of deviation

1. The angle denoting the apparent change in direction of an incident ray measured between its refracted ray and apparent path of the original ray, usually expressed in degrees (Figure 3).
2. Amount an eye deviates from its straight ahead position as the other eye remains straight and fixates normally, usually expressed in prism diopters or degrees.

angle of incidence The angle formed between an incident light ray striking a surface, and the perpendicular (normal) to the surface at that point, usually measured from the normal to the incident ray (see Figure 3).

angle of reflection The angle formed between a reflected light ray and a perpendicular (normal) to the surface at point of incidence, usually measured from the normal to the reflected ray (see Figure 3).

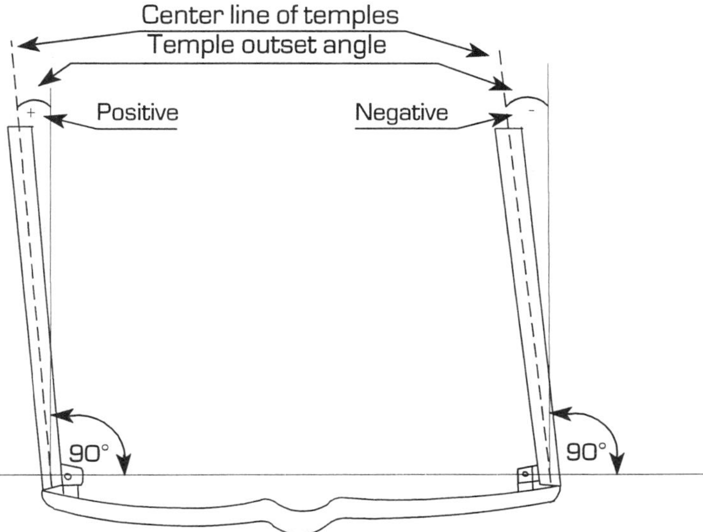

Figure 4 Set-back angle.

angle of refraction The angle formed between a refracted ray and a perpendicular (normal) to the surface at the point of refraction, usually measured from the normal to the refracted ray (see Figure 3).

angle of view See *angle, viewing.*

angle, set-back, temple The angle formed by a spectacle front and temple with the temples in the open position as viewed from above. The numerical value in degrees is determined by measuring the angle between the center line of the temple and a line perpendicular to the horizontal line joining the centers of the hinge barrel holes; also called *temple outset* (Figure 4).

angle, splay The horizontal angle formed by the side plane of the nose with a straight anterior–posterior plane that would bisect the nose vertically. The nose is wider as it approaches the nostrils or nares (cf. *angle, frontal*).

angle, temple fold The angle formed between spectacle temples in the folded position and the horizontal line joining the hinge centers, as viewed from the back of the frame; also called *cross angle.*

angle, viewing The orientation of the eyes with respect to the viewed object. The angle formed by the intersection of the fixation axis with the horizontal plane bisecting the pupil. Angles measured above the horizontal plane are considered plus (+), and angles measured below the horizontal are termed minus (–).

angle, visual The angle formed at the nodal point of an eye and subtended by the extremities of an object or visual stimulus; usually measured in degrees or minutes of arc.

angle, wetting

1. The relative value between the forces of adhesion and cohesion of a drop of liquid on a solid surface. A lower wetting angle allows a liquid to spread more evenly over the solid's surface. Water droplets placed on a newly waxed surface exhibit a high wetting angle.
2. In contact lens science, the angle formed between the edge of a drop of water and the surface of the contact lens on which it is resting; the smaller the angle, the greater the spreading of the tear film on the contact lens material.

Ångström, Å (ang'strom) A linear unit used to describe the wavelength of light and other electromagnetic radiations; 1/10 of a nanometer; this term has generally been superseded by the unit "nm," nanometer. Named for Swedish physicist Anders Jonas Ångström (1814–1874), University of Uppsala.

angular magnifying power See *power, angular magnifying.*

aniridia (an″i-rid′e-ah) Total absence of the iris; rarely complete because a rudimentary peripheral iris stump is usually visible on gonioscopy; better described as irideremia; associated with photophobia, secondary glaucoma, and sometimes Wilms' tumor of the kidney.

aniseikonia (an″i-si-kō′ne-ah) Unequal size of images formed on the two retinas. When symptomatic, may be corrected by prescribed iseikonic lenses. Term developed in 1932 by Walter B. Lancaster (1863–1951) Boston ophthalmologist and authority in physiological optics. See *eikonometer.*

aniso- Prefix meaning uneven, unequal, or dissimilar.

anisocoria (an-ī″so-kō′re-ah) Unequal diameters of the two pupils.

anisometropia (an-ī″so-me-trō′pe-ah) Unequal refractive errors in the two eyes.

anisometropic (an-ī″so-me-trop′ik) Relating to or having anisometropia.

anisophoria (an″i-so-fō′re-ah) Heterophoria in which the degree of the phoria varies with the angle of gaze; may be neuro-anatomical in origin or optically induced.

anisophoria, optical (induced) Pseudo-imbalance of the muscles of the two eyes induced by spectacle correction of anisometropia as the line of fixation moves from the optical axes of the spectacle lenses to the periphery of the lenses.

anisopia (an″i-sō′pe-ah) A defect of unspecified origin that causes unequal vision in the two eyes.

anisotropic (an″i-so-trop′ik)

1. Unequal turning of the two eyes. (incomitant heterotropia).
2. Unequal or multiple refracting powers in a transparent medium; sometimes, multiple polarizing powers as seen on inspection of lens materials between two sheets of Polaroid film with their axes placed at right angles to each other. (cf. *isotropic.*)

ankyloblepharon (ang″ki-lō-blef′ah-ron) Adhesion of the ciliary edges of the eyelids to each other; may be extensive or limited to small filamentous strands. (cf. *symblepharon.*)

annealing

1. The process of heating glass and then slowly cooling to relieve strain and avoid brittleness. Sometimes applied to similar process with methylmethacrylate. See *lehr.*
2. In molecular genetics, heating to produce separation of nucleic acid molecules containing paired strands of DNA and cooling to attain pairing of molecules that have segments with complementary base pairs; a critical thermal process.

annular design contact lens See *lens, contact, annular design.*

anodize To put a protective, often colored, oxide film on a light metal by an electrolytic process in which the metal acts as the anode; used for aluminum spectacle frames.

anomaloscope (a-nom′a-lo-skōp″) (Nagel anomaloscope) Optical device for critical measurement of color vision defects by requiring the observer to mix lithium red and thallium green to match a standard sodium yellow. The Nagel anomaloscope was introduced between 1899 and 1907 by W.A. Nagel (1870–1911), ophthalmologist of Rostock, Germany. (cf. *Nagel interference filter anomaloscope.*)

anomaly A deviation from the usual or the norm.

anophthalmos (an″of-thal′mos) Absence of the eyeball. Rarely may be a congenital defect; commonly is post-surgical following enucleation.

anoxia (a-nok'se-ah) A pathologic condition of total oxygen deprivation to the body or its parts; long duration causes permanent damage to the affected parts (cf. *hypoxia*).

antagonist

1. A muscle or substance having opposite primary action to that of another; an opposing muscle.
2. A drug that binds to a cell receptor without eliciting a biological response.
3. A substance that tends to nullify the action of another. (cf. *agonist.*)

anterior chamber See *chamber, anterior.*

anterior optical zone (AOZ) See *zone, anterior optical* (AOZ).

anterior segment See *segment, anterior.*

anthropo- Prefix meaning human, or denoting a relationship to a human being.

anthropometry (an"thro-pom'e-tre) The study of human measurements; for example, size, breadth, girth, and distance between anatomical points such as interpupillary distance.

anti- Prefix meaning against.

anti-glare filter See *filter, anti-glare.*

anti-reflective coating See *coating, anti-reflective.*

antibiotic A drug to inhibit or kill pathological organisms; generally derived from a strain of microorganisms.

antibody An immune system protein (immunoglobulin) induced by a specific foreign antigen.

antigen Substance entering or within the body, usually protein or polysaccharide, that stimulates the production of specific antibodies.

antimetropia (an"ti-me-trō'pe-ah) Opposite refractive errors in the two eyes—one plus, one minus.

antimony A crystalline metallic element with a bluish luster; chemical symbol Sb, atomic number 51; as antimony oxide (Sb_2O_3) sometimes used as a component of heat-resistant optical glass. Originally described and studied by Baghdad physician Rhazes (c. 845–c. 930).

AO Disc Trade name for a preservative-free, platinum-coated device used in the stem of the AOSept contact lens cup holder as a neutralizer of the oxidation/chemical AOSept disinfectant solution for soft contact lenses.

AOZ Mnemonic for zone, anterior optical; q.v.

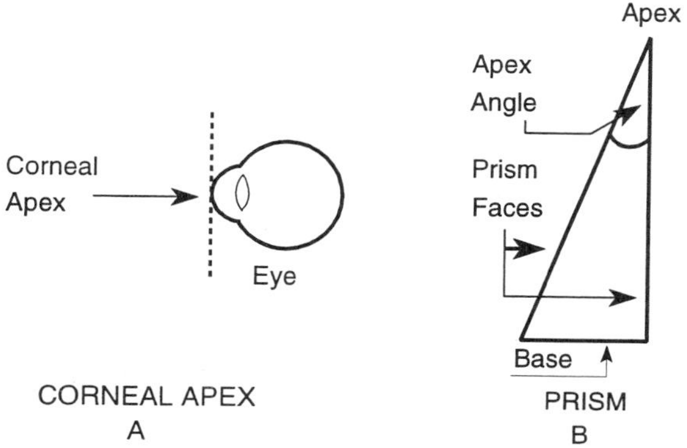

Figure 5 Apex and base. (A) Corneal apex. (B) Apex angle; prism faces; prism apex; and prism base.

APC Mnemonic for curve, anterior peripheral; q.v.

aperture

1. The opening in a spectacle front into which a lens is inserted. Aperture dimensions (in millimeters) do not include the depth of the lens groove.
2. In an optical system, the opening or orifice in an opaque component designed to transmit a given cone diameter of light from a point source ('f' stop in a camera; pupil in the iris); numerical aperture (abbreviated A.) is a measure of the resolving efficiency of the objective lens in a microscopic lens system, or the (adjustable) diameter of the iris diaphragm in the dioptric system of a camera.

aperture of lens Angle formed at a luminous point, between the most divergent rays that are capable of passing through a lens; angle of aperture, or angular aperture.

aperture ratio See *ratio, aperture.*

apex The vertex of an angle, cone or pyramid; the tip (Figure 5, Part B).

apex, corneal The location on the front surface of the cornea which is most anterior when the eye is in a straightforward or primary position; the most steeply curved area of the anterior corneal surface. Sometimes referred to as corneal crest (Figure 5, Part A).

apex, prism The thin edge of a prism where its two faces intersect opposite to its base; the edge toward which the apparent image is displaced (Figure 5, Part B).

aphakia (a-fā'ke-ah) Absence of the crystalline lens. Commonly is post-surgical following cataract extraction; rarely congenital.

aphakic (a-fā'kik)
1. One who has aphakia.
2. Pertaining to or having aphakia, or absence of the crystalline lens from the eye.

aphakic lens See *lens, aphakic.*

apical alignment See *alignment, apical.*

apical bearing See *bearing, apical.*

apical clearance See *clearance, apical.*

apical zone See *zone, apical.*

apostilb (a-post'ilb) A European psychophysical unit for brightness; 1/10 millilambert; an equivalent lux; used in quantification of target stimulus in static perimetry (cf. *nit*); also called a Blondel for the French physicist André Eugène Blondel (1863–1938). Abbreviation, asb. One apostilb equals 0.318 nit.

applanation tonometry See *tonometry, applanation.*

apprentice optician See *optician, apprentice.*

approach magnification See *magnification, approach.*

aqueous flare See *flare, aqueous.*

aqueous humor See *humor, aqueous.*

Ar Chemical symbol for the gaseous element argon; q.v.

arbor press See *tool, staking.*

arc welding See *welding, arc.*

ARC See *coating, anti-reflective*; *anomalous retinal correspondence*; also *American Red Cross.*

arcus An arched, curved or bow-like configuration.

arcus lipoides (lip-oi'des) A gray or white arc in the periphery of the cornea, characteristic of age or fatty deposits; arcus senilis or gerontoxon; less common in early life (arcus juvenilis) when it is usually related to elevated fat concentration in the blood.

arcus senilis See *arcus lipoides.*

Arden plates See *plates, Arden.*

area endpiece See *endpiece, area.*

area, pad The section of a spectacle front where the nosepads are normally located.

argon An inert gaseous element, chemical symbol Ar, atomic number 18; used as a lasing medium in ophthalmic lasers particularly for the destruction of abnormal blood vessels in the ocular fundus; discovered in the earth's atmosphere and named argon in 1894 by Lord John W.S. Rayleigh (1842–1910), English physicist and 1904 Nobel Prize winner, and Scottish chemist Sir William Ramsey (1852–1916).

arm, guard See *arm, pad.*

arm, Numont A portion of a semi-rimless spectacle mounting, extending upwards from the connecting strap at the bridge along the posterior upper edge of the lens to the endpiece temple hinge, providing a flexible lens mounting.

arm, pad That part or extension of a spectacle frame or mounting that connects the pad retainer to the bridge or the front; guard arm.

Armati, Salvina degli A nobleman of Florence, Italy (d. 1317) given inaccurate and legendary credit for the invention of spectacles as an aid to vision early in the fourteenth century. Though the time may be approximately correct, there is little evidence to support Armati's invention.

artificial eye See *eye, artificial.*

artificial tears See *tears, artificial.*

asb Abbreviation for apostilb; q.v.

aspheric In geometric optics, an optical surface which departs slightly from a fixed radius of curvature and hence is free from or has reduced spherical aberrations (e.g., ellipse, parabola, hyperbola curves or mirrors).

aspheric pole See *pole, aspheric.*

aspheric surface See *surface, aspheric.*

assembled lens See *lens, assembled.*

Association for Research in Vision and Ophthalmology (A.R.V.O.) A major professional society for investigative research, established in 1928; originally, Association for Research in Ophthalmology; 6000 members, publishes *Investigative Ophthalmology and Visual Sciences,* formerly (1962–1978) *Investigative Ophthalmology.* Thirteen (13) issues per year. Office: Bethesda, Maryland 20814.

Association of Technical Personnel in Ophthalmology (A.T.P.O.) Designated as ACAHPO until 1988; membership consists of

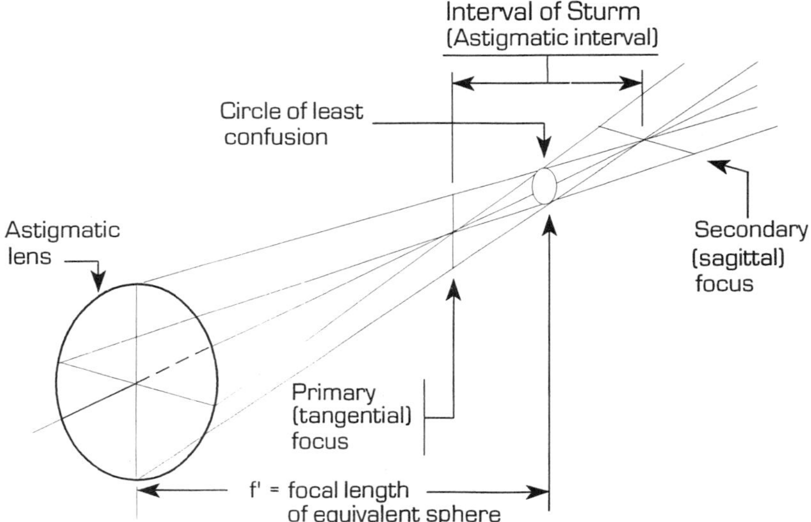

Figure 6 Astigmatism as demonstrated by Sturm's conoid.

J.C.A.H.P.O.-certified ophthalmic assistants, technicians, and technologists; about 1100 members; Publishes *Viewpoints* twice a year. Office: 36 Lee Rd., Chestnut Hill, Massachusetts 02167.

Association of University Professors of Ophthalmology (A.U.P.O.) A voluntary educational association established in 1966 for chairmen of medical school departments of ophthalmology and other educational directors in ophthalmology. Office: San Francisco, California 94101-0369.

asthenopia (as"the-no'pe-a) Ill-defined eye discomfort, eyestrain, or tired eyes. Aggravated by use of the eyes, and sometimes manifested by headache, brow ache, or occipital ache. A descriptive, rather than a diagnostic term, introduced c. 1830 by Glasgow ophthalmologist William Mackenzie (1791–1868).

astigmatic aberration See *aberration, astigmatic.*

astigmatic interval See *interval, astigmatic.*

astigmatic lens See *lens, astigmatic.*

astigmatism (ah-stig'mah-tizm) An imperfect condition of refraction in which rays emanating from a single luminous point are not focused at a single image point by an optical system, but instead are focused

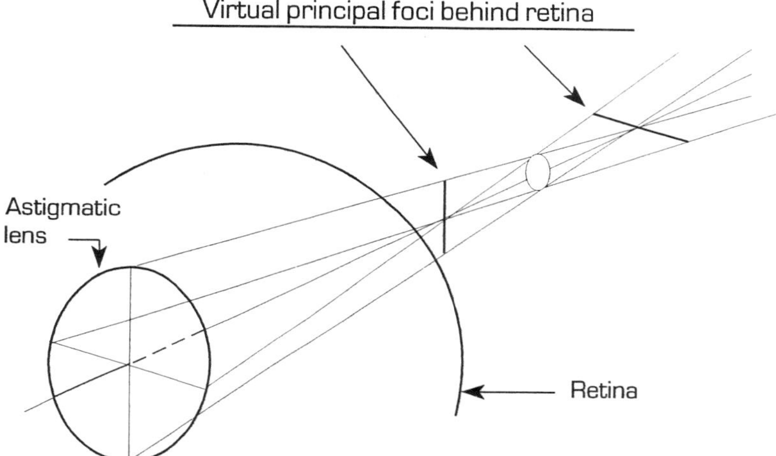

Figure 7 Compound hyperopic astigmatism.

as two line images, generally at right angles to each other and at different distances from the object point. In the eye, a refractive defect due to unequal refraction of incident light by the dioptric system, in different meridians. Generally caused by a toroidal anterior surface of the cornea, but can also be caused by the crystalline lens surface, tilting of the lens, or tilting of a lens implant. Term introduced in 1829 by the mathematician and philosopher Rev. William Whewell (1794-1866) of Trinity College, England, for his own refractive aberration (Figure 6).

astigmatism, against the rule

1. An abnormal refractive condition of an eye in which the meridian of greatest refractive power is at or near the horizontal (0° to 180°) meridian of the eye, wherein the correcting astigmatic cylinder lens power has its minus (–) axis at or near (i.e., within 30°) the vertical (90°) meridian, or has its plus (+) axis at or near (i.e., within 30°) the horizontal meridian.
2. A corneal astigmatism in which the flattest corneal curve meridian is found within 30° of the vertical plane.

astigmatism, compound hyperopic (hī″per-op′ik) An abnormal refractive condition of an eye in which both principal meridians appear to focus behind the retina at two separate image lines. Corrected by a plus spherocylindrical (toric) lens (Figure 7).

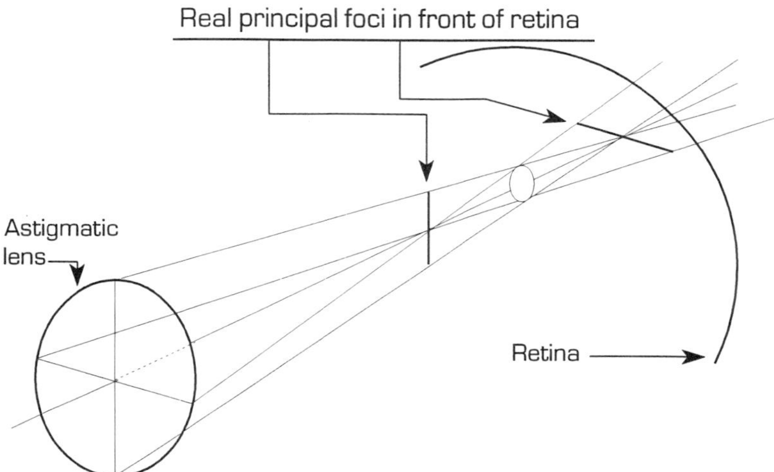

Figure 8 Compound myopic astigmatism.

astigmatism, compound myopic (mī-op'ik) An abnormal refractive condition of an eye in which both principal meridians focus in front of the retina as two separate image lines. Corrected by a minus spherocylindrical (toric) lens (Figure 8).

astigmatism, corneal An astigmatic error of the eye usually deriving from the anterior corneal surface; a minor component may derive from the posterior corneal surface.

astigmatism, irregular An optical defect in which refractive power is unequal in the major meridians and also not uniform along a meridian; unsuitable for correction by a spectacle lens, but may be improved by a contact lens.

astigmatism, lenticular (len-tik'yu-lar) An abnormal refractive condition of an eye in which the refractive power of the crystalline lens is unequal in various meridians; may derive from an unwanted tilting of a surgically implanted intraocular lens.

astigmatism, mixed An abnormal refractive condition of an eye in which one principal meridian focuses at an image line in front of the retina and the other focuses at an image line behind the retina. Corrected by a mixed power spherocylindrical lens (Figure 9).

astigmatism, oblique

1. An abnormal refractive condition of an eye wherein the correcting astigmatic cylinder lens power has its minus (–) axis meridian

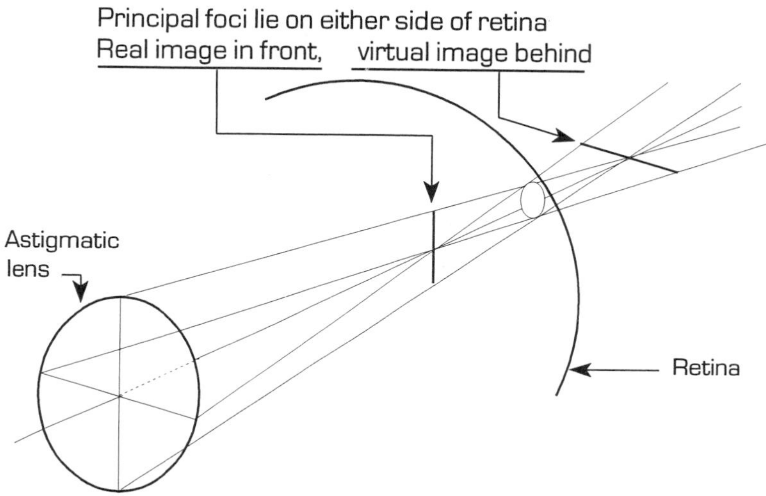

Figure 9 Mixed astigmatism.

within 30° to 60° or 120° to 150° measured from the 0° to 180° meridian.

2. An abnormal refractive condition of an eye in which the principal meridians focus at lines other than the horizontal or vertical orientation; marginal astigmatism.

astigmatism, radial A monochromatic aberration of spherical surfaces, refracting or reflecting as a result of small bundles of incident rays being oblique to the optic axis, forming two line images of a point source.

astigmatism, regular An abnormal refractive condition of an eye in which there is unequal refraction in different meridians but the refractive power is consistent along the axes of the meridians.

astigmatism, residual That portion of ametropia remaining after spherical correction of a refractive error; generally stated for a cylindrical error remaining after spherical (non-toric) contact lens fitting.

astigmatism, simple hyperopic An abnormal refractive condition of an eye in which one principal meridian focuses an image line on the retina and the other principal meridian appears to focus behind the retina, but 90° away from the first meridian. Corrected by a simple plus (+) cylindrical lens (Figure 10).

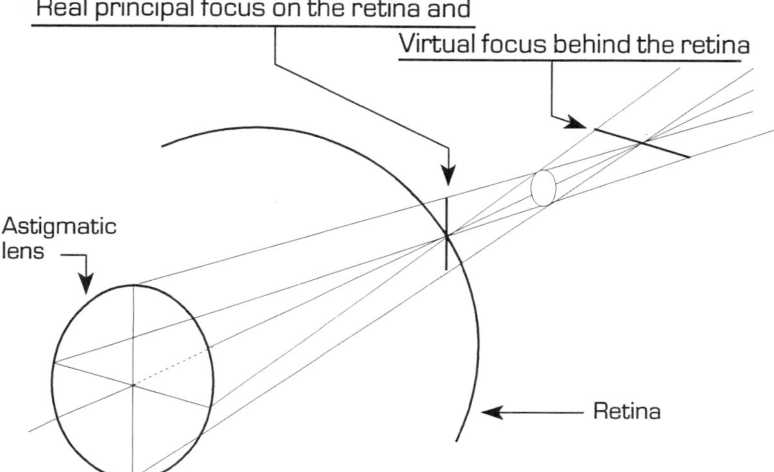

Figure 10 Simple hyperopic astigmatism.

astigmatism, simple myopic An abnormal refractive condition of an eye in which one principal meridian focuses an image line on the retina and the other principal meridian is focused in front of the retina, but 90° away from the first meridian. Corrected by a simple minus (–) cylindrical lens (Figure 11).

astigmatism, with the rule

1. An abnormal refractive condition of an eye in which the meridian of greatest refractive power is at or near the vertical (90°) meridian of the eye, wherein the correcting astigmatic cylinder lens power has its minus (–) axis meridian at or near (i.e., within 30°) of the 0° to 180° meridian, or has its plus (+) axis at or within 30° of the vertical meridian; the most frequent or usual orientation of astigmatic errors in early and adult life.
2. A corneal astigmatism in which the flattest corneal meridian is found within 30° of the horizontal plane.

astronomic telescope See *telescope, astronomic.*

asymptomatic (ā″simp-to-mat′ik) Having no subjective evidence, personal complaints, or perception by the patient of disorder or abnormality.

atomic number See *number, atomic.*

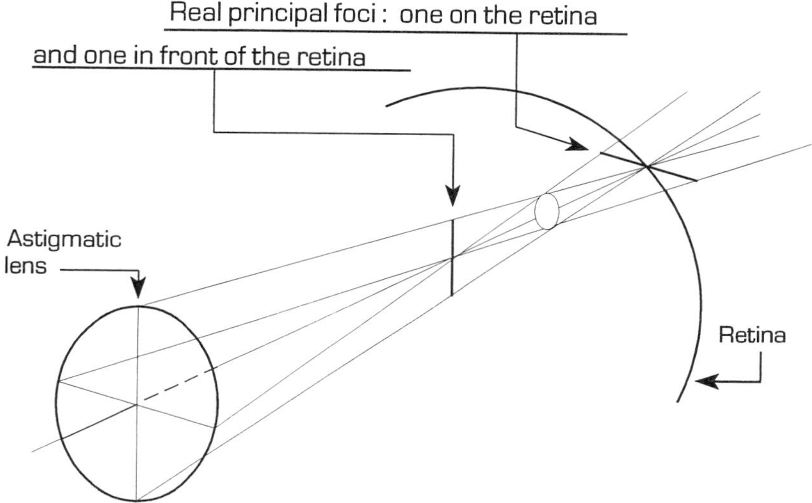

Figure 11 Simple myopic astigmatism.

atrophy (at'ro-fe) A wasting away of a tissue or organ, with reduction of its size and function.

atrophy, optic Degeneration of the optic nerve (Cranial N II); may follow injury, inflammation, tumor, impaired blood supply, or occur without apparent cause.

atropine (at'ro-pēn) Chemical name of an alkaloid originally derived from belladonna plants and used in ophthalmology to give prolonged dilation of the pupil and paralysis of accommodation; an anticholinergic cycloplegic. Although known as a deadly poison in the time of the ancient Hindus and the Roman Empire, Carolus Linnaeus (1707–1778), Swedish physician and taxonomist, named its shrub of origin, Atropa belladonna.

attenuate To reduce in force, intensity, effect, quantity, or value; in light science, sometimes referred to as extinction (or extinction coefficient), or absorption (or absorption coefficient); usually due to absorption or to scattering. See *law, Lambert's.*

Au Chemical symbol for the metallic element gold; q.v.

auto- Prefix meaning self, same.

auto refractor See *refractor, auto.*

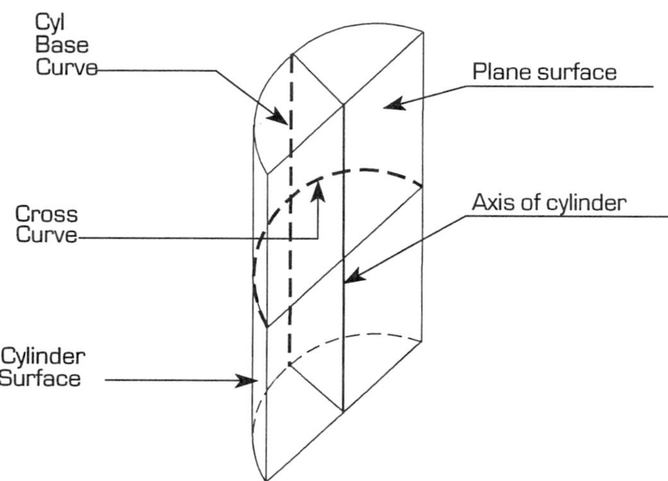

Figure 12 Cylinder axis

automated perimeter See *perimeter, automated.*

axial Pertaining to, or along an axis.

axial hyperopia See *hyperopia, axial.*

axial length See *length, axial.*

axial myopia See *myopia, axial.*

axis

1. An imaginary straight line passing through a body or a system with respect to symmetry of such body or system.
2. An imaginary line passing through a body or an object about which the body or object rotates.
3. A line of reference corresponding to a unique diametric dimension of a body or system.

axis aligner See *aligner, axis.*

axis, cylinder That principal meridian of an astigmatic lens which contains the least curvature in the meridian which is 90° from the meridian containing the full cylinder power (Figure 12).

axis drum See *drum, axis.*

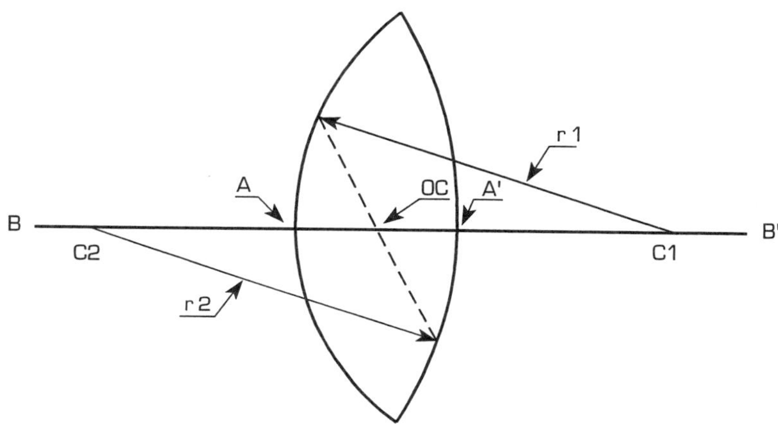

Figure 13 B, B' = Optical (principal) axis; A, A' = Lens vertices.

axis, fixation An imaginary straight line passing from the point of regard in the visual field to the presumed center of rotation of the globe. *Note*: Center of rotation is theoretical and shifts with movement of the globe. (cf. *axis, visual*.)

axis, optic In physiologic optics, a straight line passing through the centers of curvature of the cornea and the lens in the eye.

axis, optical In geometric optics, a straight line perpendicular to both faces of a lens, along which path rays of light will pass through a lens without deviation. It represents the locus of the lens at which the prism power is zero. In most lenses, there is only one line normal to both faces. In a plus spherical lens, the optical axis penetrates the thickest part; in a minus spherical lens, it penetrates the thinnest part. If the lens has prism power, the optical axis may lie outside the lens. If the two surfaces are concentric in a given meridian, any line that is normal to both surfaces in such a meridian may be selected to represent an optical axis. If the surfaces are concentric in all meridians, any line may be elected to represent the optical axis (Figure 13).

axis, principal In geometric optics, a straight line passing through the vertex points and nodal points of a lens system (see Figures 13, 33).

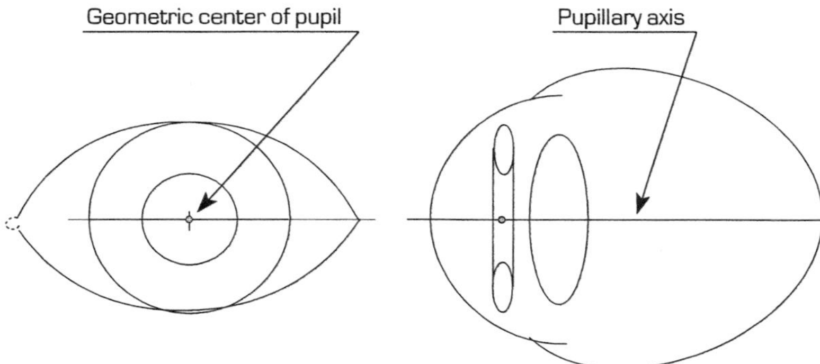

Figure 14 Pupillary axis

axis, pupillary (pyoo'pi-lah-re) An imaginary line that passes through the geometric center of the entrance aperture (pupil) of the eye; commonly does not coincide with the visual or fixation axis (Figure 14).

axis, secondary In geometric optics, a straight line passing through a lens system but outside the principal axis (Figure 15).

axis, visual An imaginary straight line from the point of regard in the visual field to the corresponding point on the retina (normally the fovea centralis of the macula), passing through the nodal points of the eye. (cf. *axis, fixation*).

axis, x of Fick

1. An imaginary straight line lying horizontally in Listing's plane, and intersected by the fixation axis or y axis of Fick; originally described in 1854 by Zurich ophthalmologist Adolph Eugen Fick (1829–1901).
2. Cf. x axis in spectacle optics, an imaginary straight line connecting the geometric centers of a pair of spectacle lenses.
3. In Cartesian coordinates, the x axis is the horizontal coordinate, designated the axis of abscissa.

axis, y of Fick

1. An imaginary straight line extending anteroposteriorly through the anterior and posterior poles of the globe; described in 1851

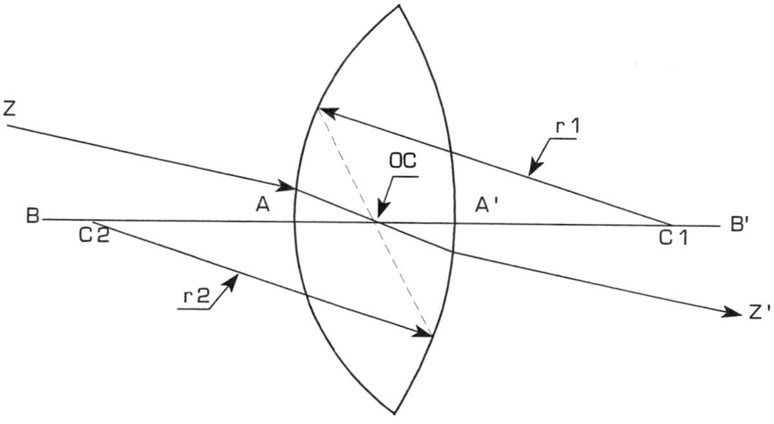

Figure 15 Example of a secondary axis, Z, Z'.

by Zurich ophthalmologist Adolph Eugen Fick (1829–1901); commonly referred to as the fixation axis.

2. Cf. y axis in spectacle optics, an imaginary straight line in the plane of an ophthalmic lens, joining the 90° to 270° axis.
3. In Cartesian coordinates, the y axis is the vertical coordinate or axis of the ordinate.

axis, z of Fick

1. An imaginary straight line lying vertically in Listing's plane and intersected by the y axis or fixation axis; originally described in 1854 by Zurich ophthalmologist Adolph Eugen Fick (1829–1901).
2. In spectacle optics, an imaginary straight line lying in a horizontal plane coincident with the visual axis and passing through the theoretical center of rotation of the eye.
3. In three-dimensional Cartesian coordinates, the z axis indicates depth as a perpendicular to the plane of polar coordinates (x and y) at the pole or intersection.

axon That part of a nerve cell through which impulses travel away from the cell body.

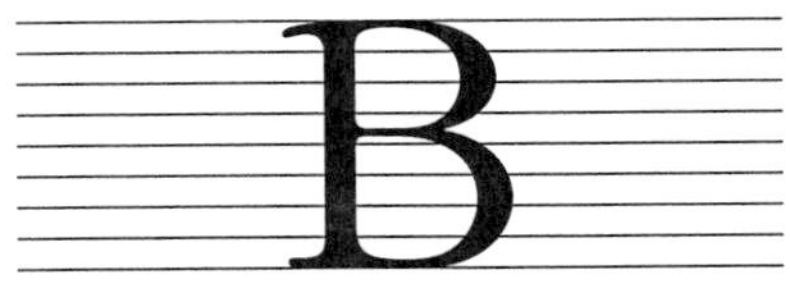

B **1.** Chemical symbol for the non-metallic element boron, atomic number 5; q.v.
2. Abbreviation for Bel; q.v.
3. The vertical distance in millimeters between the superior and inferior horizontal tangents to the apex of the rim groove in a spectacle frame front (see Figure 19); vertical distance in millimeters between the superior and inferior horizontal tangents to the apex of the bevel of a spectacle lens (see Figure 20).

B.B. Small metallic sphere or shot, usually lead, standardized at 0.177-inch in diameter; commonly fired from an air gun. Agent of serious eye injury by contusion or performation.

B.S.S. Abbreviation for solution, balanced salt; q.v.

Ba Chemical symbol for the metallic element barium; q.v.

back focal distance See *distance, back focal.*

back focal length See *distance, back focal.*

back vertex power See *power, back vertex.*

balanced salt solution (B.S.S.) See *solution, balanced salt.*

Balgrip Trade name for a spectacle frame with tension mounting of the lenses located at notches above the horizontal lens bisector; patented by Bausch and Lomb.

balsam, Canada An adhesive used to cement lenses. Obtained from the sap of the North American balsam fir tree; has an index of refraction similar to crown glass; now generally superseded by clear epoxy resins.

bandage lens See *lens, bandage.*

bar, brow

1. A protective component formed or molded at the top of an impact-resistant safety frame front, shielding the open space between the top of the front and the wearer's forehead; usually contoured to conform to the forehead and intended to reduce or avoid injury to the wearer's eyes from above.
2. A metallic, plastic covered bar component of a dress metallic spectacle frame front connecting the top of one eyewire to the other, conforming to the contour of the forehead to maintain an open space between eye brows and frame to aid structural strength, and reducing the accumulation of perspiration on the lenses during normal wear or sporting activities; sweat bar.
3. Spectacle front design with each lens and its eyewire hinged to the center of a horizontal bar to eliminate the nasal bridge and contact with the nose. Trade name: Multiframe (Priestly and More, London, England).

bar code See *code, bar.*

barium A chemical element of the alkaline earths; chemical symbol Ba, atomic number 56; its oxide is used in the segment glass of a glass multifocal lens to raise the index of refraction without creating undesirable levels of dispersion. First isolated in 1808 by English chemist Humphry Davy (1778–1829).

barrel distortion See *distortion, barrel.*

barrel

1. The component of a hinge that interlocks with the mating component of the hinge set.
2. A threaded closure device attached to a metal eyewire (eyewire tube). Abbreviated bbl.

base curve See *curve, base.*

base-down Vertical placement of prism so that the base of the prism is toward the bottom of an ophthalmic lens or at 270° on a 360° scale. Abbreviation b.d.

base-in Horizontal placement of prism so that the base is toward the nose along the 0° to 180° line—for the right eye, at 0° on a 360° scale; for the left eye, at 180° on a 360° scale. Abbreviation b.i.

base-out Horizontal placement of prism so that the base is toward the side of the head along the 0° to 180° line—for the right eye, at 180° on a 360° scale; for the left eye, at 0°on a 360° scale. Abbreviation b.o.

base, prism The thick edge of a prism, opposite the apex or thin edge; the direction toward which a light ray is refracted by a prism. (See Figure 5, Part B.)

base-up Vertical placement of prism so that the base of the prism is toward the top of an ophthalmic lens or at 90° on a 360° scale. Abbreviation b.u.

BAT Acronym for Brightness Acuity Tester; q.v.

bath, bead A heated container filled with glass spheres to provide uniform warming of a spectacle frame placed in it; a frame warmer.

bath, potassium nitrate A heated ion-exchange immersion chamber used for increasing the impact resistance of glass lenses by chemical exchange of surface ions.

Baumé scale See *scale, Baumé.*

Be Chemical symbol for the metallic element beryllium; q.v.

bead bath See *bath, bead.*

beads, glass Small (e.g., 1 millimeter) spheres of glass used in a frame warmer to provide even, constant heat to a frame; larger spheres are sometimes used as surgical implants to restore volume in an injured or enucleated orbit of the eye.

bearing, apical An area of contact between the posterior surface of a contact lens with the steepest point of the cornea; usually evaluated with sodium fluorescein solution placed on the cornea and viewed with the lens in situ.

bedewing, corneal (kor'ne-al be-doo'ing) Clouding or swelling from small collections of fluid in the anterior layers of the corneal epithelium due to hypoxia, death of epithelial cells, or breakdown of endothelial cells and the passage of aqueous through the cornea; visible with a biomicroscope; also referred to as Hubert's or Sattler's veil, or central corneal clouding; sometimes designated as Fick's phenomenon (1888). Extensively studied by German ophthalmologist C. Hubert Sattler (1844-1928).

Bel A unit of relative power or intensity based on log scale; used in static perimetry; named in 1921 for Alexander Graham Bell (1848–1922), naturalized U.S. citizen born in Edinburgh, Scotland, and inventor of the telephone. Abbreviated B.

below An inappropriate term used to describe the amount of displacement in millimeters that a multifocal segment top must be shifted vertically (i.e., up or down) with respect to the horizontal lens bisector, to accommodate the desired segment height at the time of surfacing or finishing layout. (See Figure 22.) See also *VSP; position, vertical segment.*

bend, down The drop or downward curve of the tip end of a spectacle earpiece (temple) to fit over and around the ear; also known as ear bend.

bend, ear See *bend, down.*

bend, mastoid The curvature in the tip end of a spectacle earpiece (temple) adapting to the mastoid curvature behind the ear.

benzalkonium chloride (bens-al-kō′ne-um) A rapidly acting surface disinfectant, detergent, and wetting agent of the quaternary ammonium compounds; effective against a wide variety of gram-negative and gram-positive bacteria, fungi, and viruses; will not kill spores, *Mycobacterium tuberculosis*, and some *Pseudomonas* species.

beryllium (ber-il′le-um) A metallic element; chemical symbol Be, atomic number 4; used in spectacle frame construction particularly as an alloy with copper; as a dust or fume, causes toxic reaction in the lungs and (less often) on the skin. First recognized within the gems beryl and emerald at the end of the eighteenth century by French chemist Louis Nicolas Vauquelin (1763–1829).

beta B, β

1. The second letter in the Greek alphabet.
2. The second item in a series or system of classification.

Better Vision Institute (B.V.I.) A voluntary organization funded by Vision Industry Council of America (V.I.C.A.) with a goal "to keep the public aware of the need for more adequate vision care," initially established in New York in 1929; merged with Vision Council of America (V.C.O.A.) in 1989; the voice of the ophthalmic community. Office: 1800 N. Kent St., Suite 1210, Rosslyn, Virginia 22209.

bevel A slanted or angled edge, generally not a right angle; in spectacle lens manufacture, an edge configuration of "V" shape with the apex directed outward from the lens.

bevel, CN Technique for reducing edge thickness of a high minus (–) power hard contact lens; developed c. 1949 by, and named for, Charles Nishamora (c. 1915–), Chicago contact lens technician.

bevel finish, Con-Lish A contraction of the words *contact* and *polish* to describe an edging technique for contouring and polishing the edge of high minus (–) power rigid contact lenses; designed to reduce edge thickness and lid interaction by using select sequential conical tools, such as 60°, 90°, 120°, and 150° with low speed (i.e., within 100 to 500 rpm), each for a specified number of seconds, first holding the concave surface down, then up; introduced in 1959 by Gilberto Cepero, M.D., of Havana, Cuba, and Miami, Florida. Alternate spelling Conlish.

bevel, lens The periphery of an edged lens having an angular cross section.

bevel, pin A chamfer ground on an otherwise sharp edge of an ophthalmic lens to minimize chipping of the lens edge and reduce possible injury to the wearer; improperly called safety bevel.

bevel, rimless Flat or faceted edge design of an ophthalmic lens for rimless, semi-rimless, nylon cord retention, or other mountings not having a lens groove. See *groove.*

bevel, safety A slope ground on a lens edge to prevent chipping of the edge; a flattening of the back bevel edge to provide facial clearance, or removal of the sharp edge to minimize injury if facial contact should occur.

bevel, V See *bevel.*

beveling A machining process intended to alter contours.

bi- Prefix meaning two, twice, or double; also written as bin- when before a vowel (e.g., binocular).

bicentric grinding (bī-sen'trik) See *grinding, bicentric.*

biconcave lens See *lens, biconcave.*

biconcave Having two concave surfaces. See *surface, concave.*

biconvex Having two convex surfaces. See *surface, convex.*

biconvex lens See *lens, biconvex.*

bicurve. A contact lens design containing two concentric curves on its posterior surface.

bid Abbreviation of Latin "bis in die," twice a day.

bifocal See *lens, bifocal.*

bifocal, diffractive A rigid or non-rigid multifocal contact lens of simultaneous design. The lens is composed of a series of concentric rings with small facets that diffract 50% of the light rays into a separate focus. The faceted rings are on the posterior surface, and increase in number as near addition power increases.

bifocal, straight-top See *lens, straight-top bifocal.*

bilateral Affecting or pertaining to the two sides or halves of the body with reference to the midsagittal plane; in common ocular use, referring to both eyes.

binocular (bin-ok'yu-lar) Referring to or involving both eyes; the use of both eyes simultaneously in such a manner that each retinal image contributes to the final, single perception.

binocular field See *field, binocular visual.*

binocular fusion See *fusion, binocular.*

binocular PD measurements See *distance, interocular.*

binocular vision See *vision, single binocular.*

binocular visual acuity See *acuity, binocular visual.*

binocular visual field See *field, binocular visual.*

binocularity (bin-ok"yu-lar'i-te) Ability to use both eyes together.

biomicroscope (slit lamp) Optical examining instrument with a binocular microscope of 6 to 40 power and an articulated light source that can be adjusted to various slit sizes, intensities, and configurations. One of the most important and fundamental ophthalmic diagnostic instruments; used in contact lens fitting (e.g., to evaluate lens-corneal relationship); Gullstrand slit lamp. Originally designed in 1902 by Swedish ophthalmologist Allvar Gullstrand (1862–1930), who received the 1911 Nobel Prize in medicine.

bipolar cells See *cells, bipolar.*

biprism Optical device consisting of two equal prisms placed base to base; used to analyze extraocular muscle balance; invented in 1890 by British ophthalmologist Ernest Edmund Maddox (1860–1933); Maddox biprism.

birefringence (bī"re-frin'jens) Unequal refraction of incident light by a non-isotropic optical material, such as the crystalline structure of Iceland Spar; double refraction. Usually assessed in polarized light.

birefringence strain See *strain, birefringence.*

bisector A straight line that divides an angle, line segment, or plane object into two equal parts.

bisector, horizontal lens (HLB) A straight line passing through the geometric center of a finished spectacle lens in the x axis of the Cartesian coordinate system; horizontal center line; datum line (British term); mounting line; geometric center line (all now lesser used or obsolete terms). (See Figure 20.)

bisector, vertical lens (VLB) A straight line passing through the geometric center of a finished spectacle lens in the y axis of the Cartesian coordinate system (see Figure 20).

bisector, vertical segment (VSB) A straight line through the geometric center of a segment in the y axis of the Cartesian coordinate system (see Figure 20).

BITA Acronym for bilevel telemicroscope apparatus. See *telemicroscope.*

bitoric contact lens See *lens, contact, bitoric.*

bitoric lenses See *lens, bitoric.*

blank, major The basic lens substrate to which segments of different refractive power may be added to produce a multifocal lens.

blank, molded The basic lens stock of a lens manufacturer, which may be obtained in pressed form from chunk optical glass or as pressings made directly from molten optical glass. Plastic lenses are molded by casting, injection, or other techniques to finished (uncut) or semi-finished form.

blank, multifocal semi-finished Lens blank that is designed after surfacing to provide two or more corrective powers over different areas. Before surfacing, one face of such blanks is a finished surface and the other face is unfinished. This includes blanks with blended segments.

blank, pattern A flat piece of hard plastic or metal material, usually rectangular, round or oval, approximately 1 to 2 millimeters thick, drilled with a 0.302-inch centering hole and two sets of smaller horizontal alignment holes; used manually or by machine to make a form or template to edge the desired lens shape.

blank, progressive power semi-finished Lens blank that is designed after surfacing to provide a continuous change rather than discrete changes of corrective power over a part or whole of the surface. Before surfacing, one face of such blanks is a finished surface and the other face is unfinished. Some lens designs incorporate characteristics of both multifocal and progressive power blanks. In these cases, tolerances apply according to the manufacturer's specifications.

blank, semi-finished A lens blank in which one face is a finished surface and the other face is unfinished.

blank, single vision semi-finished Lens blank that is designed after surfacing to provide a single corrective power for a single viewing distance; before surfacing, one face is a finished surface and the other face is unfinished.

blank size See *size, blank.*

blend curve See *curve, blend.*

blended lens See *lens, blended.*

bleph- Prefix meaning eyelid.

blepharitis (blef″ah-rī′tis) Inflammation of the eyelids.

1. Marginal: eyelid infection manifested by redness, crusty debris, and scales on the lid borders.
2. Allergic: itching but painless swelling of the eyelids due to sensitivity or contact reaction to irritants or allergenic proteins; sometimes attributed to spectacle frames (spectacle dermatitis).
3. Infectious: due to invasion of bacteria, and less commonly, virus or fungi into the lids.

blepharochalasis (blef″ah-ro-chal-ā′sis) Relaxation and redundancy of upper lid tissues that may cover the lid margin and interfere with vision. (cf. *dermatochalasis*).

blepharoplasty (blef″ah-ro-plas′te) Surgical correction of a defect in the eyelid.

blepharoptosis (blef″ah-ro-tō′sis) See *ptosis.*

blepharospasm (blef′ah-ro-spazm″) Persistent or repetitive involuntary contraction of the orbicularis oculi muscle, generally due to unidentified or unknown cause (essential blepharospasm). May be unilateral, but tends to become bilateral.

blind spot, normal A physiologic scotoma in the temporal visual field of each eye, corresponding to the position of the optic disc; Blind Spot of Mariotte; named after Edme Mariotte (1620–1684), French philosopher and mathematician who published its description in 1668.

blindness, color A non-specific term for congenital or acquired impairment or absence of color discrimination; incorrectly applied to any or minor deviations from normal perception of hues.

blindness, cortical Loss of vision due to a defect in the visual area (occipital pole) of the brain; usually Brodmann's area 17.

blindness, flash (actinic keratitis) Visual impairment, usually temporary, caused by viewing bright light; welder's flash (actinic), painful visual impairment due to ultraviolet damage to the epithelial cells of the cornea.

blindness, legal Loss of vision to a best corrected visual acuity of 20/200 or less, in the better eye, utilizing conventional ophthalmic or contact lenses, or loss of visual field to a diameter of 20° or less in the better eye, or total homonymous hemianopia. For information on legal blindness or total homonymous hemianopia, write to Social Security Administration, Division of Disability Determination, for listings 2.02, 2.03, and 2.05, respectively.

blink rate See *rate, blink.*

blink reflex See *reflex, blink.*

blocker

1. A mechanical device, usually of table top design, for affixing an ophthalmic lens blank to a plastic or metal lens carrier (i.e., blocking body); used in lens edging and lens surfacing.
2. A drug that inhibits the entry of a biological chemical into the surface or interior of a living cell (e.g., beta blocker).

blocking

1. The procedure of attaching a lens to a metal or plastic body for the purpose of surfacing or finishing.
2. Injection of a local anesthetic drug to interrupt the transmission of sensation from that site or region.
3. Administration of drugs designed to compete for a receptor site on a cell and prevent other compounds from acting on that cell.

blocking body See *body, blocking.*

Blondel Eponym for apostilb; q.v.

blue blockers Generic term for spectacle lenses that absorb or reflect wavelength of light from 415nm to 470nm.

blue light injury mechanism The potential for photochemical or phototoxic damage to the retina resulting from irradiance in the narrow band width of 415nm to 470nm. This is distinct from thermal damage of infrared light.

blue sclera See *sclera, blue.*

blur circle See *circle, blur.*

blur, color See *aberration, chromatic.*

blur, spectacle A transient impairment of visual acuity on changing from contact lenses to spectacle corrections usually due to induced epithelial edema lasting from a few minutes to a few hours; prolonged blur suggests a poor contact lens fit.

body, blocking A plastic or metal base to which a lens is attached for the purpose of surfacing or finishing.

body, ciliary (sil'e-ah-re) Portion of the vascular coat (uvea) between the iris and the choroid of the eye; consists of ciliary processes and the ciliary muscle; source of elaboration of the aqueous humor of the eye.

body, foreign A particle or mass of material that is not normal to the anatomic location where it is found; e.g., a cinder in the eye, a B.B. in the vitreous, and the like.

body, lateral geniculate (je-nik'yu-lāt) Part of the visual system that relays nerve impulses from the optic tract to optic radiations within the brain.

Boley gauge See *gauge, Boley.*

boron A non-metallic element occurring as crystals and powder; chemical symbol B, atomic number 5; used as a major component of ophthalmic glass. First isolated in elementary form in 1808 by French chemist Joseph Louis Gay-Lussac (1778–1850).

bow Anything bent or curved; in spectacle components, properly referred to as earpiece (temple). See *temple; curve, temple head.*

bow, temple The combined outward and inward curvature of a spectacle earpiece (temple), designed to eliminate contact with the head in front of the ear.

box, drop back A rigid, protective case commonly constructed of wood, leather, or hard paper, double-hinged over the spine to protect a book; clam shell box; (British) fall down back box; Solander Box invented in late 1770s by Daniel Charles Solander (1736–1782), a botanist at the British Museum in London.

box, Yerkes discrimination A maze with a series of doors; used in laboratory study of visual and color discrimination in animals; rewards are produced by opening correct door, and electric shocks are delivered by opening incorrect door; developed after World War I by Robert M. Yerkes, Ph.D. (1876–1956), psychologist at Harvard and Yale.

Box-o-graph Trade name for a mechanical device used for measuring the horizontal (i.e., "A" dimension) and the vertical (i.e., "B" dimension) of ophthalmic lenses.

boxing system See *system, boxing.*

Br Chemical symbol for the element bromine; q.v.

brace bridge See *bridge, brace.*

break-up time test (BUT) See *test, break-up time.*

bridge The supportive structural member connecting the two rims of an ophthalmic front; the two lenses in a rimless mounting, sometimes referred to as "center" with rimless mountings.

bridge, brace Metal embedded in a plastic front to reinforce the bridge area; an extra member for styling purposes or reinforcement, or both, used to improve alignment retention of a spectacle front.

bridge inset See *inset, bridge.*

bridge, keyhole A bridge designed for a spectacle front that does not permit continuous contact between the nose and the front in the nasal crest area; a bridge taking the appearance of a "keyhole" when viewed frontally.

bridge on plane A condition where the bridge fitting surface of a spectacle front is located in the same plane as the lenses.

bridge outset See *outset, bridge.*

bridge, saddle A bridge design for a spectacle front that permits continuous contact between the nose and the front in the nasal crest area, immediately below the glabella.

bridge, sculptured An individually designed bridge area of a spectacle front that conforms to an unusual nasal anatomical variation.

bridge size See *size, bridge.*

Brightness Acuity Tester (BAT) Trade name for a hand-held optical instrument that presents a bright hemifield to a patient through an opening in which the patient observes any elected resolving symbol; three intensities of glare may be presented—40, 340, or 1370 Cd/m^2; manufactured by Mentor O. & O., Inc., of Massachusetts.

brightness In psychophysical photometry, the measure of light from a unit area or surface; commonly expressed in Lamberts (1 lumen per square centimeter of area).

broach A mechanical reaming tool, tapering to a point, used as an awl or cutting file to smooth, enlarge or remove material from a previously drilled hole in an ophthalmic lens; a pointed awl.

broken ring test chart See Figure 17; see also *optotype.*

bromine One of the silver halides in phototropic (photochromatic) glass; chemical symbol Br, atomic number 35. A reddish-brown liquid element extracted from seawater; intermediate in properties between chlorine and iodine; first isolated in 1826 by French chemist Anton J. Balard (1802–1876).

brow bar See *bar, brow.*

Bruch's membrane See *membrane, Bruch's.*

bulbar Relating to the ocular globe, bulbus oculi.

bulbar conjunctiva See *conjunctiva, bulbar.*

bullous keratopathy See *keratopathy, bullous.*

Bureau of Radiologic Health (B.R.H.) Former name of division of the U.S. Food and Drug Administration charged with safety performance standards for all electromagnetic energy sources. Name changed to Center for Devices and Radiological Health (C.D.R.H.). Laser products were included in 1976. Located in Rockville, Maryland.

Burton lamp See *light, Wood's.*

butt joint See *joint, butt.*

butt, temple Proximal end of a spectacle temple that joins with an ophthalmic frame front.

B.V.I.

1. Abbreviation for Better Vision Institute; q.v.
2. Trade name for French commercial house BioVision International, in field of ultrasound and lasers for ophthalmic use.

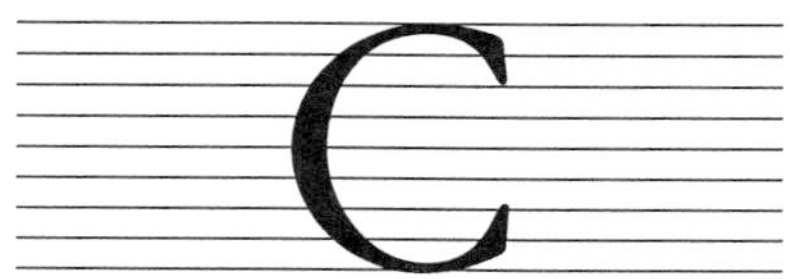

c. Abbreviation for "circa," about; used to indicate approximate dates, time, etc.

C **1.** Chemical symbol for the element carbon; q.v.
2. Symbol for degree on the Celsius temperature scale; fresh water freezes at 0°C and boils at 100°C, under normal atmospheric pressure; developed in 1742 by Anders Celsius (1701–1744), Swedish astronomer from Uppsala.

CAB Abbreviation for cellulose acetate butyrate; q.v.

CAcTS Abbreviation for clockwise add, counterclockwise subtract; q.v.

CAC Abbreviation for curve, central anterior; q.v.

CAD Abbreviation for computer-assisted design.

CAM Abbreviation for computer-aided manufacturing.

C.E.N. *Comité Européen de Coordination des Normes*; board that establishes and maintains scales and obligatory standards binding for all member nations in the European Community of Nations; also called Comité Européen de Normalisation.

CEU Abbreviation for continuing education unit. See *continuing education credit.*

C.I.E. Abbreviation for Commission Internationale de l'Eclairage; q.v.

C.I.H. Abbreviation for Certified Industrial Hygiene technologist; see *technologist, Certified Industrial Hygiene.*

C.L.A.O. Abbreviation for Contact Lens Association of Ophthalmologists; q.v.

C.L.M.A. Abbreviation for Contact Lens Manufacturers Association; q.v.

C.L.S.A. Abbreviation for Contact Lens Society of America; q.v.

C.O.A. Abbreviation for:
1. Commission on Opticianry Accreditation; q.v.
2. Canadian Orthoptic Association; q.v.
3. Certified Ophthalmic Assistant; q.v.

C.O.M.T. Abbreviation for J.C.A.H.P.O.-certified ophthalmic medical technologist; q.v.

C.O.S. Abbreviation for Canadian Ophthalmological Society.

C.O.T. Abbreviation for J.C.A.H.P.O.-certified ophthalmic medical technician; q.v.

c-sizer A mechanical device for measuring the circumference of a lens by using a flexible tape measure (i.e., circumference sizer); measurements taken in this manner afford more precise sizing than those taken with a Box-o-graph.

Ca 1. Chemical symbol for the yellow, metallic element calcium; q.v.
2. The abbreviation for cancer.

cable temple See *temple, cable.*

cadmium A bivalent metal, similar in appearance and properties to tin; chemical symbol Cd, atomic number 48. Used as corrosion-resistant coating and in alkaline storage batteries. Highly poisonous and toxic; fumes are irritating to the conjunctiva and respiratory passages. Named and identified in 1817 by German chemist Friedrich Strohmeyer (1776–1835).

cadmium oxide A chemically active compound of cadmium with oxygen; chronic exposure to fumes produces severe conjunctival and lung inflammation.

cadmium sulfide A coloring compound producing rich yellow color in glass; fumes are toxic and cause epithelial cell damage.

calcite A mineral consisting of calcium carbonate crystallized in hexagonal form; valuable in optics as a naturally polarizing medium.

calcium A silvery yellow metal, the base element of lime (calcium oxide); chemical symbol Ca, atomic number 20; the basic element in calcium fluoride lenses that have very low dispersion and low index of refraction (1.4 to 1.5). First isolated in 1808 by English chemist Humphry Davy (1778–1829).

calibration The adjustment of a machine or measuring device relative to a working standard test object that has accuracy traceable to a fundamental standard.

caliper, lens A hand-held (usually) mechanical measuring instrument in the form of pliers, having two legs or jaws that can be adjusted to determine thickness, diameter, caliber, and/or distance between surfaces. Thickness gauge for lenses; optical calipers formerly were calibrated in "points" (i.e., 0.2mm = 1 point) but are now more frequently made calibrated in tenths of millimeters; available as inside calipers and as outside calipers. In contact lens optics, thickness gauges are made an integral part of the radiuscope, utilizing the gauges to read the center thickness of the rigid contact lens held between the base and rod attached to the movable upper portion of the radiuscope.

caliper, thickness See *caliper, lens.*

caliper, vernier A hand-held precise measuring instrument made up of a graduated beam with a fixed arm at right angles to it and a right-angled fixed leg on a movable arm graduated in the linear (i.e., English or Metric) system, which slides along the beam to measure diameter of various objects (e.g., lens or frames). The beam is graduated so that ten (10) units (if metric) on the beam are equal to only nine (9) units on the movable arm. When measurements are taken, only one graduated mark on the beam aligns itself with one mark on the movable arm scale, providing accurate measure. Devised in 1631 by the French mathematician Pierre Vernier (1580–1637).

cam An eccentric disc fastened on and revolving with a shaft for converting regular rotary motion into irregular rotary or reciprocating motion.

camera An opaque box or similarly shaped enclosure to exclude the entry of light except from a small shutter-controlled aperture made of a pinhole or a diaphragm. Used to time the exposure on internal light sensitive substance (i.e., film) of the image so formed following the laws of rectilinear propagation.

campimeter A mechanical or optical apparatus to measure the central portion (usually within a radius of 30°) of the visual field; term introduced in 1875 by Julius Hirschberg (1843–1925), ophthalmologist of Berlin. Also called tangent screen (1886) of J.P. Bjerrum (1851–1920); stereo campimeter (1920) of Ralph Lloyd (1875–1968); Harrington-Flocks screener (1954), David Harrington (1904–1990); Allain Friedmann analyzer (1966); B & L Autoplot.

Canada balsam See *balsam, Canada.*

canal, lacrimal (lak′ri-mal) The tubular passage from the lacrimal sac into the nose; the nasolacrimal duct.

canal of Schlemm (shlem) Complex drainage channel for outflow of aqueous humor from anterior chamber of the eye; named in 1831 for Berlin anatomist Friedrich S. Schlemm (1795–1858), who described the canal after observing it filled with blood in a hanged man in 1827.

canaliculi (kan″ah-lik′yu-lī) Plural of canaliculus.

canaliculitis (kan″ah-lik″yu-lī′tis) Inflammation of the small lacrimal drainage tube in the nasal portion of either eyelid between the lacrimal punctum and the lacrimal sac.

canaliculus, common (lacrimal) (kan″ah-lik′yu-lus) A short and narrow membranous tubular passage, part of the lacrimal drainage system, joining the superior and inferior canaliculi with the lacrimal sac.

candela (kan-dē′lah) An SI base unit of luminous intensity superseding in 1948 the "new candel"; a source of one candela emits one lumen per steradian; abbreviated cd.

Candida A common, yeast-like fungus often found in the mouth, skin, intestinal tract, and vagina; opportunistically may invade the cornea; of several known types, *Candida albicans* is the most usual pathogen. May cause keratitis or other infection, particularly in the immunocompromised patient. Disinfection of contact lenses always is aimed at removing this organism, as well as other common skin and oral bacteria.

candlepower The luminous intensity of a light source expressed in candelas.

canthi Plural of canthus; q.v.

canthus The angle formed at either end of the eyelids at their point of union; commonly referred to as inner and outer, or medial and lateral canthi. Term used in English language medical literature since about 1600 A.D.

canthus, lateral (outer) The angle joining the upper and lower eyelids close to the temple.

canthus, medial (inner) The angle joining the upper and lower eyelids close to the nose.

cap, lens

1. A plus lens fitted over the objective lens of a simple Galilean telescope for use in the reading range; usually about +10D power.
2. A protective device to cover the lens shielding it from dust, impact, and debris.

capsule, lens A normally clear, elastic membrane entirely surrounding the crystalline lens and of varying thickness; consists of an inner (main or cuticular) layer and a thin, outer or zonular lamella; attaches to the zonules of Zinn and contributes to the accommodative process.

capsule, Tenon's (bulbar fascia) A membranous-appearing fibrous network of connective tissue encapsulating the ocular globe and blending with the sheaths of the extraocular muscles; first described in 1806 by Jacques René Tenon (1724–1816), Parisian anatomist and surgeon.

capsulectomy (kap"su-lek'to-me) Surgical removal of all or part of the capsule of the crystalline lens.

capsulotomy (kap-su-lot'o-me) Incision of a capsule; e.g., such as of the crystalline lens in cataract surgery.

carbon A non-metallic element having a valence or oxidation number 4, found nearly pure in diamond; chemical symbol C, atomic number 6; major component of charcoal, graphite, and the like; used in carbon fibre graphite frames, golf clubs, and tennis rackets.

cardinal points See *points, cardinal.*

cardiopulmonary resuscitation (CPR) A coordinated forcing of cardiac compression and mouth-to-mouth ventilation for an unconscious patient without heart or lung activity.

carpal tunnel syndrome (CTS) See *syndrome, carpal tunnel.*

carrier lens See *lens, carrier; lens, lenticular.*

Cartesian lens See *lens, Cartesian.*

caruncle, lacrimal (lak'ri-mal kar'ung-kl) A small, pink, fleshy structure situated in the medial canthus between the upper and lower lids of the eye. From the Latin diminutive of "caro," flesh.

cast To form from liquid material into a particular shape by injecting, pouring or pressing into a mold.

casting, glass lens The process of forming rough glass lens blanks by pouring and pressing molten glass into lentiform molds and subsequent annealing.

casting, plastic lens The process of forming polymerized lenses by injecting liquid monomer into highly polished lentiform molds allowing appropriate time for curing.

cataract Any opacity of the normally clear crystalline lens or its capsule; partial or complete loss of transparency. Morphologically graded as incipient, immature, mature and hypermature.

cataract, cortical spoke Radially arranged opacities or lines at the outer layers of the crystalline lens.

cataract extraction See *extraction, cataract.*

cataract, hypermature A fully developed opacity of the lens with fluid degeneration and swelling of the lens volume.

cataract, immature A partially cloudy crystalline lens that has clear areas remaining.

cataract, incipient Early or partial lens opacity with limited effect on vision; common in aging.

cataract lens See *lens, aphakic.*

cataract, mature A fully opaque lens; candidate for surgical removal.

cataract, nuclear sclerotic Opacification and hardening of the central portion of the crystalline lens. Often requiring additional minus (–) spectacle power to compensate for the thickening and therefore additional plus (+) power of the crystalline lens.

cathode ray tube See *tube, cathode ray.*

catoptrics The division of optical physics dealing with reflected light and reflected images.

caustic

1. In geometric optics, the designation of or relating to the configuration of rays of light emanating from a point source and reflected or refracted by a curved solid or curved surface; a basis of optical aberration.
2. A burning or corrosive chemical that can destroy tissue, particularly hazardous to the cornea.

cc

1. Abbreviation for cubic centimeter; component of the SI-derived unit for volume, the cubic meter.
2. Abbreviation for "with correction."
3. Abbreviation for "chief complaint," the introductory unit in a patient's medical history.

Cd Chemical symbol for the metallic element cadmium; q.v.

Ce Chemical symbol for the metallic element cerium; q.v.

cell The fundamental structural and functional unit of living organisms; consists of a nucleus, cytoplasm, organelles, and an enclosing membrane. Concept and term introduced in 1663 by Robert Hooke (1635-1703), English experimenter, early developer of single lens microscope, and author of *Micrographia*, 1665.

cells, bipolar Nerve cells in the inner nuclear layer of the retina connecting the photoreceptors (rods and cones) with the ganglion cells; consisting of a nucleus, cytoplasm, organelles, and enclosing membrane.

cells, ganglion (gang'gle-on) Large nerve cells in the retina; axons of the ganglion cells form the optic nerve fiber layer and lead to the optic nerve.

cells, goblet Small, unicellular glands found in epithelium of various mucous membranes, particularly in the conjunctiva where they contribute mucin to the posterior layer of the pre-corneal tear film.

cellulose acetate A clear, thermoplastic polymer commonly used in the manufacture of fashion and ophthalmic frames; low flammability; easily polished; durable; easily colored. Commonly called "Zyl" or "Kodapak."

cellulose acetate butyrate (CAB) (byoo'ti-rāt) An isotropic organic ophthalmic plastic of low flammability used in the manufacture of safety spectacle frames; first used in 1974 as gas-permeable hard contact lens material. Accidentally discovered in 1938 by research scientists at Eastman Kodak Company, Rochester, New York.

cellulose nitrate or zylonite (zī'lo-nīt) A highly flammable derivative of guncotton, voluntarily banned from use in the manufacture of spectacle frames and camera film; polishes extremely well, but subject to spontaneous combustion under heated conditions.

cellulose propionate (prō'pe-o-nāt) An organic plastic material incorporating a salt of propionic acid used in the manufacture of frames. It is similar to Optyl in that frames are molded rather than being cut from a flat sheet. Propionate is light and strong. The molding process reduces waste and manufacturing cost.

Celsius Unit of a temperature scale in which 0° is the freezing point of fresh water and 100° is the boiling point at normal atmospheric pressure; devised in 1742 by Swedish astronomer Anders Celsius (1701–1744); before 1948 the degree Celsius was called the degree centigrade.

cemented segment See *segment, cemented.*

center

1. The point at an average distance from all exterior angles, points, and lines of a geometric figure or body.
2. A point, pivot, or axis around which something or some system rotates, revolves, or from which activity emanates.

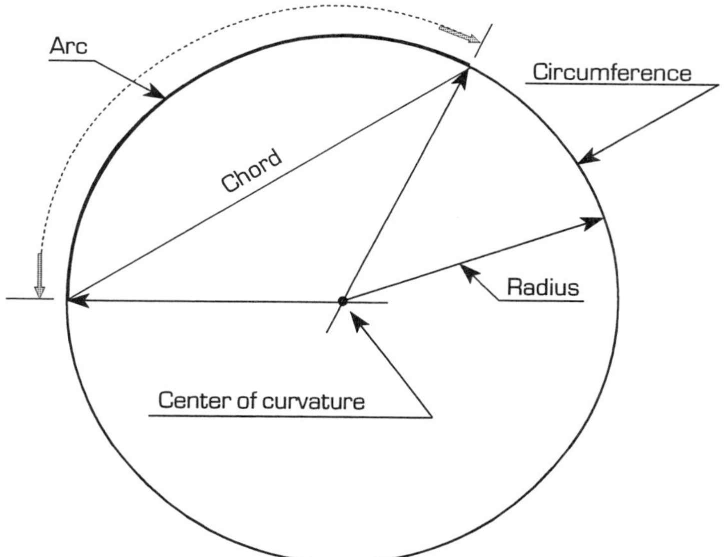

Figure 16 Center of curvature of circle or arc.

center, geometric In the boxing system, the intersection of the horizontal and vertical lens bisectors or the intersection of the diagonals joining opposite corners of a box that circumscribes the finished lens or lens shape. (See Figures 19 and 20.)

center, grinding See *center, surfacing.*

center line, geometric See *line, geometric center.*

center line of temple A straight line through the middle of the proximal or front portion of a spectacle earpiece, and extending horizontally through the length of the earpiece, past the bend, if any. (See Figures 2, 4, 35, and 36.)

center of curvature The intersection of two perpendiculars to an arc of a circle or a spherical surface (Figure 16).

center of rotation In ocular physiology, a theoretic conceptualization of a locus somewhere behind the posterior pole of the crystalline lens (usually taken as approximately 12mm to 14mm behind the corneal apex, variably near the center of the eyeball, but shifts with different degrees of ocular rotation) about which a human eye was formerly considered to rotate; does not exist as an identifiable or fixed point due to convergence-divergence and torsional movements in addition to those of basic Cartesian coordinates.

center, optical

1. One of the intersection points on the optical axis of a lens commonly referenced to the lens surfaces. When the image of a focimeter target is centered on the cross hairs, the optical center of the lens being measured is also considered to be at the point along the optical axis at which the lens has no prism power. There are special cases in which no unique pair of points represents the optical centers. For example, in the combination of a concentric spherical and a toric surface in one meridian, the prism power is zero at any point along this meridian.
2. The point on a lens through which the principal optical axis passes; characteristically the thickest point on a plus lens and the thinnest point on a minus lens.
3. The point on a lens through which extra axial (abaxial) rays pass undeviated. (See Figures 13, 15, and 24 through 27.)

center piece See *piece, center.*

center, resultant optical

1. The point of zero prism power occurring when two or more lenses are superimposed with their optical axes separated, such as a bifocal segment over the distance portion of a carrier lens. The location of the resultant optical center within the superimposed lens area depends on the lens size, distance of optical axes separation, and dioptric power of each lens. The resultant optical center is sometimes displaced outside the superimposed lens area, and may not be located with the focimeter without use of auxiliary prisms.
2. A point through a multifocal segment combined with a distance correction where a ray of light will pass undeviated or where no prismatic effect is present. The resultant optical center will coincide with the optical center of the segment alone with a plano distance component, or when the distance optical center is ground in coincidence with the optical center of the segment.
3. When the distance correction is plus power in the 180° meridian, the resultant optical center will be displaced temporally from the geometric center of the segment. If minus power exists in the 180° meridian of the distance correction, the resultant optical center will be displaced nasally from the geometric center of the segment. The vertical position of the resultant optical center will be altered correspondingly depending upon the dioptric power of the lens in the 90° meridian. The resultant optical centers are

a primary consideration in the fitting of high power lenses, anisometropic corrections, and patients with convergence insufficiencies in order to produce base in prism power assisting single binocular reading vision.

center, segment optical The point through a segment where a ray of light will pass undeviated, without regard to the carrier lens power. The optical center of a round bifocal segment will be found at the center of the circle. The optical center of a flat-top bifocal is midway between the horizontal margins of the segment and may vary in vertical position depending upon the manufacturer's design. To determine accurately the optical center of the segment alone, the manufacturer's schematic diagram should be consulted. The distance prescription may cause the segment optical center to be displaced. (See Figure 20; see also *center, resultant optical.*)

center, surfacing That point on a progressive power lens where the lens manufacturer designates that prism power is to be ground and determined.

center thickness See *thickness, center.*

Center for Devices and Radiological Health (C.D.R.H.) A recent division of the U.S. Food and Drug Administration responsible for safety and efficacy of over 1,000 different medical devices in Risk Classification I (least), II, or III (most), covering lenses, sunglasses, optical products, and the like.

centi- Prefix meaning 100.

centimeter Abbreviated cm. A unit of linear measurement in the metric system; one-hundredth of a meter; ten millimeters.

central anterior curve (CAC) See *curve, central anterior (CAC).*

central corneal clouding See *bedewing, corneal.*

central posterior curve (CPC) See *curve, central posterior (CPC).*

central visual acuity See *acuity, central visual.*

centration In spectacle optics, the process of locating the major reference point of an ophthalmic lens within a frame according to prescription requirements and physical characteristics of the patient.

cerium (sēr'i-um) A metallic element of the rare earth series, chemical symbol Ce, atomic number 58; emits low radioactivity; discovered in 1803 by Swedish chemists Jans Jacob Berzelius (1779–1848) and Wilhelm Hisinger (1766–1852).

cerium oxide A polishing compound used on glass lenses derived from the metallic element cerium (Ce); cerium oxide is pink in color; is added to ophthalmic glass as an ultraviolet absorber; introduced in 1909 as "Euphos" glass by Drs. Schanz and Stockhausen of Dresden, Germany.

certified optician See *optician, certified.*

Certified Occupation Health and Safety Technologist (O.H.S.T.) See *Technologist, Certified Occupational Health and Safety.*

Certified Ophthalmic Assistant (COA) The initial or entry level of the three levels of JCAHPO certification; certified ophthalmic medical assistant, as established in 1969.

cf. Abbreviation for compare.

chalazion (kah-lā'ze-on) Inflammatory granuloma of a Meibomian gland in the tarsal plate of the eyelid.

chamber, anterior The space in the eye between the front surface of the iris and inner surface (endothelium) of the cornea; space is filled with aqueous humor.

chamber, posterior The space in the eye between the back surface of the iris and the suspensory ligaments of the lens; space is filled with aqueous humor.

chamber, vitreous (vit're-us) The large or major cavity of the eye between the lens and the retina; cavity is filled with vitreous humor.

chamfer

1. A bevel or slope put on a lens edge or on the edge of a hole in a lens to minimize chipping of the edge.
2. To make a groove or fluting in a material.
3. The surface formed by cutting away the angle at the intersection of two faces of a solid.

chart A simplified graphic representation of a function or variable; the use of a printed display of letters or figures at a distance to evaluate visual acuity; introduced in 1843 by German ophthalmologist Heinrich Küchler (1811–1873).

chart, Amsler See *grid, Amsler's.*

chart, Bailey-Lovie test A visual acuity test display based on the Snellen 1-minute visual angle, but with equal numbers of letters on each line with letters sized in regular geometric progression from line to line; introduced c. 1976 by Australian optometrists, Ian L. Bailey and J. E. Lovie.

chart, ETDRS test (Early Treatment Diabetic Retinopathy Study) A 1980 modification of the 1976 Bailey-Lovie chart, using 10 letters on each row, with letter size on each row being 1.2589 times the

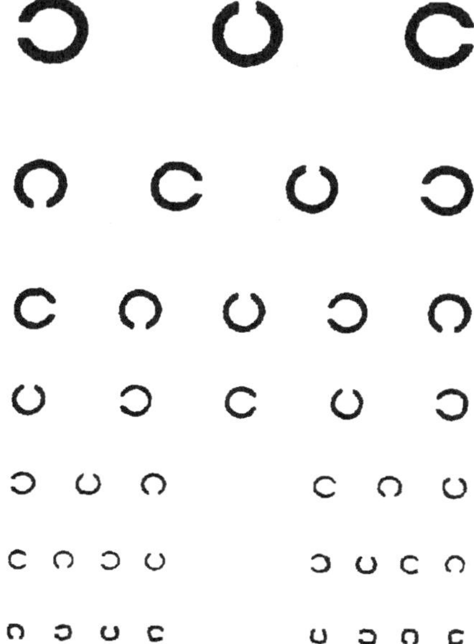

Figure 17 Landolt C, broken-ring test chart.

height of the next smaller line (0.1 log unit). Space between letters is one letter wide.

chart, geometric test A gradation and logarithmic notation. A highly standardized series of optotypes for quantifying central visual acuity; derived in 1966 from earlier geometric letter size in equal steps. Popularized by Chinese ophthalmologist Tian-Yung Mizo.

chart, Landolt C (broken ring) test A standard test for grading central visual acuity with one uniform optotype in graded Snellen sizes presented in four different positions of rotation requiring the patient to identify the direction of the break (Figure 17); introduced in 1888 by Parisian ophthalmologist Edmond Landolt (1846–1926).

chart, Pelli-Robson Test for contrast sensitivity presenting subtle gradations in greyness between test object and background; introduced in 1988 by Dennis G. Pelli, Ph.D., and J.G. Robson; manufactured by Metropia Ltd. of Cambridge, England.

chart, Regan A simplified visual function test of 5 charts printed with low contrast optotypes approximating mid-range spatial frequencies (3 to 5 cycles/degree) in sine wave grating tests of contrast sensitivity; initial plate is full contrast; 4 successive plates present contrast reduced to 64%, 35%, 22%, and 10%; devised in the mid-1970s by Canadian visual scientist David Regan, D.Sc.

chart, Snellen's A standardized test chart used to measure central visual acuity. Test letters are designed to subtend a 5-minute angle with 1-minute components at the eye and are most commonly used at a distance of 20 feet or 6 meters. Visual acuity is expressed as a fraction (e.g., 20/20 in feet or 6/6 in meters) in which the numerator reflects the test distance and the denominator indicates the distance at which a person with normal eyesight can resolve the letters. Introduced in 1862 by Utrecht ophthalmologist Hermann Snellen (1834–1908). See *letters, Snellen's.*

chassis In ophthalmic frames, the metal rims and bridge components of a combination front that holds the lenses.

cheiroscope (kī'ro-skōp) An orthoptic instrument used to train coordination of visual capability and hand movement; the patient uses one eye to visualize a picture and the other eye to direct hand motions to trace the picture. Made in table and hand-held models; introduced by Scottish ophthalmologist Ernest E. Maddox (1860–1933).

chem-hardened lens See *lens, chem-tempered.*

chemical disinfection See *disinfection, chemical.*

chemosis (kē"mo'sis) Swelling or edema of the conjunctival tissue, generally due to exposure to chemical agents, irritants, or local trauma.

chiasma, optic (kī-az'mah) Neuroanatomic structure located above the pituitary gland and formed by the junction and partial crossing-over of the optic nerves from each eye. The fibers from the nasal half of the retina of the left eye cross over to join the fibers from the temporal half of the right retina to make up the right optic tract and vice versa. Optic chiasm; named for the shape of the Greek letter chi (χ).

chipping goggles See *goggles, chipping.*

chord length See *length, chord.*

choroid (kō'roid) The middle of the three anatomic layers (retina, choroid, and sclera) constituting the wall of the eye; consists of a pigment layer and blood vessels in three different sizes supplying nourishment to the outer layers of the retina.

choroiditis (ko-roid-ī'tis) Inflammation of the pigmented vascular layer of the eye between the retina and the sclera.

chroma- Prefix meaning color or hue.

chromatic aberration See *aberration, chromatic.*

chromatic dispersion See *dispersion, chromatic.*

chromatic Pertaining to color.

chromatology That part of optics which treats the properties of color; science of color; chromatics.

chromatopsia (kro"mah-top'se-ah) A visual defect in which colored objects appear unnaturally colored, or colorless objects appear tinged with color. Most commonly caused by drugs.

chromium A bluish-white brittle metal, chemical symbol Cr, atomic number 24; an essential trace element in nutrition, also used in alloys of steel to increase weather resistance as in some spectacle frames. First discovered in a Siberian mineral in 1797 by Louis Nicolas Vauquelin (1763–1829), French chemist.

chronic conjunctivitis See *conjunctivitis, chronic.*

cilia (sil'e-ah) Plural of cilium; the eyelashes.

ciliary body See *body, ciliary.*

ciliary muscle See *muscle, ciliary.*

ciliary processes See *processes, ciliary.*

cilium (sil'e-um) A single eyelash.

circle, blur A circular area viewed as a cross-section of a bundle of focused rays from a point source, centered along the optical axis of a lens. The higher the index of refraction of the lens material, the smaller the diameter of the blur circle; diffusion circle.

circle, distant verification The circular area centered by the distant reference point on a progressive power spectacle lens where the manufacturer designates the distant power of the lens should be verified. The distant verification circle is centered over the focimeter aperture providing verification at the distant reference point. The prismatic power cannot be checked in this area but must be verified at the major reference point. (See Figure 29.) See also *lens, progressive power.*

circle of least confusion

1. A disc-like, near focal plane of light intermediately between the two line images of a bundle of rays emerging from a spherocylindrical lens system and forming Sturm's conoid.

2. The smallest cross-section of a circular (non-astigmatic) bundle of rays, thereby yielding the smallest and clearest image. (See Figures 6 through 11.)

circumcorneal Relating to the area around the corneal perimeter.

cladding A layer of one substance bonded to another; formerly in rolled gold spectacle frames; now commonly a layer of relatively low refractive index material surrounding fiber optics.

cleaner, contact lens, enzymatic A cleaning solution to remove protein deposits on contact lenses; contains a protein molecule that catalyzes chemical reactions of lipoprotein deposits without itself being destroyed. Enzymes are described and classified by the International Commission on Enzymes (established 1956) and the Nomenclature Committee of the overseeing International Union of Biochemistry. For contact lenses these include fat-splitting enzymes (lipase), hydrolytic enzymes (hydrolase), and proteolytic enzymes (protease). Enzymes particularly useful in contact lens cleaning are papain (hydrolase class) that breaks proteins and peptides by cleavage of amino acid bonds (papain is obtained from the latex of the plant papaya); subtilisin, a proteolytic enzyme that catalyzes the hydrolysis of peptide bonds (subtilisin is isolated from the soil bacteria, *Bacillus subtilis,* and contains 274 amino acid residues. These products are used in water in addition to cleaning and sterilization processes.

clearance, apical The linear distance between the most anterior corneal surface (the corneal epithelium), and the posterior surface of a contact lens.

clinical diagnostics See *diagnostics, clinical.*

clock, Geneva segment A mechanical instrument designed to measure the sagitta of a segment curve on an ophthalmic multifocal lens, usually calibrated to express the measurement in dioptric tool surface power, consisting of three (3) pins in line, spaced 13mm apart, rather than 21mm as on the Geneva lens measure, enabling the pins to be completely encompassed by the segment area.

clock, lens (or lens measure) A mechanical instrument designed to measure the sagitta of a lens curve; usually calibrated to express the measurement in dioptric surface power for a given index of refraction, usually that of crown glass ($n = 1.523$); based on two fixed pins 21mm apart and a movable third pin in straight line between them; Geneva lens clock. Invented and patented in 1891 by optician J.C. Brayton of Geneva, New York.

clockwise add, counterclockwise subtract (CAcTS) Mnemonic. In contact lens fitting, a procedure used to compensate for axis and/or power caused by the misorientation of a toric contact lens.

CN bevel See *bevel, CN.*

Co Chemical symbol for the element cobalt; q.v.

coat An outer, external, or surface layer of any substance covering another.

coating, 4-C A trade name for four coatings applied to a lens to combine both safety and visual purposes.

coating, anti-fog A thin, silicon-based, grease-like layer applied to both sides of a lens to reduce or prevent the adhesion of moisture to the lens surface under changes of temperature from cold to hot.

coating, anti-reflective A single or multi-layered application of magnesium fluoride to a refracting surface designed to reduce by interference the amount of light normally reflected from the surface. When applied to ophthalmic lenses, such coatings increase light transmittance and cause the medium to be less apparent; commonly deposited on the lens in a vacuum to a thickness corresponding to 1/4 wavelength of Fraunhofer's sodium "D" line. Trade name: Mirage, reflection-free coating. Developed and refined before World War II by optical scientists at California Institute of Technology and Massachusetts Institute of Technology.

coating, edge Application of an opaque color to the edge of a spectacle lens for the purpose of decreasing edge visibility and internal reflections that create the appearance of concentric rings in high minus power lenses.

coating, electrically conductive (CEC) A reflective metallic layer applied to the front surface of protective or filter lenses to avoid excessive temperature rises as in infrared absorptive filters.

coating, scratch resistant (SRC) Various materials bonded in thin layers to the surface of most types of plastic lenses to reduce susceptibility to pitting and scratching (e.g., polysiloxane); q.v. See also *coating, abrasion-resistant.*

cobalt A metal, chemical symbol Co, atomic number 27; used to produce blue color in glass; a deficiency in humans leads to anemia. First isolated about 1730 from a copper-like ore by George Brandt (1694-1768), Swedish chemist and physician.

cobalt blue filter See *filter, cobalt blue.*

cocaine A crystalline alkaloid derived from coca plant leaves or by chemical synthesis; an efficient topical anesthetic; initially applied to the eye in 1884 by Carl Koller (1858–1944), ophthalmologist of Europe and New York City. Koller received the first Howe Medal from the A.O.S. (1922) and the first Medal of Honor of the New York Academy of Medicine (1930) for his discovery of a method to render ocular surgery painless.

code, bar A symbol system that conveys information encoded in parallel bars and spaces; the code information is read by an optical scanning device, usually hand-held or mounted beneath a working surface, that recognizes the difference between dark bars and lighter spaces; in 1993, the Optical Industry Association (O.I.A.) endorsed a product code system (UPC-A) for its frame division; in 1986, a product code system (OPC) was established for its spectacle lens division.

coefficient A numerical factor multiplying a term in an algebraic equation.

coefficient, reverse thermal A numerical factor indicating the inhibition by heat on the speed of a chemical reaction.

coefficient, thermal A numerical factor indicating the acceleration by heat upon the speed of a chemical reaction.

coherence In light science, the property of a highly monochromatic light beam, usually laser generated, in which the photons in the beam are in corresponding phases; in holography there must be both transverse and longitudinal coherence.

collagen The protein substance of the fibrils that comprise most of the corneal stroma, Bowman's membrane, sclera, tendons, cartilage, and similar connective tissues; composed of molecular units about 1.4nm wide and 280nm long (tropocollagen); a helical structure consisting of 3 polypeptide chains each composed of about 1,000 amino acids coiled about each other to form a spiral. Rich in glycine, proline, hydroxyproline, and hydroxylysine. May be converted into gelatin by boiling.

collagen shield See *shield, collagen.*

collimation In optical science, the processes used to minimize or eliminate diverging or converging rays in a beam, thus approaching or achieving light rays that are parallel or aligned with the optical axis.

colloid

1. Resembling glue.
2. A state of matter in which one component (the disperse phase) is distributed throughout another medium (the dispersion me-

dium) in particles larger than ordinary crystalloid molecules, but not large enough to settle out under the influence of gravity; said of gold introduced into glass to yield a red or ruby color. Both the name and the class of substances introduced about 1850 by Scottish chemist Thomas Graham (1805–1869).

collyrium (ko-lir′e-um) A soothing lotion or eyewash; generally containing no significant ocular medication (non-medicinal).

colmascope (kol′mah-skōp) See *polariscope, plane.*

coloboma (kol′o-bō″mah) An absence of some ocular tissue usually resulting from congenital defects in closure of the fetal intraocular fissure, but may be subsequent to surgery or injury.

color The visual sensation resulting from stimulation of cone cells of the retina by light waves of various length between 380nm and 800nm; hue; chroma; measurements and standards based on 3 primary colors; (red, green, and blue) formalized in 1913 by Albert Henry Munsell (1858–1918), U.S. artist and inventor of instruments for color measurements, but related to several earlier schemes.

color blindness See *blindness, color.*

color blur See *aberration, chromatic.*

Colormatic Trade name for a photosensitive lens coating that may be applied to plastic lenses. When activated, changes color from light brown to a darker blue-gray.

com- Prefix meaning with.

coma

1. A state of unconsciousness from which a patient cannot be aroused.
2. See *aberration, coma.*

coma aberration See *aberration, coma.*

combination frame See *frame, combination.*

comfort cable temple See *temple, comfort cable.*

Commission Internationale de l'Eclairage (C.I.E.) A voluntary standard-setting agency established in 1913 with offices in Geneva, Switzerland; develops international standards of light, illumination, light sources, color, and the like; established tristimulus color-value diagram in 1931 that was revised in 1964.

Commission on Opticianry Accreditation (C.O.A.) Accredited in 1985 by the U.S. Department of Education, the sole agency in the United States to accredit two-year ophthalmic dispensing and one-year ophthalmic laboratory technology post-secondary educational programs.

common canaliculus See *canaliculus, common.*

community, ophthalmic A term describing the combination of industrial, commercial, and professional groups concerned with the policies, products, and care of ophthalmic patients.

compensated lap See *lap, compensated.*

compensated segments See *segments, compensated.*

compensation Adaptation or departure from the normal to alleviate an undesirable condition. See *segments, compensated.*

compensation, image size The change of form of a pair of ophthalmic lenses worn for the correction of aniseikonia to reduce the image-size difference produced by two ophthalmic lenses of different powers to a tolerable amount. See *lens, iseikonic.*

compensation, instrument A modification made to the normal settings of a device to correct for external factors not otherwise accounted for.

compensation, lens An allowance in lens power, lens surface power, or lens thickness made when designing ophthalmic lenses to provide for differences in ophthalmic lens indices or lens power changes caused by lens thickness.

compensation, vertex distance The change in power of an ophthalmic lens necessary to provide the same effective power at the wearing vertex distance that was determined at a different refracting vertex distance. See *distance, vertex.*

compound hyperopic astigmatism See astigmatism, compound hyperopic.

compound lens See *lens, compound.*

compound myopic astigmatism See Figure 7; *astigmatism, compound myopic.*

con- Prefix meaning with.

Con-Lish bevel finish See *bevel finish, Con-Lish.*

concave lens See *lens, concave.*

concave surface See *surface, concave.*

concentric Having a common center of curvature or symmetry.

concomitance (kon-kom'i-tans) In visual physiology, a condition in which the two eyes move in concert with each other so as to maintain a relatively constant angle between the lines of sight for all directions of gaze; also concomitant.

concomitant (kon-kom'i-tant) Pertaining to or having concomitance.

concomitant strabismus See *strabismus, concomitant.*

conditioning solution See *solution, conditioning.*

cone

1. In solid geometry, a flat-based, single-pointed solid formed by a rotating straight line that traces out a closed curve base from a fixed vertex that is not in the same plane as the base.
2. Anatomical, photoreceptor cell in the retina, consisting of an outer and an inner zone in the layer of rods and cones, a nucleus in the outer nuclear layer, and a cone fiber and cone foot in the outer plexiform layer. They synapse with a bipolar cell and are involved in color vision, high visual acuity, and photopic vision. The human eye has 6 to 7 million cone cells.

cone, McGuire A rigid contact lens design for keratoconus patients, employing a series of three different diameter lenses—by name: 8.1mm (nipple), 8.6mm (oval), and 9.1mm (globus)—having multiple radii on the secondary curvature resulting in an optical zone approximately 0.26mm less than the respective original diameter; mimics an aspheric edge design. The deep central curve on the posterior surface vaults the apex of the cornea in patients with keratoconus. Developed c. 1960 by James McGuire (c. 1926–), Minneapolis contact lens technician.

cone monochromacy See *monochromacy, cone.*

cone, Soper A rigid contact lens design for keratoconus patients, employing a series of three different diameter lenses approximating 7.5, 8.5, and 9.5mm and corresponding o.z. diameters of 6.0, 7.0, and 8.0mm. The CPC varies with each series while maintaining a constant peripheral curve; developed in 1969 by Joseph W. Soper and Allen Jarret, opticians of Houston, Texas; Soper bicurve (cf. *cone, McGuire*).

confocal Having the same foci, real or virtual, independent of other functions in an optical system; as in microscopes using narrow or precisely limited laser illumination to visualize very thin levels of tissue.

conformer A plastic shell sometimes used as a temporary stent to maintain eyelid position after enucleation and before an artificial eye is fitted; usually made of methyl methacrylate or polyethylene.

congenital A condition that exists at the time of birth; may or may not be heritable.

conjugate foci See *foci, conjugate.*

conjugate movement (con"juh-git) Concurrent parallel movement of the eyes in the same direction; version, as dextroversion, levoversion, and the like.

conjunctiva (kon"junk-tī'vah) A thin mucous membrane that covers the inner surface of the eyelids and extends over the exposed surface of the sclera.

conjunctiva, bulbar The portion of the conjunctiva that covers the scleral (white) surface of the eye.

conjunctiva, tarsal The portion of the conjunctiva that covers the inner surface of each eyelid.

conjunctival injection See *injection, conjunctival.*

conjunctivitis (kon-junk"ti-vī'tis) Inflammation of the conjunctiva; pink eye; generally marked by pain, redness and photophobia.

conjunctivitis, allergic Inflammation and edema of the conjunctiva following previous exposure to an antigen and later antigenic challenge; sometimes occurs seasonally and called vernal conjunctivitis, a relative contraindication to wearing contact lenses. First described in 1876 by German ophthalmologist Edwin T. Saemisch (1833–1909).

conjunctivitis, chronic Episodic or continuing inflammation of the conjunctival and underlying tissue.

conjunctivitis, follicular (fo-lik'yu-lar) Inflammation of the palpebral conjunctiva characterized by small mounds of elevated lymphatic tissue. Often confused with giant papillary conjunctivitis.

conjunctivitis, giant papillary (GPC) A form of allergic conjunctivitis characterized by hard flattened papillae arranged in a cobblestone pattern on the inside surface of the eyelids. Often related to wearing contact lens with surface deposits.

conjunctivitis, papillary Inflammation of the conjunctiva marked by rounded elevations of the conjunctiva usually about a small blood vessel and found in some forms of allergic or sensitivity reaction conjunctivitis.

Con-Lish bevel finish See *bevel finish, Con-Lish.*

conoid (kō'noid) A solid, geometric configuration or shape resembling a cone or having a circular base and tapering in hyperboloid, paraboloid, or ellipsoid curvature toward a crest or apex; used in lenses for indirect ophthalmoscopy and low-vision aids. See *lens, Volk.*

conoid of Sturm The changing appearance of a bundle of light rays at different distances after passing through a toric lens system; commonly characterized by two ellipses at right angles to each other and an intervening circle of least confusion. Described in 1845 by Parisian mathematician Jacques Charles Francois Sturm (1803-1855). (See Figures 6 through 11.)

constringence A British term; the reciprocal of the dispersive power of an optical medium. A high value means low dispersion. (cf. *Abbé number; Nu value.*)

Consumer Product Safety Commission (C.P.S.C.) An independent federal agency in Bethesda, Maryland, established in 1973, reporting to the president of the United States; develops safety standards for non-automotive and non-medical related products; operates the National Electronic Injury Surveillance System (N.E.I.S.S.) which records product-related (e.g., spectacle or contact lens) injuries in hospital emergency rooms.

contact dermatitis See *dermatitis, contact.*

contact hypersensitivity See *hypersensitivity, contact.*

contact lens base curve See *curve, central posterior (CPC).*

contact lens See *lens, contact.*

Contact Lens Association of Ophthalmologists (C.L.A.O.) A voluntary group of professional individuals particularly interested in the subject of contact lenses; established in 1962; membership 2,000; publishes quarterly *C.L.A.O. Journal.* Office: 523 Decatur St., New Orleans, Louisiana 70130.

Contact Lens Manufacturers Association (C.L.M.A.) A trade association of major contact lens producers organized in 1963. Office: 2000 M. St., NW., Suite 700, Washington, DC 20036-5503.

Contact Lens Society of America (C.L.S.A.) A voluntary professional association established in 1955 for educational and technical advancement of individual contact lens technicians. Office: 11735 Bowman Green Dr., Reston, Virginia 22090.

Contactoscope Trade name of an optical instrument used for quality control inspection of a contact lens under magnification.

continuing education credit (CEC) A unit of instruction credit awarded to a professional for attending a one-hour (usually) seminar, workshop, classroom instruction, etc. in a topic germaine to the professional field and approved by appropriately involved agencies, such as state licensing boards or credentialing bodies for the purpose of relicensure or recertification, respectively. Similarly applicable to recertification of ophthalmic assistants, technicians, and technologists.

contra- Prefix meaning against.

contraindication A condition which renders some particular type of management or treatment undesirable.

contrast The brightness relationship of two adjacent surfaces viewed under the same illumination and in the same immediate surroundings; increasing contrast generally increases visibility; commonly expressed as a ratio or as a percentage.

contrast ratio See *ratio, contrast.*

contrast reversal See *reversal, contrast.*

contrast sensitivity See *sensitivity, contrast.*

contusion Blunt injury in which the skin is not broken; usually results in a bruise; on the eye may disrupt the corneal epithelium, cause bleeding within the eye, or classical "black eye."

convergence

1. In geometric optics, the directional property of a bundle of light rays turned or bent toward a real image point (positive vergence).
2. In visual physiology, simultaneous inward movement of both eyes by action of the internal rectus muscles turning the visual axes to intersect an approaching object.

convergence, accommodative The portion of ocular convergence reflexively stimulated by the act of focusing the eyes in the near range.

convergence, amplitude Amount in prism diopters (Δ), that the two eyes can simultaneously turn inward (nasally) before double vision occurs.

convergence, fusional That portion of convergence either positive (increasing the angle) or negative (decreasing the angle) needed to maintain single binocular vision by turning the visual axes precisely to the same fixation point. Is commonly measured in prism diopters (Δ), with graduated base-out prisms.

convergence insufficiency See *insufficiency, convergence.*

convergence, voluntary Amount that both eyes can be turned in (adducted) at the will of the patient; usually estimated in arc degrees or prism diopters (Δ).

convex lens See Figures 25 and 27; *lens, convex.*

convex surface See *surface, convex.*

coordinates, chromaticity A tri-stimulus system based on reference values of 1) hue, 2) saturation, 3) brightness, to relate any designate color value. See *color.*

copolymer A polymer constituted of monomers of more than one kind.

copper A malleable metallic element, chemical symbol Cu, atomic number 29; as an ocular foreign body is chemically active and destructive and should be removed promptly; used in some brown-based, mirrored sunglasses.

core- A combining form indicating relation to the pupil.

core

1. A central strand around which other wires are wound in a core temple.
2. Wire reinforcement embedded in plastic temples (core wire).

corectopia (kor-ec-tōp'ia) Abnormal position or eccentric location of the pupil; the farther the ectopic pupil from the fixation axis, the more acuity is degraded by optical aberrations.

coreometry (ko're-om"e-tre) See *pupillometry.*

coreoplasty (ko're-o-plas"te) Also pupilloplasty. The altering or making of a pupil by reshaping the iris aperture; this is usually done surgically, but in the aphakic patient may be done by laser intervention.

Corlon lens See *lens, Corlon.*

cornea The transparent structure forming the anterior part of the fibrous layer of the eye which overlies the iris and pupil. Appears horizontally elliptical in contour from the front and circular in contour when viewed, in surgical specimen, from behind.

cornea, artificial A test sphere of precisely known radius of curvature, usually made of polished steel; used to establish standardized readings of a keratometer or ophthalmometer. See also *keratoprosthesis.*

cornea guttata (goo-ta'ta) A common and often age-related breakdown or dystrophy of endothelial cells lining the inner surface of the cornea; appears predominantly in females; leads to corneal edema; usually a bilateral process.

corneal abrasion See *abrasion, corneal.*

corneal apex Also corneal crown. See Figure 5; *apex, corneal.*

corneal astigmatism See *astigmatism, corneal.*

corneal bedewing See *bedewing, corneal.*

corneal dellen Also Fuchs dimple. See *dellen, corneal.*

corneal desiccation See *desiccation, corneal.*

corneal deturgescence See *deturgescence, corneal.*

corneal endothelium See *endothelium, corneal.*

corneal epithelium See *epithelium, corneal.*

corneal erosion See *erosion, corneal.*

corneal graft See *keratoplasty, penetrating.*

corneal hydrops See *hydrops, corneal.*

corneal limbus See *limbus, corneal.*

corneal molding See *molding, corneal.*

corneal opacities See *opacities, corneal.*

corneal reflex See *reflex, corneal.*

corneal reflex pupillometer See *pupillometer.*

corneal rehabilitation Process used to allow a molded cornea to return to its normal corneal curvature usually after long-term rigid contact lens wear or wearing warped lenses.

corneal-scleral junction See *junction, corneo-scleral.*

corneal stroma See *stroma, corneal.*

cornpicker's pupil See *pupil, cornpicker's.*

corrected curve See *lens, corrected curve.*

corrective power See *power, corrective.*

corridor, lens The 2 to 5mm wide, 12 to 18mm high variable channel of an ophthalmic progressive lens joining the superior distance viewing area and the inferior usable near visual space between the nasal and temporal edges of the lens.

corrosion resistance See *resistance, corrosion.*

cortex, visual That part of the brain that receives the nerve impulses of the visual pathway; located at the posterior tips of the occipital lobes; Brodmann's area 17; primary visual projection area.

cortical blindness See *blindness, cortical.*

cosmesis (koz-mē′sis) The study and art of beautifying or improving appearance (aesthetics).

cosmetic Pertaining to beautifying, improving appearance; aesthetics.

cosmetic contact lens See *lens, cosmetic contact.*

couching A primitive mechanical technique for dislocating an opaque (cataractous) crystalline lens from the visual axis by pressing it downward with the aid of a sharp needle; reclination.

counts fingers An approximation used in evaluating visual acuity of the partially sighted patient; the patient is asked to count the number of fingers displayed by the examiner at a given distance.

cover lens See *lens, cover.*

CPC Mnemonic for curve, central posterior; q.v.

CPR Abbreviation for cardiopulmonary resuscitation; q.v.

CR-39 Trade name for a liquid allyl resin material, allyl diglycol carbonate, from which plastic lenses are cast; about half the weight of crown glass, with an index of refraction of 1.498 compared to 1.523 for crown glass; not as brittle as glass, thus is more impact resistant, but more susceptible to scratching; a registered trademark of P.P.G. Industries; common name for "plastic" lenses. Number indicates the successful 39th trial in 1942 to create a high optical quality resin lens material by organic chemists at Columbia Southern Corporation.

crazing A cracked or spider-web appearance on a lens surface resulting from exposure of surface coatings to heat or chemicals.

crest, nasal See *nasion.*

cribbing The breaking or chipping of excess glass from an uncut lens or lens blank.

cross angle See *angle, temple fold.*

cross curve See *curve, cross.*

cross cylinder See *cylinder, cross.*

cross-eyed See *esotropia.*

cross, fitting The location on a progressive addition lens that is normally fit in front of the pupil center, denoted by two 1/4-inch lines crossed at right angles to each other. It is usually 2mm to 4mm above the major reference point of the lens. The intersection of the fitting cross arms is the fitting point. (See Figure 29.) See also *lens, progressive addition.*

cross, optical A diagram consisting of two straight lines crossing each other at right angles oriented to represent the principal refractive meridians of an ophthalmic prescription lens; used to chart the axes and refractive powers in the principal meridians (Figure 18).

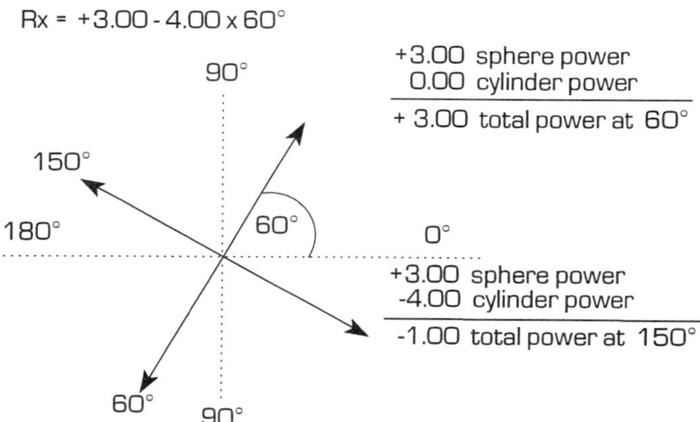

Figure 18 Optical cross.

crown glass See *glass, crown.*

CRP Mnemonic for corneal reflection pupillometer; see *pupillometer, corneal reflection.*

CRT Abbreviation for cathode ray tube. See *tube, cathode ray.*

crutch, ptosis (tō'sis) An attachment to a spectacle front to support and elevate a drooping upper eyelid, often made of spring steel with a single anchor point near the lateral extremity of the bridge; Masselon's spectacles, described by French ophthalmologist Michel Julien Masselon (1844–1917).

Cruxite lens See *lens, Cruxite.*

cryptophthalmos (krip'tof-thal"mos) A very rare congenital defect in which the skin is continuous over the eyeballs without formation of lid structure; classified as primary or secondary in origin.

crystal optics See *optics, crystal.*

crystalline lens See *lens, crystalline.*

Cu Chemical symbol for the metallic element copper; q.v.

cul-de-sac, conjunctival In ocular anatomy, the loose conjunctival fold covered by epithelial tissue forming the junction of the lid conjunctiva with the bulbar conjunctiva, both above the upper tarsal plate and below the lower tarsal plate; also called the conjunctival fornix. Literally, "a blind pouch."

cup goggles See *goggles, cup.*

cupped disc See *disc, cupped.*

curvature A continuous bending of a line or surface without angles. The angle through which a surface turns in a unit length of arc. (See Figure 16.)

curvature hyperopia See *hyperopia, curvature.*

curvature myopia See *myopia, curvature.*

curvature of field An optical aberration of refractive and reflective optics in which a curvilinear image surface results from a plane object, because each object point is a different distance from the refracting or reflecting surface; Petzval curvature of field of view; described in 1843 by Jozsef Miska Petzval (1807–1891), Hungarian mathematician; may be corrected by Petzval surface. Also occurs with A-scan and B-scan ultrasound examination directed through the lens of the eye.

curvature of field aberration See *curvature of field.*

curvature, surface The smooth optical face of a lens without linear or angular component. The reciprocal, R, of the radius of curvature, r (in meters)—i.e., $R = 1/r$; often (although not universally) and incorrectly expressed in diopters.

curve A continuously bending line without angles; any curved outline, form, thing or part.

curve, base A manufacturer-marked (or nominal) surface power for the first side curve to be ground and polished on a series of finished or semi-finished corrected or uncorrected lenses, which, when combined with the second side ground and polished curvature, produces the desired lens power. Base curves, for a given range of powers, can be of a common marked value, either plus or minus, spherical or toric (i.e., cylindrical) in configuration depending on the correction(s) for which the series of lenses were designed. See *lenses, corrected curve.*

curve, blend A contour modification to the ocular side of a rigid corneal contact lens smoothing out the circular edge or rings to allow for a smooth transition between posterior peripheral curvatures.

curve, central anterior (CAC) In contact lens design the front surface area of a corneal contact lens commonly referred to as the diopter power curve that determines the actual power of the lens when used in conjunction with the central posterior curve, lens thickness, and index of refraction of the lens material; not specified by the fitter, but determined by the fabricator.

curve, central posterior (CPC) In contact lens design, the optical component of the back surface of a corneal contact lens often referred to as the base curve or CPC; expressed as a radius in millimeters.; the fitting curve of a contact lens, CPC expressed to nearest 0.01mm.

curve, cross The maximum surface power of a toric (cylindrical) surface (90° from the toric base curve meridian). (See Figure 12.)

curve, fractal In mathematical schemes, a curve that retains a consistent pattern of irregularity or subdivision regardless of how many times it is multiplied or subdivided; an idiosyncracy in mathematical curves in which the length or perimeter approaches infinity, but the enclosed area is always less than that of the original figure.

curve, intermediate A blending curve on a rigid contact lens surface between the optical zone and the lens periphery.

curve, intermediate peripheral (IPC) A curvature on the posterior surface of a contact lens that serves as a transitional curve between the CPC and the lens edge. The IPC has a specified radius of curvature and designated width. The width is specified to 1/10mm.

curve, peripheral One or more concentric curves generated at the periphery of a rigid contact lens to match more closely the flattening of the cornea in its transitional and peripheral zones; the radius of curvature is specified in units of 0.01mm; the width of the peripheral curve is specified to 0.1mm.

curve, peripheral anterior (PAC) A bevel applied to the edge of the front surface of a contact lens to reduce edge thickness, lid awareness, and dislocation by lid border forces.

curve, peripheral posterior (PPC) The outermost curve on the concave surface of a contact lens specified to the nearest 0.10mm. The peripheral posterior curve is always flatter than the central posterior curve, and the intermediate posterior curve.

curve, second surface In an ophthalmic lens, the other or opposite face from the base curve, sometimes called the combining surface.

curve, temple head The curvature in a spectacle earpiece to conform to the contour of the human head; also called head bend or head bow.

curve, toric base See *curve, base.*

curve, Tscherning's (chern'ings) A nomogram displaying on an elliptically plotted curved line the optimal front curvature of an ophthalmic lens for its dioptric power to minimize oblique astigmatic aberration; the basis for so-called corrected curve lenses (Orthogon, Tillyer, etc.). Developed in 1904 by Marcus Hans Eric Tscherning (1854-1939), ophthalmologist of Paris and Copenhagen; Tscherning's ellipse.

curvilinear Enclosed by a bent line having no straight or angular part.

cutaneous (kyoo-tā'ne-us) Pertaining to the skin.

cutter, lap A precision electromechanical machine for generating convex or concave spherical, toric, or flat cylindrical surface curvatures on spectacle lens grinding or polishing laps made from cast iron, aluminum or brass; may be computer-driven and may perform cribbing.

cutting line An archaic term. See *bisector, horizontal lens.*

cycle A revolving or recurring that repeats itself in the same order and at the same intervals.

cyclitis (sik-lī'tis) Inflammation of the ciliary body, usually accompanied by an inflammation of the iris (iritis); when the ciliary body alone or principally is affected, a reduction of aqueous formation and reduced intraocular pressure tends to occur. Term introduced in 1844 by Parisian ophthalmologist Francois Louis Tavignot (b. 1818).

cycloplegic drug See *drug, cycloplegic.*

cylinder A solid body shaped in the form of a column.

cylinder axis See *axis, cylinder.*

cylinder, cross An optical examining device composed of two cylindrical lenses of different powers with their axes at right angles to each other (often ground as a spherocylinder). Commonly a plus (+) cylinder and a minus (–) cylinder of equal dioptric strength; used during refraction to refine or verify cylinder power and axis location. Jackson Cross Cylinder, popularized 1887–1907 by Edward Jackson (1856–1942), Philadelphia and Denver ophthalmologist.

cylinder foci See *foci, cylinder.*

cylinder lens See *lens, cylinder.*

cylinder, minus An expression of optical power in which the cylindrical component of a written formula has more minus power than the spherical component, or a lens that has its toric surface on the ocular side of the lens.

cylinder, plus An expression of optical power in which the cylindrical component of a written formula has more plus power than the spherical component, or a lens that has its toric surface on the front side of the lens.

cylinder power See *power, cylinder.*

cyst A sac, especially one having a distinct membrane and containing fluid.

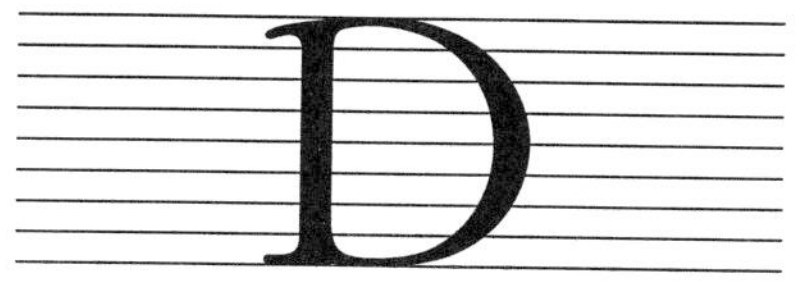

d Symbol used for the expression of optical density.

D **1.** Abbreviation for the unit of refractive power, the diopter. **2.** Abbreviation for dexter (right).

D.I.N. Abbreviation for Deutsches Institut für Normung, the German standard-setting agency, similar to A.N.S.I. in the United States. Headquartered in Berlin.

DL Abbreviation for diameter of laser beam at given range (n).

D.V.S. Abbreviation for Descriptive Video Service; q.v.

dacryo- Prefix meaning tear.

dacryoadenitis (dak″re-o-ad″e-nī′tis) Inflammation of the lacrimal gland.

dacryocanaliculitis (dak″re-o-kan″ah-lik″yu-lī′tis) An inflammation of the lacrimal canaliculus or canaliculi between the tear points and the tear sac (commonly canaliculitis); frequently due to fungus infection.

dacryocystitis (dak″re-o-sis-tī′tis) Inflammation of the lacrimal sac.

Daltonism Eponym for red-green colorblindness; classical description published in 1798 by John Dalton (1762–1844), British chemist who suffered red-green colorblindness as a congenital defect.

datum line A British term used in specification of ophthalmic lens characteristics; mounting line; 180° line; superseded by boxing system. See *bisector, horizontal lens* (HLB).

Db Abbreviation for decibel; q.v.

DBGC Mnemonic for distance between geometric centers; q.v.

DBL Mnemonic for distance between lenses; q.v.

DBMRP Mnemonic for distance between major reference points; q.v.

DBOC Mnemonic for distance between optical centers; q.v.

DBSC Mnemonic for distance between segment centers; q.v.

de- Prefix meaning removal, separation, negation, reversal.

decenter To place the optical center or major reference point of an ophthalmic lens away from the geometric center of the lens in the process of fabricating an ophthalmic lens. The major reference point may be moved horizontally or vertically in relation to the geometric center, or in combination of the two. See *centration; decentration.*

decentration, distance (DD) Specific displacement of the OC along the horizontal meridian for the purpose of locating the major reference point (MRP) coincident with the patient's visual axis when viewing to infinity. The amount is based on the formula:

$$DD = \frac{FCD - DIOD}{2}$$

where

FCD = frame center distance in millimeters (i.e., A + DBL)
DIOD = distant interocular distance in millimeters
DD = distance decentration in millimeters for each lens (see Figure 20).

decentration The act of decentering an ophthalmic lens; usually expressed in millimeters. Decentration may be employed to achieve desired prismatic effects. Improper or inadvertent decentration will produce unwanted prism which should be kept within ANSI tolerances. See *centration; decenter.*

decibel (dB) A unit of relative power intensity expressed in log unit scale; one-tenth of a Bel; specifically used to express acoustic power, but also applied to retinal sensitivity to a target stimulus; somewhat comparable to the perception of loudness in relation to a specified sonic stimulus intensity to the ear. Thus, if decibel sensitivity is low, a high lux or apostilb stimulus will be required for perception. See *Bel.*

decongestant, ocular A drug used to relieve redness (congestion) in the conjunctiva, usually by vasoconstriction.

decussation A crossing over, as in the chiasm of the optic fibers from each eye; in the shape of X from the Roman numeral 10, "deca."

degeneration Older term used for a complex and poorly understood process of impaired anatomical structure and functional capacity deterioration (e.g., macular degeneration); macula involution.

degeneration, macular (mak'yu-lar) Partial or total loss of central vision, most commonly age-related; generally classified as wet (edematous) or dry (ischemic); involution of the macula; may be accompanied by hemorrhage or the development of a sub-retinal neovascular network; macular involution.

degree A 360th part of the circumference of a circle. The unit is used to specify the position of the axis of a cylinder or the location of the base of a prism. Also, a unit of measure of temperature, indicated by the sign (°).

dellen, corneal Localized area of corneal thinning associated with dehydration (tear deficiency), exposure, or extensive wear of contact lenses, and usually found near the limbus in the interpalpebral area.

delta, δ, Δ

1. Fourth letter of the Greek alphabet.
2. A triangular area.
3. A mathematical increment in a variable.

demi- From the French, a prefix meaning half, as in half eyeglasses or demi-glasses.

demi-glasses Spectacles or eyeglasses with only the lower half of the ophthalmic lenses used for near focal distance only; pulpit spectacles.

density, optical A measurement of the transparency of a medium. It is related to light transmission through the equation:

$$d = \log_{10} \frac{(I_i)}{(I_t)}$$

where

I_i = the intensity of incident light
I_t = the intensity of transmitted light

Note: Optical density is not expressed in units, but either a percent transmission or a log notation of attenuation may be used.

density, power A measurement of energy per unit area, per unit time; used in reference to the delivery of laser energy within the eye; energy flosan; term introduced at the 1974 International Congress of Radiation.

deposits, lens Surface film or aggregates of organic or inorganic materials on or into the matrix of contact lenses. May include lipids, calcium, protein, mucin, other byproducts of lacrimation, or foreign material.

depression

1. Movement in a downward direction; movement of the eye by the extraocular muscles to look down (infraduction).
2. A dellen or surface excavation as on the cornea.

depressor An extraocular muscle responsible for downward movement of the eye (e.g., the superior oblique and the inferior rectus muscles).

depth of focus The axial linear distance between the farthest points on either side of the focal point of a lens or optical system where a clear image is attained.

depth perception See *perception, depth* and *stereopsis.*

depth, sagitta Sagitta value. Straight line distance between the back surface of a contact lens at its vault and the chord diameter of the lens; apical height; vertex depth of a lens. May be computed by using the formula

$$s = r - \sqrt{[r^2 - (D/2)^2]}$$

in which

s = the sagitta value
r = the radius of curvature in millimeters
D/2 = the semi-diameter (radius) of the lens in millimeters

derma- Prefix meaning skin.

dermatitis, contact Local inflammation of the skin in an area having direct contact with drugs, chemicals, cosmetics, or spectacle components to which an individual is sensitive.

dermatochalasis A relaxation and redundancy of the skin, particularly as seen on the eyelids, following atrophy of elastic tissue; may create an obstructive fold over the upper lid margins. (cf. *blepharochalasis.*)

dermis The layer of skin deep to the epidermis and containing a dense bed of vascular connective tissue; the corium.

Descemet's membrane See *membrane, Descemet's.*

Descriptive Video Service (D.V.S.) A technical modification of commercial and public television broadcasting and receiving including a Second Audio Program (SAP) feature through which scenes and silent interludes on the screen are vocally described for visually impaired viewers; developed and marketed in 1990 in Boston, Massachusetts.

desiccation, corneal Drying of the anterior surface of the cornea, often caused by reduced tear production, particularly in advancing age; may result from impaired blinking or poor lid closure as in facial nerve (cranial nerve VI) paralysis.

design, translating An optical arrangement or pattern in which a lens divides and refracts incident light into two or more separate foci.

detachment A separation of one ocular tissue from the adjacent or underlying tissue; e.g., retinal detachment (or separation).

detachment, vitreous Physical separation of the gel-like vitreous from the surface of the retina; may contribute to retinal tears or detachment.

deturgescence, corneal (dē'ter-jes"ens) The normal state of relative dehydration maintained by the healthy, intact cornea which enables it to remain transparent.

deuter- A combining prefix from the Greek, meaning second or second in order; also *deutero-*.

deuteranomaly (doo"ter-a-nom'ah-le) A mild color deficiency of green receptors.

deuteranope An individual with green color perception deficiency.

deuteranopia A major absence of the ability to perceive the color green; an absence of the second or green sensitive pigment, chlorolabe.

Deutsches Institut für Normung (D.I.N.) The German standard-setting agency counterpart to A.N.S.I. in the United States; headquartered in Berlin; originally (1917) Deutsche Industrie Norm.

deviation

1. The change in direction of light due to the action of a prism or optical system without a change in vergence.
2. A departure from a normal or expected course of behavior.
3. A misalignment of one or both eyes associated with extraocular muscle imbalance (a heterotropia). (See Figure 3.)

di-, diplo- Prefix meaning two; double.

dia- Prefix meaning passing through.

diagnosis, differential The science and art of determining which one of two or more diseases or abnormalities a patient is suffering.

diagnostics The science and art of distinguishing one disease from another or determination of the nature of a disease. In the United

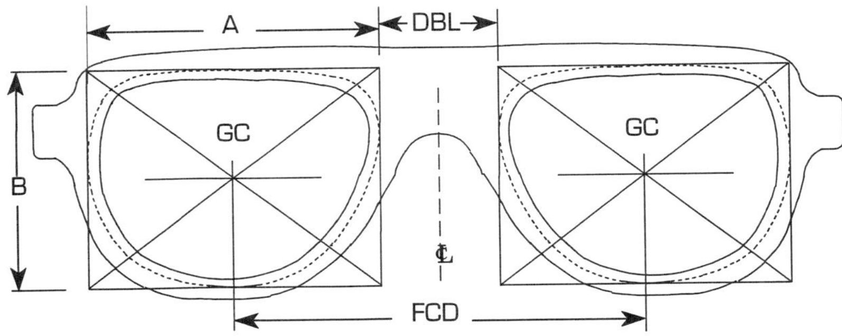

Figure 19 Boxing system frame measuring diagram. (All measurements are in millimeters.)

States, generally a judgmental responsibility exercised under statutory authority in each of the fifty states on behalf of a patient.

diagnostics, clinical Diagnoses based on signs, symptoms, and laboratory findings during life.

diagnostics, pathological Diagnoses based on tissue findings from removed portions of the body (biopsy) or by examination of the body after death, (autopsy).

diagonal, longest The greatest linear measurement of a finished lens from bevel apex to bevel apex passing through the geometric center, not in the 90° or 180° meridian. Not to be confused with effective diameter.

diagram, boxing system frame measuring A drawing illustrating the basic frame measurements (Figure 19) in accordance with the boxing system of measurement adopted January 1, 1962 by the Optical Manufacturers Association (O.M.A.). For easy reference, definitions of terms used in the diagram follow:

A = The horizontal distance between vertical tangents to the apex of the rim groove of a lens opening on the temporal and nasal sides of a spectacle frame. **B** = The vertical distance between the superior and inferior horizontal tangents at the apex of the rim groove in a spectacle frame front. **DBL** = Distance between lenses; the horizontal linear measurement between vertical tangents at the apices of the nasal rim grooves of a spectacle frame, or between tangents to lens nasal edges of rimless mounting. **GC** = Geometric center; the intersection of the horizontal and vertical bisectors of a frame front lens

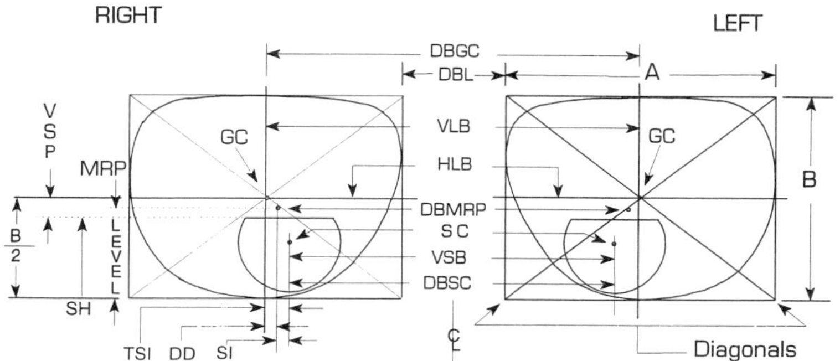

Figure 20 Boxing system multifocal lens measuring diagram. (All measurements are in millimeters.)

opening, or of the diagonals joining opposite corners of a box that circumscribes the spectacle rim groove. **FCD** = Frame center distance; the horizontal linear measurement between the GCs of the lens openings of a spectacle front; for rimless mountings, the horizontal measurement between GC, or vertical lens bisectors (VLB) of the mounted lenses.

diagram, boxing system lens A drawing illustrating the basic lens measurements (Figure 20) in accordance with the boxing system of measurement adopted January 1, 1962, by the Optical Manufacturers Association (O.M.A.). For easy reference, definitions of terms used in the diagram follow:

A = The horizontal distance between vertical tangents to the apex of the bevel on the temporal and nasal edges of a spectacle lens. **B** = The vertical distance between the superior and inferior horizontal tangents to the apex of the bevel of a spectacle lens. **DBL** = Distance between lenses; the horizontal linear measurement between vertical tangents at the apices of the nasal bevel of a pair of mounted or inserted spectacle lens. **GC** = Geometric center; the intersection of the horizontal and vertical lens bisectors or the intersection of the diagonals joining opposite corners of a box that circumscribes the finished lens. **DBGC** = Distance between geometric centers.; the horizontal linear measurement between GCs or VLBs of a mounted pair of spectacle lenses. Such measurement would equal the sum of the A + DBL dimensions; also FCD. **LD** = Lens difference (A – B); the horizontal measurement less the vertical measurement of a spectacle lens; pattern difference. **HLB** = Horizontal lens bisector; a straight (horizontal) line passing through the GC of a finished spectacle lens in the x axis of the Cartesian coordinate system; lesser used now or obsolete are: horizontal center line, datum line (British term), mounting line, and geometric center line. **VLB** = Vertical lens bisector; a straight (vertical) line passing through the GC of a finished spectacle lens in the y axis of the Cartesian coordinate system. **SC** = Segment center; the optical center location of a multifocal addition. **VSB** = Vertical segment bisector; a straight (vertical) line through the optical center of a segment in the y axis of the Cartesian coordinate system. **DBSC** = Distance between segment centers; the horizontal linear measurement between the segment optical centers (or VSB) of a pair of mounted multifocal spectacle lenses; measurement normally equals the near interocular distance (NIOD). **MRP** = Major reference point; that location on an ophthalmic lens at which the specified distance prescription requirements should apply (commonly, but less precisely, referred to as OC); when no prism is prescribed, the OC is the MRP. **DBMRP** = Distance between major reference points; the horizontal linear measurement between vertical MRP bisectors of a pair of mounted spectacle lenses; measurement should equal the distant interocular distance (DIOD). **SH** = Segment height; the vertical distance from a tangent horizontal to the apex of the bevel of the lower finished lens edge to the tangent horizontal to the top of the segment; the top of the trifocal segment is specified in locating trifocal SH. **VSP** = Vertical segment position; the vertical location of the horizontal tangent to the top of a multifocal segment measured from the HLB, being:

a = a zero value, coincident with the HLB, stated: on . . .;
b = a positive value (e.g., +4mm) below the HLB, stated: 4B;
c = a negative value (e.g., –4mm) above the HLB, stated: 4A; formerly, but inaccurately, referred to as "below" and algebraically determined by the formula

$$VSP = \frac{B}{2} (-) SH$$

SI = Segment inset.; the horizontal distance between the vertical MRP bisector and the VSB; based on the formula

$$SI = \frac{(DIOD - NIOD)}{2}$$

where

DIOD = distant interocular distance
NIOD = near interocular distance
TSI = Total segment inset; the sum of the segment inset and distance decentration for each lens; the horizontal distance between the VLB and the VSB based on the formula

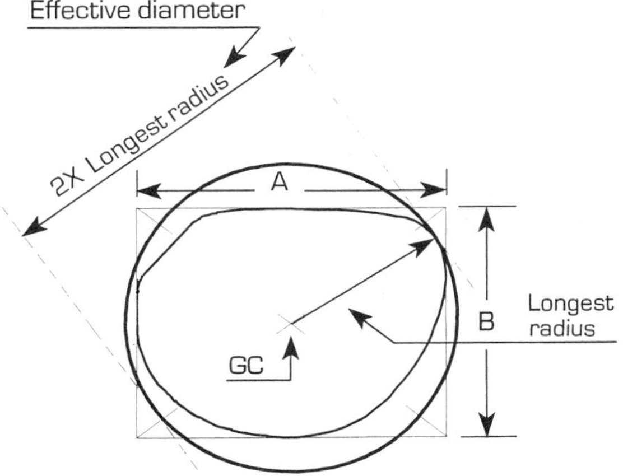

Figure 21 Effective diameter (ED).

$$TSI = \frac{(FCD - NIOD)}{2}$$

where

FCD = frame center distance

NIOD = near interocular distance

DD = Distance decentration; specific decentration of the MRP along the horizontal meridian for the purpose of locating it coincident with the patient's DIOD when viewing to infinity, the amount based on the formula

$$DD = \frac{(FCD - DIOD)}{2}$$

where

FCD = frame center distance

DIOD = distant interocular distance

DD = distance decentration for each lens

diameter A straight line passing from side to side and through the center of any figure or body (Figure 21). See *diameter, effective; size, blank.*

diameter, effective A linear measurement expressed in millimeters, equal to twice the distance of a radius measured from the geometric center to the farthest finished apex edge of an ophthalmic lens (see Figure 21).

diameter, pupil A linear measurement of pupil size in millimeters, usually performed in a normally lighted room.

diameter, thread The overall outside diameter of a screw thread measured across thread peaks.

diameter, visible iris (VID) A convenient, horizontal straight line measurement in millimeters of the maximum iris width as seen clinically through the corneal periphery; sometimes used to determine contact lens diameter; usually greater than a 6 to 12 o'clock measurement.

dichroic filter See *filter, dichroic.*

dichromat (di'kro-mat) A patient with partial impairment of color vision, limiting visual response to two primary colors; usually yellow-green or yellow-red; inability to respond to one of the three primary colors.

dicoria (di-ko're-ah) A condition in which there are two pupils in one iris; double pupil or polycoria; may be a congenital defect or the result of intraocular surgery or a perforating injury.

didymium Obsolete name applied to a metallic component of the rare earth group. Recognized since 1885 as the two elements neodymium and praseodymium, isolated and named by Austrian chemist Karl Auer, Baron von Welsbach (1858–1929). Used in the production of colored glass filters.

dif-, dis- Prefix meaning apart or away.

difference, lens opening (LOD) Numerical difference expressed in millimeters between the A and B dimensions of the lens opening of an ophthalmic frame front. (See Figure 19.)

difference, lens In spectacle optics, the numerical difference expressed in millimeters between the horizontal A, and vertical B, finished spectacle lens dimensions. (See Figure 20.)

differential diagnosis See *diagnosis, differential.*

diffraction

1. A phenomenon of wave motion when a full wave front is not brought to a focus, as when light passes the edge of an opaque body or through narrow slits or is reflected from a ruled surface or grating, creating a concentric series of light and dark fringes; discovered by Francesco Maria Grimaldi (1618–1663), a Jesuit physicist of the University of Bologna.
2. The bending of light rays when passing by the opaque edge of an aperture, creating a concentric series of light and dark rings, or passing by an opaque straight edge causing a series of light

and dark parallel fringes; Fraunhofer diffraction, named for its discoverer, Joseph von Fraunhofer (1787–1826), a German optician for whom solar spectral lines "A" to "H" are named (1814); von Fraunhofer also invented a machine for mathematically uniform polishing of lenses.

diffraction grating See *grating, diffraction.*

diffractive bifocal See *bifocal, diffractive.*

diffuse illumination See *illumination, diffuse.*

diffusion In optical science, the scattering of light by irregular reflection at a surface, or within an optical medium. See *light, scattered.*

dilatation (dil′ah-tā″shun) The condition of an orifice or tubular structure in being stretched or increased beyond its diameter.

dilation The act of stretching or enlarging the pupil (mydriasis) beyond its normal diameter; mydriatic drugs are pharmacologic agents which dilate the pupil, but do not affect accommodation.

dilator In anatomy of the iris, a radially oriented smooth muscle innervated by sympathetic nerve fibers; contraction of the muscles enlarges the pupil.

dimension, longest The greatest linear measurement of a finished lens from bevel apex to bevel apex. This measurement is usually less than the effective diameter.

dimer A compound formed by combining two identical simple molecules; when existing in their excited state are called excimers, a contraction of the words excited and dimers, coined by B. Stevens and E. Hutton in 1960.

DIOD Mnemonic for distant interocular distance; q.v.

diode A two-terminal (cathode and anode) electronic device containing a semiconducting crystal which may emit electrons when a positive voltage is applied to the anode; used as a solid state rectifier and useful in laser trabeculoplasty and in cyclophotocoagulation.

diopter (dī-op′ter) A positive (or negative) optical unit of measurement, the reciprocal of the secondary focal length in meters, used to express the power of a lens. A plus (or minus) one diopter lens will converge (or diverge) parallel rays of light to a real (or virtual) focus at 1m. The diopter equivalent is also used to express the curvature of surfacing tools and the refracting power of curved surfaces for a specific optical material. The symbol D is used to designate the diopter. Term and concept introduced in 1872 by Felix Monoyer (1836–1912), French ophthalmologist. (See Figure 34.)

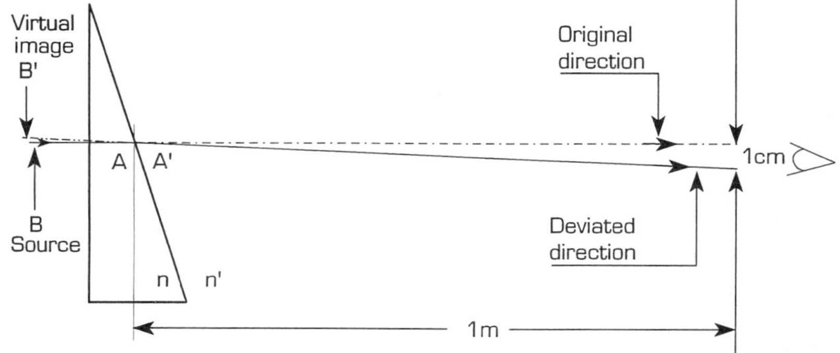

Figure 22 One-diopter prism (drawing not to scale).

diopter, prism An optical unit of measurement used to express the angle of deviation of a ray of light by a prism or lens. One prism diopter (Δ) will deviate parallel rays of light 1cm at a distance of 1m. Prism power in these units is measured as the displacement of the ray, in centimeters, perpendicular to its line of incidence at a distance of 1m. The symbol (Δ) is used to designate the prism diopter. Introduced in 1890 by Charles E. Prentice (1854–1946), ophthalmic engineer of New York City, to supersede earlier terms such as centune, centrad, etc. (Figure 22).

dioptric power See *power, refractive.*

dioptrics (dī-op'triks) The science of transmitted and refracted light.

DIP Acronym for distance intersection point; q.v.

diplopia (di-plō'pe-ah) Double vision; perception of two images from a single object. Rarely, may occur in one eye only (monocular), but more commonly in an abnormal positioning of the two eyes in relation to each other.

diplopia, transitory A variable occurrence of double vision, at times associated with myasthenia gravis, fatigue, alcoholic intoxication, oxygen deprivation, or poorly compensated heterophoria.

direct illumination See *illumination, direct.*

dis- See *dif-.*

disc A circular or rounded flat plate.

disc, Airy The actual image of a point light source which at best is slightly blurred due to diffraction; a fine line is spread into a slightly elongated blur, described in 1827 by George B. Airy (1801–1892), professor of mathematics and astronomy at Cambridge, England.

disc, cupped Depression or excavation in the appearance of an optic nerve head usually due to increased intraocular pressure.

disc, optic Portion of the optic nerve which is formed by the meeting of all the retinal ganglion cell axons exiting through the scleral foramen at the back of the eye.

disc, Placido's A hand-held test disc or keratoscope used to visualize the curvature characteristics of the anterior surface of the cornea by reflection of alternating black and white concentric circles. Named for Antonio Placido (1848–1916), Portuguese ophthalmologist who introduced this instrument between 1880 and 1882. (cf. *keratoscope.*)

disc, stenopaic (sten″o-pā′ik) An opaque disc mounted in a trial lens rim and containing a narrow opening or slit aperture; used in detecting and measuring astigmatism of the eye.

disciform ulcer See *ulcer, disciform.*

disinfection, chemical The elimination or killing of harmful, pathogenic organisms by the use of soaking or treating with "cold" antibacterial and antibiotic agents; not a means of true sterilization.

disinfection, contact lens A physical or chemical procedure which substantially reduces common pathogenic organisms which come in contact with the eye. Contact lens disinfection does not completely eradicate all organisms, and may permit non-pathogenic organisms to survive.

disinfection, hydrogen peroxide The use of a 3% solution of H_2O_2 in sterile water (3% H_2O_2 U.S.P.) to kill harmful ocular pathogen, present in hydrophilic contact lenses.

disinfestation The elimination or extermination of insects, mites, or other animal forms which transmit infection, and which may be found on the person or clothing of an individual carrying such organisms. On the eyelash, infestation of the sucking lice of the *Pediculus* genus may be found; more commonly the small worm or mite, *Demodex,* may be found in hair follicles, particularly of the lids, face, and nose.

disjunction Movement of the two eyes in opposite directions. See *vergence.*

dislocated lens See *lens, dislocated;* see also *subluxation of the crystalline lens.*

dispenser, ophthalmic See *optician, dispensing.*

dispensing optician See *optician, dispensing.*

dispersion In physical optics, the breaking up of white or polychromatic light into its component colors (i.e., wavelengths); dispersion is the cause of chromatic aberrations; normal dispersion; chromatic dispersion.

dispersion, mean The difference between the refractive indices for the partial dispersion of light for the Fraunhofer spectral lines "F" (blue 486.1nm) and "C" (red 656.3nm), i.e.,

$$n_F - n_C,$$

where

n_F = the index of refraction for the "F" line
n_C = the index of refraction for the "C" line

For example, if $n_F = 1.6287$ and $n_C = 1.6142$, then the mean dispersion is $1.6287 - 1.6142$, or 0.0145.

dispersion power See *power, dispersive.*

dispersion, reciprocal relative See *number, Abbé.*

dispersion, relative δ A significant measure or quotient (a value always less than unity, i.e., 1), expressing the mean dispersion of a given optical material divided by the excess refractive index at the sodium D line. Stated algebraically as

$$\delta = \frac{(n_F - n_C)}{(n_D - 1)}$$

where

n_D = the index of refraction for radiation wavelength 589nm (i.e., yellow or sodium D line on the Fraunhofer scale).
n_C = the index of refraction for radiation wavelength 656nm (i.e., red line on the Fraunhofer scale).
n_F = the index of refraction for radiation wavelength 486nm (i.e., blue line on the Fraunhofer scale).

displacement, image

1. In lens optics, the linear deviation of an image from the viewed object.
2. In visual physiology, the linear deviation of the apparent binocularly perceived image from the viewed object, described in 1935 by Boston ophthalmologist F.H. Verhoeff (1874–1968), as "lateral displacement"; discretional difference.

display The presentation of information from a device or system in a form designed to be seen or heard by a human operator; the component of a VDT used to present information to the user visually. Display technologies can be cathode ray tubes (CRT), liquid crystal displays (LCD), light emitting diodes (LED), and others.

display, light emitting diode (LED) An electronic display using solid crystal semiconductors to emit light.

dissimilar segments See *segments, dissimilar.*

distal Away from.

distance The amount of space between two things or points, usually measured in a straight line; a gap or interval between two lines or objects.

distance, back focal The horizontal linear measurement in the metric system along the optical axis from the back vertex of an ophthalmic lens or lens system to its secondary focal point.

distance between centers (DBC) Imprecise term.

1. See *distance, frame center.*
2. See *distance between major reference points.*
3. See *distance between geometric centers.* (See also Figures 19 and 20.)

distance between geometric centers (DBGC) The horizontal linear measurement in millimeters between vertical lens bisectors of a mounted pair of spectacle lenses. Such measurement would equal the sum of the A + DBL dimensions. (cf. *frame center distance.*) See also Figures 19 and 20.

distance between lenses (DBL) The horizontal linear measurement in millimeters between vertical tangents at the apices of the nasal bevel of a pair of mounted spectacle lenses; abbreviated DBL. (See Figures 19 and 20.)

distance between major reference points (DBMRP) The horizontal linear measurement in millimeters between vertical lines through the major reference points of a pair of mounted spectacle lenses; measurement equals the distant interocular distance, DIOD. (See Figure 20.)

distance between optical centers (DBOC) The horizontal linear measurement in millimeters between the optical centers of a pair of mounted spectacle lenses.

distance between segment centers (DBSC) The horizontal linear measurement in millimeters between the segment optical centers (or vertical segment bisectors) of a pair of mounted multifocal spectacle lenses; measurement equals the near interocular distance, NIOD. (See Figure 20.)

distance, distant interocular (DIOD) The horizontal linear measurement in millimeters between the reflexes on the visual axes of the two eyes measured at the plane of the spectacles with the head in the primary position (i.e., the eyes focused at infinity). Loosely and incorrectly referred to as "distant interpupillary distance" (DPD), or distant PD. Equal to the distance between major reference points. (See Figure 20.)

distance, frame-center (FCD) The horizontal linear measurement in millimeters between the geometric centers of the lens openings of a spectacle front. For rimless mountings, the horizontal measurement between the geometric centers or vertical lens bisectors (VLB) of the mounted lenses. Improperly referred to as distance between center (DBC) and/or frame (PD). (See Figure 19.)

distance, frame pupillary Abbreviated frame PD; inaccurate and confusing term superseded by frame-center distance, FCD; q.v. (See Figure 19.)

distance, intermediate interocular (IIOD) The horizontal measurement in millimeters between the reflexes on the visual axes at the plane of the spectacles when the eyes are focused at an intermediate distance (i.e., between the reading distance and infinity). Incorrectly referred to as "intermediate PD."

distance, interocular (IOD) The horizontal linear measurement in millimeters between the reflexes of the visual axes of the wearer's two eyes; loosely referred to as the interpupillary distance (i.e., distance between the centers of the pupillary openings). Should be measured for distant, intermediate and near (reading) positions DIOD, IIOD and NIOD.

distance, interpupillary See *distance, interocular.*

distance, monocular The individual measurement in millimeters from the median sagittal plane to the point where the visual axis of either eye intersects the plane of the lens as indicated from the corneal reflex. Important to be measured in the presence of facial or nasal asymmetry; noted as right (R), (O.D.) or left (L), (O.S.), distant (D), intermediate (I), or near (N); e.g., (RDMD), i.e., Right Distant Monocular Distance, (RIMD), (RNMD), etc.

distance, near interocular (NIOD) Near IOD. The horizontal linear measurement in millimeters between the reflexes of the visual axes of the two eyes, measured at the plane of the spectacle front when the eyes are focused on a near object. Equal to the distance between segment centers. (See Figure 20.)

distance, vertex The straight line measurement in millimeters (z axis) from the back or ocular surface vertex of a mounted spectacle lens to the apex of the cornea. Abbreviated V.D.

distance, viewing The linear measurement, in either the English or metric system, between the eye and the viewed object.

distant Far away or widely separated in space or time.

distant intersection point (DIP) See *point, distant intersection.*

distant power See *power, distant.*

distant reference point See Figure 29; *point, distant reference.*

distant verification circle See Figure 29; *circle, distant verification.*

distometer, interpupillary (in"ter-pyu'pi-lah-re dis-tom'i-ter) An optical or mechanical instrument to measure the linear distance between the centers of the two pupils.

distometer, vertex A hand-held mechanical caliper for the measurement of the distance from the back surface of a spectacle lens to the front surface of the eyelid or cornea, which is then read as vertex distance in millimeters. See *distance, vertex.*

distortion An aberration that results in straight lines being imaged as curved. In ophthalmic optics, "barrel" distortion occurs with minus lenses whereas "pin-cushion" distortion occurs with plus lenses; these are inherent in the optical characteristics of simple plus or minus lenses. Distortion evidenced by waves or ripples in the image of a line viewed through a lens held remotely from the eye can be induced by local surface irregularities resulting from improper processing.

divergence

1. In visual physiology, movement of the eyes turning away from each other so that the lines of sight intersect behind the eyes; negative vergence, the opposite of convergence.
2. In geometric optics, the directional property of light rays which are spreading apart or radiating from a common source.

dividing line See *line, dividing.*

Dk Expression of the diffusion coefficient of oxygen in relationship to the solubility of oxygen within a contact lens material. D is the diffusion coefficient for oxygen; k is the solubility of oxygen in the material. This is independent of lens thickness. Range extends from 5 to 100 in current contact lens materials. Polarographic method for determination is expressed in X units at a given pressure and temperature.

Dk/L Formula expressing the oxygen transmissability of a contact lens in relation to its thickness. The permeability relates the diffusion coefficient (Dk) of the material to the lens thickness (L) in millimeters. For a rigid lens, a high Dk with minimum thickness presents ideal oxygen transmissability. For soft lenses, the ideal values would be a high Dk with high water content, and minimum thickness; L is elevated with increasing temperature.

DL Abbreviation for the diameter of a laser beam.

dominant eye See *eye, dominant.*

dot, Hartinger A small opaque spot placed on an objective lens in the light pathway of a fundus camera to eliminate the central light spot reflex in early fundus photographs. Developed in 1929 by H. Hartinger (b. 1891) of Zeiss, Jena.

dot, Mittendorf A small white or grey congenital opacity on the back surface of the human lens, usually just inferonasally to its posterior pole; represents remains of the lenticular attachment of the hyaloid artery and does not affect vision; described in 1892 by New York ophthalmologist William F. Mittendorf (d. 1919).

dot, random A printed display of computer generated non-uniform patterns for stereoacuity test charts of geometric figures free of all monocular cues; developed and computer generated in 1959 by Hungarian-born Bela Julesz (b. 1928), experimental psychologist working in New Jersey (Bell Laboratories); may be used with no glasses or with stereoscopic glasses; trade name, Randot. When double printed in complementary red and green, as anaglyphs, may be seen more easily with correlated red filter for one eye and green for the other.

double D lenses See *lens, double D.*

double refraction See *birefringence, double refraction.*

double slab-off contact lens See *lens, contact, double slab-off.*

double vision See *diplopia.*

doublet A pair of lenses placed together to reduce aberrations (e.g., a chromatic doublet to reduce chromatic dispersion); a Huygens eyepiece constructed of two plano convex lenses with the plane faces closest to the observer's eye.

down bend See *bend, down.*

dress-hardened lenses See *lens, impact resistant for dress eyewear.*

dress ophthalmic frame See *frame, dress ophthalmic.*

drop ball test See *resistance, impact; test, drop ball.*

drop, segment The manufacturer's specification for the vertical distance from the horizontal lens blank bisector to the horizontal tangent at the top of the segment (or the highest point of a curved top segment) on a semi-finished, ophthalmic multifocal lens blank supplied by the manufacturer.

drug A chemical compound intended for the diagnosis or treatment of a disease.

drug, cycloplegic (sī"klo-plē'jik) A chemical compound which paralyzes the ciliary and sphincter pupillae muscles of the eye, resulting in a loss of ability to accommodate and to constrict the pupil; e.g., atropine, homatropine, cyclogyl (cyclopentolate HCL).

drug, miotic (mī-ot'ik) Chemical compound which constricts the pupil, e.g., pilocarpine, eserine, phospholine iodide (ecothiophate).

drug, mydriatic (mid"re-at'ik) Chemical compound which dilates the pupil, e.g., neosynephrine, epinephrine. May cause acute, angle-closure glaucoma in sensitive patients with narrow filtration angles at the periphery of their anterior chambers; may also trigger cardiac arrhythmia in sensitive patients.

drug, photosensitizing Chemical compound which increases the sensitivity of the eye and skin to light (especially the ultraviolet wavelengths), e.g., sulfa drugs, tetracyclines, phenothiazides, psoralens, etc. See *Food and Drug Administration, U.S.*

drum, axis Locating device on a manual focimeter for noting the axis of a lens; a rotating wheel which is calibrated in 1° increments. It rotates the target to be coincident with the cylinder axis of the lens.

drum, power

1. A rotating wheel on a manual focimeter which is calibrated in 1/8 (0.125) and 1/4 (0.25) diopter units. It moves the target into focus and allows the lens power to be read.
2. Rotating drums on a keratometer to determine horizontal and vertical radii of corneal curvature by conversion to millimeters or diopters.

dry cell

1. A small transparent plastic lens container used to hold a soft contact lens while evaluating its power.
2. A portable electric battery without fluid contents.

Duane's rule See *rule, Duane's.*

duct, nasolacrimal (nāz"o-lak'ri-mal) A membranous tube of the lacrimal apparatus through which tears drain from the lacrimal sac into the nasal cavity.

duction The movement of one eye by the extraocular muscles under monocular conditions. Adduction, inward rotation; abduction, outward rotation; supraduction, upward rotation; infraduction, downward rotation.

duochrome test See *test, duochrome.*

dys- Prefix meaning ill or bad.

dyschromatope (dis-krō'mah-tōp") A general term for an individual having imperfect discrimination of colors; incomplete or partial color blindness.

dyschromatopsia (dis-krō'mah-top"se-ah) A general term for disorder of color vision.

dyscoria (irregular pupil) (dis-kō're-ah) Abnormality in the shape of the pupil.

dyslexia A neurological impairment of reading, characterized by the ability to see letters clearly but inability to interpret them as letters or words or to understand written material. Term developed in 1877 by Prof. Rudolph Berlin (1833–1897), ophthalmologist of Stuttgart, Germany.

dysnomia (dis-nō'me-ah) A neurologic impairment of interpreting numbers when visually displayed, though there is ocular ability to see numbers clearly.

dystrophy (dis'tro-fe) Inherited bilateral disease connected with abnormal development or faulty nutrition, commonly applied to the cornea.

dystrophy, Fuchs (fyooks) A pathologic condition of the cornea, with epithelial edema, stromal clouding, reduced sensitivity and pain following loss of integrity of the endothelium (cornea guttata); occurs bilaterally especially in older female population and is slowly progressive; combined dystrophy of Fuchs; originally described in 1910 by Ernst Fuchs (1851–1930), ophthalmologist of Germany and Austria.

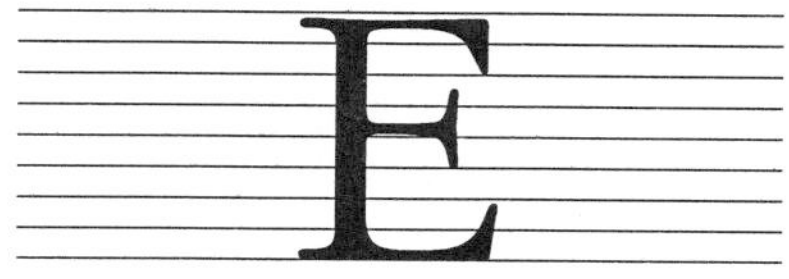

earpiece A component of a spectacle frame designed to assist its stabilization by extending over the external ear; introduced in the early eighteenth century by Edward Scarlett (1677–1743) of Soho, London, England, optician to King George II.

ecchymosis (ek″i-mō′sis) Small hemorrhages within or beneath the skin or mucous membrane; about the eye and eyelids, commonly designated as black eye.

echography Synonym for ultrasonography; q.v.

ECORA Acronym for European Community Ophthalmic Research Association; q.v.

ectasia (ek″tā-sē′ah) Thinning or stretching of the cornea or sclera as a result of a congenital defect, inflammation of the anterior segment, immune complex diseases such as rheumatoid disease, or dystrophic diseases.

ecto- Prefix meaning outer, outside, external.

-ectomy Suffix meaning excision of.

ectopia (ek-tō′pe-ah) Malposition or displacement of a part.

ectopic macula See *macula, ectopic.*

ectropion (ek-trō′pe-on) Turning out of the eyelid.

edema (e-dē′mah) Swelling due to retention of fluid within tissues.

edema, lid An abnormal collection of excess watery fluid in the tissue spaces of the eyelid.

edge In lens optics, the flat or angled surface which limits the refracting surfaces of a lens; the edge determines the peripheral shape of a lens.

edgecoat See *coating, edge.*

edge, knife The periphery of a convex lens that has been surfaced thin enough to provide a cutting effect, as in a knife or razor.

edge, nasal The side of a spectacle lens closest to the nose.

edge, temporal The side of a spectacle lens closest to the ear.

edged lenses See *lens, edged.*

edger A machine used in manufacturing opticianry to reduce a lens to a desired size and shape with the desired edge contour; commonly operates from a pattern, former or template, but more recently "patternless edgers" operate from electronically automated traces.

Educational Foundation in Ophthalmic Optics (EFOO) Trust established by American Board of Opticianry to provide scholarships, student loans, and to enhance educational advancement in opticianry.

effect, confounding Extraneous and non-causally related factor that confuses, exaggerates, or obscures actual or causal factor of significance in conducting or evaluating a study.

effect, McCullough See *McCullough effect.*

effect, negative after-image A harmless temporary change of color perception after looking at objects or images of relatively intense colors (e.g., after viewing a green object or light, some people see a pink "shadow" or after-image). Yellow objects may produce a blue after-image. Rarely, used to describe or sketch "after-image visual fields" of a patient.

effect, positive after-image Temporary perseverance of an initiating color or bright light stimulus after it is extinguished. Rarely, used to describe or sketch "after-image visual fields" of a patient.

effect, Tyndall The action of a light beam passing through an atmosphere containing large particles, such as water droplets or smoke particles, that creates a foggy visibility similar to that in passing through a solution of colloids just large enough to scatter light; commonly seen with a slit lamp in the anterior chamber of the eye during inflammation of the iris; Tyndall scatter; described in 1869 by John Tyndall (1820–1893), physicist of Ireland and England.

effective diameter See *diameter, effective.*

effective power See *power, effective.*

efferent (ef'er-ent) Nerve fibers carrying impulses away from the brain; commonly motor nerves, as those controlling the muscles of the eye.

efficiency, refracting See *number, Abbé.*

EFOO Acronym for Educational Foundation in Ophthalmic Optics; q.v.

eikonometer (ī″ko-nom′i-ter) An optical instrument used to measure differences in retinal image sizes and shapes (aniseikonia), sometimes referred to as "space eikonometer." Originally produced by the American Optical Company, but discontinued. Developed in the 1940s by Paul Boeder, Ph.D. (b. 1902) of Iowa and Massachusetts, expert in physiologic optics; superseded in 1982 by "new aniseikonia test" of S. Awaya and M. Sugawara of Japan, using booklet of 25 pairs of red or green hemidiscs, each differing by 1% in printed size and viewed through red and green filter lenses.

electromagnetic spectrum See *spectrum, electromagnetic.*

ellipse (conic section) A closed curve formed by the section of a cone cut by a plane less steeply inclined than the side of the cone; first defined and described in extensive detail by the Greek mathematician and geographer Apollonius (c. 262 B.C.–c. 190 B.C.).

ellipsoidal A structural shape, as in a compensated curve lens, resembling a spindle, ellipse, oval, or end of an egg.

emerald A variety of the mineral beryl ($BeAl_2Si_2O_{16}$), a silicate of beryllium and aluminum with great hardness; appears green in color because of the presence of chromium. Used in solid state or crystal lasers.

emergent ray See *ray, emergent.*

-emia Suffix referring to the state of the blood.

emmetropia (em″e-trō′pe-ah) The normal ocular refractive condition in which the principal focal point of the dioptric system of the eye lies exactly in the plane of the retina. Theoretically normal refractive status.

endo- Prefix meaning inside, within.

endophthalmitis (en″dof-thal-mī′tis) Inflammation of the tissues of the internal structures of the eye, commonly bacterial or viral, but may be fungal.

endothelium, corneal (en″do-thē′le-um) Posterior or inner layer of the cornea—very sensitive to injury and only one cell thick.

endpiece The portion of a spectacle front where the temple and front are normally joined; also called area endpiece. On a rimless mounting, the device attached to the temporal lens edge to which the temple is joined.

endpiece, area The portion of a spectacle front where the temple and front normally are joined; also called endpiece.

English hinge See *hinge, English.*

enophthalmos (en"of-thal'mos) Abnormal inward displacement of eyeball; recession of the eye into its orbit. May be seen after fracture of orbital bones or with extensive weight loss.

entropion (en-tro'pe-on) Turning in of the eyelid.

entropy A quantity that is a measure of the amount of energy in a system or the efficiency of the system to do useful work.

enucleation (e-noo"kle-ā'shun) Complete surgical removal of the eyeball. Usually the extraocular muscles are spared and left within the orbit for attachment to an orbital implant. First practiced in 1841 and reported in London in 1851 by ophthalmologist George Critchett (1817–1882).

enzymatic contact lens cleaner See *cleaner, contact lens, enzymatic.*

Eonite Trade name of Schott Optical Glass, Inc. for a lens material rapidly and effectively strengthened by ion exchange (S-8000).

epi- Prefix meaning on, outer.

epicanthus (ep"i-kan'thus) A fold of skin partially covering the inner canthus.

epidermis The outer, nonvascular, nonsensitive layer of the skin, covering the dermis or corium.

epikeratophakia (ep'i-ker"ah-to-fā'ke-ah) Relating to a button of prepared corneal tissue shaped as an optical onlay to be surgically anchored to the front of the cornea for reduction of extreme refractive error. Technique originally introduced in 1979 for surgical correction of aphakia and hyperopia by U.S. ophthalmologists H. Edward Kaufman and T. Paul Werblin.

epiphora (e-pif'o-rah) An excessive flow of tears commonly over the lid border and onto the cheek due to impairment or stricture in the lacrimal drainage passages (puncta, canaliculi, lacrimal sac and nasolacrimal duct). (cf. *hyperlacrimation.*)

episclera A loose interlayer between the sclera and bulbar conjunctiva consisting of connective tissue and small blood vessels.

epistemology The study of the theory, nature, sources, methods and validity of knowledge.

epithelium (ep"i-thē'le-um) A cellular covering layer of internal and external surfaces of the body.

epithelium, corneal Cellular front layer of the cornea consisting of stratified squamous cells between the tear film and Bowman's glass-like membrane; normally about five cells thick.

eponym (ep'o-nim) The name of a person, inventor, or discoverer as used to identify a disease, a device, a unit, or the like.

epoxy A thermosetting resin in which oxygen atoms are joined to each of two attached atoms, usually carbon (epoxy group), characterized by high adhesibility, toughness and chemical resistance.

equation, lens maker's A Gaussian calculation to determine lens power through infinitely thin lenses where:

F_t = Total lens power.
n = index of refraction of medium surrounding lens (usually air)
n' = index of refraction of lens material
r_1 = radius of curvature (in meters) of first surface
r_2 = radius of curvature (in meters) of second surface

Measurements are taken from appropriate lens vertex to centers of curvature, object or image. Measurements taken against incoming light direction are negative, and measurements made in the same direction of incoming light are positive.

$$F_t = (n' - n)\,[(1/r_1) - (1/r_2)]$$

equi- Prefix meaning equal.

equivalent oxygen percentage The total amount of oxygen which passes through a finished contact lens to reach the cornea in a given period of time; this measurement is done in vivo (on the eye), and therefore has more clinical significance than Dk/L.

equivalent power See *power, equivalent.*

equivalent, spherical A mathematical expression of the dioptric power of a spherocylindrical lens as the spherical power of the lens plus half the cylindrical power.

Er Chemical symbol for the metallic element erbium; q.v.

erbium A rare metallic element, chemical symbol Er, atomic number 68, sometimes used as a filter in lenses to protect against radiation; recently patented and introduced as a rod in plasmaforming lasers at 1.228nm operating wavelength; yields precise cutting. Discovered in early 1840s by Carl Gustav Mosander (1797–1858), Swedish physician and chemist.

ergonomics (er"go-nom'iks) Human factors or human-factors engineering; the study of work (tasks, technology and environment) in relation to the psychological and physiological capabilities of people; the evaluation and design of the facilities, environments, jobs, training methods, and equipment to match the capabilities of users and workers; reduction of the potential for fatigue, error, or unsafe acts while maximizing increased productivity.

ergonomics, visual The proper assessment of visual needs and design of optically correct appliances for eye safety, comfort, and efficiency in the work place.

ergophthalmology The aspect of the science of visual function and visual disorder relating to the work place; occupational ophthalmology.

erosion, corneal An episodic, recurrent loss of epithelial cells due to failure to adhere properly to the underlying Bowman's membrane; may follow minor corneal scratch or abrasion.

error-free point See *point, error-free.*

error, peripheral power An optical aberration that occurs near the margin (periphery) of a lens that can be expressed in terms of cylinder power and of sphere power in amounts differing from those measured on the optical axis of the lens.

error, refractive Any deviation of the dioptric characteristics of the human ocular system from the normal refractive state of emmetropia. Commonly expressed as the corrective refractive power, in diopters, needed to return a patient's refractive state to clear focusing of distant light onto the retina. May be the cause of symptoms or may be without symptoms.

error, tangential Optical distortion or field of view aberration, present in all lenses, but especially with high dioptric power, seen in off-axis viewing; because the field of view is essentially circular, the lines of distortion occur as tangential to such a circle.

erythropsia (er″e-throp′se-ah) Visual abnormality in which all objects appear to be tinted red; particularly associated with excessive exposure to ultraviolet light, as in climbing snow-covered mountains; often enhanced by aphakia.

es- Prefix meaning into; eso-.

esophoria (es″o-fō′re-ah) Tendency of the eye to turn inward or nasally; generally manifest in the absence of adequate fusional stimuli.

esotropia (cross-eyes) (es″o-trō′pe-ah) A misalignment of the eyes in which one or, less commonly, both eyes turn inward or nasally, particularly seen with hypermetropia.

esotropia, accommodative Inward or nasal deviation of the eye associated with excessive near focal activity; particularly seen with hypermetropia; commonly greater in the near than the distant focusing range.

esthesiometer (es-thē″ze-om′i-ter) A hand-held mechanical instrument used to quantitate sensitivity particularly in the corneal surface; nylon filament esthesiometer of Cochet and Bonnet, manufactured by Luneau and Coffignon of Paris, France; trade name Tactometer.

ethology The scientific study of animal behavior, particularly in its natural state, including optical signals among animals.

European Community Ophthalmic Research Association (ECORA) A voluntary professional organization to encourage basic eye investigation and research; issues an Ophthalmic Research Register listing ongoing research. Established in 1991. Office: Bonn, Germany.

evisceration (ē-vis″er-ā″shun) Surgical removal of the contents of the globe of the eye, leaving the outer protective coat or sclera, and at times leaving all or portions of the cornea; commonly a plastic sphere is inserted into the scleral shell before surgical closure. Technique introduced in 1885 by Liverpool opthalmologist Philip Henry Mules (1843–1905).

ex-, exo-, extra- Prefix meaning out from, outside.

excimer A contraction of the words *excited dimers* to indicate double molecular compounds that have added energy as a result of absorbing photons. Name coined in 1960 by B. Stevens and E. Hutton. Excimers can be used to produce laser action, as first demonstrated in 1970 by N.G. Basov and co-workers.

exenteration (eks-en″ter-ā′shun) Surgical removal of the entire contents of the orbit and lids, usually dissecting up the periosteum of the orbital bones and then amputating all remaining orbital contents at the orbital apex; usually done in treatment of a non-radiosensitive cancer within the orbit.

exophoria (eks″o-fō′re-ah) Tendency of the eye to turn outward or temporally; generally manifest in the absence of adequate fusional stimuli.

exophthalmometer (eks″of-thal-mom′i-ter) A mechanical gauge to measure the amount of proptosis (exophthalmos) of the eye in reference to the lateral orbital rim; that is, Luedde, Hertel, Mutch, Copper.

exophthalmos (eks″of-thal′mus) Abnormal forward displacement of the eyeball. (proptosis); the opposite of enophthalmos.

exotropia (eks″o-trō′pe-ah) Divergent strabismus. Turning laterally or templeward of one or, rarely, both eyes.

exposure keratitis See *keratitis, exposure.*

exposure, radiant Radiometric quantization or dose amount of radiant energy at an object level, expressed physically as joules per square meter or watts per square meter.

external rectus muscle See *muscle, lateral rectus.*

extra Preposition or prefix meaning outside; without; additional.

extraction, cataract, extracapsular Surgical removal of the cataractous crystalline lens of the eye leaving the remaining posterior lens capsule intact.

extraction, cataract, intracapsular Total removal of a cataractous crystalline lens within its surrounding lens capsule.

extraocular (eks″tra-ok′yu-lar) External to or outside of the eye. Extrinsic to the ocular globe; said of the muscles which rotate the eye along with their tendons, vessels, sheaths, and orbital portions of their nerve supply.

extravasation (eks″tra-vah-sā′-shun) The forcing out from the proper vessels as blood or other fluids so as to diffuse through the surrounding tissues.

extrinsic Outside; extraocular.

eye The organ of vision; oculus. In humans, a spheroid body approximately one inch in diameter, occurring in pairs, positioned in sockets in the front of the skull, which focus light. The peripheral component of sight.

eye, artificial A prosthesis of plastic or glass shaped and colored to resemble the front portion of a normal eye and inserted for cosmetic reasons behind the lids after surgical enucleation or evisceration.

eye, dominant (master) The eye that functions superiorly over the other in some perceptual or motor tasks; usually the eye that is used in unilateral sighting. Approximately twenty-four different tests are available to detect the preferred eye, brighter eye, sighting eye, and the like (e.g., peep-hole test, manoptoscope test, etc.).

eye, left The eyeball situated on the side of the body which is toward the west when one faces north.

eye-refractometer (Rodenstock-Kuhl) (rē″frak-tom′i-ter) Early (1922 to 1927) objective optometer based on the Scheiner (1619) principle of double pinhole apertures placed in front of the pupil (cf. Fincham Coincidence Optometer, 1937; Hartinger Coincidence Refractometer, 1955.)

eye, right The eyeball situated on the side of the body which is toward the east when one faces north.

eye, schematic A geometric model of the optical system of the human eye that is used to practice objective refraction with a retinoscope to determine the formula necessary to neutralize ametropias.

eye, standard (Gullstrand) A simplified and schematic model of the average human eye; first calculated and published (1890–1909) by Allvar Gullstrand (1862–1930), Swedish ophthalmologist and winner of the Nobel Prize in 1911 for his work in the optical imaging of the eye. Adopted by U.S. Department of Defense, Military Standardization Handbook No. 141, 1962.

eyeglasses An optical device for assisting vision or protection from undesirable light; mounted by a nasal bridge in front of both eyes (e.g., pince-nez, folding lens pairs). See *eyewear; spectacles.*

eyelashes The fringe of hair (cilia) growing on the edge of the eyelid providing protection to the eye from dust, etc.

eyelid Either of two (upper or lower) multiple layer structures which move over the surface of the eye in protective function; outer surface is a very thin layer of skin, beneath which is the orbicularis muscle which acts to close the lids; the main structure is a fibrous tarsal plate lined by conjunctiva. The upper lid is lifted by the large levator muscle and a smaller Mueller's muscle.

eyepiece A lens or combination of lenses at the sighting end of an optical instrument closest to the observer.

eyepiece, Erfle Eyepiece composed of three achromatic lens pairs to provide extra-wide field of view and good correction of aberrations; very expensive.

eyepiece, Galilean A simple concave lens giving an erect image and a narrow field of view. Used in low-power instruments such as opera glasses. Developed about 1609 by Galileo Galilei (1564–1642), Italian physicist and astronomer.

eyepiece, Huygenian Eyepiece of two simple lenses with image plane between them; commonly used in microscopes. Developed by Christian Huygens (1629–1695), Dutch physicist and astronomer.

eyepiece, Ramsden An achromatizing pair of plano convex lenses with one or both doublets having flint and crown glass components; the two lens units are separated by distance equal to 7/8 the focal length of either lens; the exit pupil (Ramsden circle or eye point) is outside the system; designed by Jesse Ramsden (1735–1800), British optician and precision instrument designer.

eyewear A generic term encompassing all ophthalmic devices and appliances worn before the eyes to assist or protect vision or to enhance appearance.

eyewire groove See *groove, rim.*

eyewire The component of a spectacle or Oxford eyeglass front which encircles and retains the lenses. Formerly was often made of silver, gold, or nickel, hence the reference to wire; now commonly made of plastic and preferably referred to as rim; q.v.

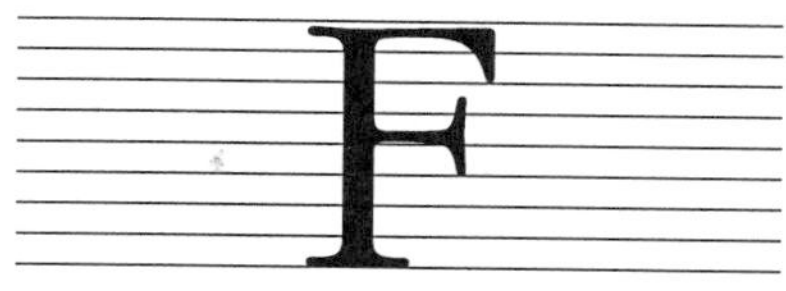

f Symbol for focal length.

F **1.** Chemical symbol for the element fluorine; q.v.
2. Symbol for temperature (q.v.) as expressed on the degrees Fahrenheit scale; q.v..

f number See *number, f.*

f stop See *number, f.*

f value See *number, f.*

F.D.A. Abbreviation for the U.S. Food and Drug Administration; q.v.

F.N.A.O. Abbreviation for Fellow of the National Academy of Opticianry; q.v.

F.T.C. Abbreviation for the U.S. government agency, Federal Trade Commission; q.v.

face form See *form, face.*

face plane See *plane, face.*

face, prism One of the flat or curved surfaces of an optical or ophthalmic prism converging from the prism base to the prism apex.

facet A small, polished plane surface as of a cut gem stone or the edge of an ophthalmic lens finished for use in a rimless mounting.

factory finished uncut lenses See *lens, stock or factory finished uncut.*

Fahrenheit scale See *scale, Fahrenheit.*

FAP In contact lenses, Mnemonic for flatter add plus; q.v.

far point sphere See *sphere, far point.*

far point See *point, far.*

Farnsworth D-15 test See *test, Farnsworth D-15.*

Farnsworth Lantern See *Lantern, Farnsworth.*

Farnsworth-Munsell 100 hue test See *test, Farnsworth-Munsell 100 hue.*

Farnsworth-Munsell 28 hue test See *test, Farnsworth-Munsell 28 hue.*

farsightedness See *hyperopia.*

fat, subcutaneous (sub″kyu-tā′ne-us) Soft pads of white or yellowish tissue under the skin and between various organs of the body that furnish a reserve supply of energy; adipose tissue; blubber.

fc See *footcandle.*

FCD Mnemonic for frame center distance; see *distance, frame center.*

Fe Chemical symbol for the metallic element, iron; q.v.

Federal Trade Commission (F.T.C.) A U.S. national agency created by the Congress in 1914 to prevent unfair methods of competition and deceptive practices affecting commerce; with the U.S. Department of Justice, it enforces federal anti-trust laws. Composed of five commissioners nominated by the president and confirmed by the Senate. Oversees trade policies in ophthalmic goods. Office: Pennsylvania Ave. at Sixth St., NW, Washington, D.C. 20580.

feldspar Any of several crystalline minerals composed of aluminum silicates with sodium, potassium, or calcium; creates birefringence or double refraction of light.

fenestration (fen″es-trā′shun) The creation of a hole or aperture in a rigid contact lens to allow for exchange of tears and oxygen; introduced in 1946 by Joseph Dallos (1905–1979), Hungarian ophthalmologist.

ferrule

1. A metal ring, cap, or coiled wire, as used in the attachment of a ptosis crutch to the nasal side of a spectacle eye wire.
2. A metal or plastic cylindroid, crimped to retain bristles at the end of a brush.

fiber optics See *optics, fiber.*

field 1. An area or space.
2. A range or area of activity.

field, binocular visual The functional field of vision when both eyes are open. Sometimes quantitated on Esterman binocular grid, as developed in 1982 by New York ophthalmologist Benjamin Esterman (b. 1906).

field, reading The area in which clear reading vision is attained at a specified distance through a bifocal segment, or near-use ophthalmic lens.

field, visual The area or extent of physical space visible to an eye in a given position; measured in degrees from central fixation (kinetic testing) or threshold and supra-threshold sensitivity in various locations (static testing); field of view, abbreviated FOV.

-filcon Combining suffix for hydrophilic (hydrogel) contact lens polymers; terminology established by U.S. Adopted Names Council, Chicago, Illinois.

film, pre-lens That portion of the tear layer and its contents distributed over the anterior surface of a contact lens.

film, tear The usually clear, pre-corneal liquid derived both from the lacrimal gland and the accessory glands; consists of an outermost or fatty (sebaceous) layer secreted by the Meibomian glands, the most voluminous or middle layer (aqueous) secreted by the lacrimal and accessory lacrimal glands, and the innermost or mucin layer secreted by the single-cell goblet glands, and other accessory glands. The film provides moistening to the cornea, smoothing of slight surface irregularities, antibacterial enzymes, and washing of debris from the corneal surface; pre-corneal tear film.

filter In optical science, a device, material or color for restricting transmission of certain light rays.

filter, anti-glare Mechanical or optical device used to reduce the intensity of eccentric light entering the eye.

filter, cobalt blue A greenish-blue light-absorbing glass or plastic lens found on most biomicroscopes used for viewing sodium fluorescein while evaluating corneal integrity or the lens/cornea relationship of the contact lens fit; usually consists of cobalt oxide and alumina; introduced as a synthetic color in 1802.

filter, dichroic (dī-krō'ik) A light attenuating device which allows some wavelengths to pass and others to be interrupted; used in welding goggles and laser shields. (cf. *A.N.S.I. Z87.1 Practice for Occupational and Educational Eye and Face Protection; A.N.S.I. Z49.1 Safety in Welding and Cutting; A.W.S. A6.2 Lens Shade Selector.*)

filter lens See *lens, filter.*

filter, neutral A tinted or absorptive lens material which reduces light transmission about the same amount throughout the visible spectrum.

filter, polarized light zero transmission (PLZT) Two polarizing elements placed in surface contact on a common axis, about which they may be rotated to reduce transmission variably to 0%.

filter, red free A green-filtering lens found on most biomicroscopes used to highlight areas of vascular growth, hemorrhages, or rust spots on the eye or contact lenses; generally transmits light only in the 410nm to 560 nm range.

filter, welding See *goggles, welding.*

Filtron Trade name for a polymerized resin containing absorptive dyes for absorption of particular wavelength laser energy; used in some laser safety lenses.

finger-piece mounting See *mounting, finger-piece.*

fining

1. Refining or clarification of liquids, metals.
2. In optical manufacturing, the grinding procedure yielding a satin smooth finish immediately prior to the polishing stage of lens surfacing.

finish To complete to the best possible condition, as the final polishing of a lens for ophthalmic use.

finished lens See *lens, finished.*

fissure, interpalpebral The space between the borders of the two eyelids in primary gaze, measured in millimeters of vertical distance, usually at the location of widest opening; generally reduced in vertical dimension with upper eyelid ptosis, and increased with exophthalmos.

fissure, palpebral Small linear breaks or cracks in the skin radiating outward from the canthi, particularly the lateral canthus, sometimes incorrectly used to designate interpalpebral fissure.

fitting cross See *cross, fitting.*

fitting cross height See *height, fitting cross.*

fitting point See *point, fitting.*

fitting system, Grolman See *system, Grolman fitting.*

fitting triangle See Figure 37; *triangle, fitting.*

fixation The condition or act of directing the eye at the object of regard, which in the normal eye causes the fixation axis to connect from the center of the fovea to the point of regard.

fixation axis See *axis, fixation.*

flair, pad The surface of the nasal bearing area of a spectacle front that conforms to the shape of the nose.

flammability The ability to support combustion, as in some organic plastics no longer used for eyewear (e.g., cellulose nitrate).

flange, safety See *lip, posterior.*

flare, aqueous The Tyndall effect of random light scattering within a light beam passing through the anterior chamber when there is increased protein, or solid particulate content in the aqueous humor; usually a sign of intraocular inflammation; described in 1869 by Irish-born English physicist John Tyndall (1820–1893).

flash blindness See *blindness, flash.*

flat lens See *lens, flat.*

flat-top See *lens, multifocal flat-top.*

flatter add plus (FAP) Mnemonic. A fitting technique for contact lenses in which the minus power created by the tears trapped between a contact lens and the corneal surface is neutralized by the addition of an equal amount of plus (opposite) power.

flatter than K Mnemonic. In contact lens fitting, the technique of fitting a rigid (usually) contact lens with a longer radius of curvature than the flattest corneal meridian.

Fleischer ring See *ring, Fleischer.*

flesh The soft muscular tissue of an animal body.

flesh, proud See *tissue, granulation.*

flexible wear contact lens See *lens, contact, flexible wear.*

flicker Periodic variation in brightness of a light source; in displayed characters on a CRT, it is caused by the alternating decay and re-excitation of the phosphors; in a fluorescent light fixture, it is the function of the Hertz (cycles per second) value of the supplied electric current. Also used as a controlled frequency luminous stimulus to evaluate retinal sensitivity (flicker fusion fields).

flint glass See *glass, flint.*

floaters (vitreous) Small opacities of varying size in the transparent vitreous which may be of embryonic origin or acquired; such floaters cast shadows on the retina as seen particularly against a uniform bright background.

fluence Flux or flow as in energy transfer by laser application commonly expressed in joules or millijoules per unit area.

fluid, lacrimal Clear, salty, slightly alkaline fluid secreted by the lacrimal glands; constitutes the major portion of the tear fluid.

fluorescein angiography See *angiography, fluorescein.*

fluorescein pattern See *pattern, fluorescein.*

fluorescein, sodium A generally non-toxic, water soluble, orange-red powder which is the simplest of the fluorane dyes. Used topically in ophthalmology because of its ability to stain Bowman's membrane when the epithelial cells have been removed by disease or trauma; also available in dry form on paper strips; used in a 10% or 25% sterile solution for intravenous injection and subsequent photography as a fluorescent pattern in the fundus of the eye; delineates vascular leaks, collections of edema, changes in the pigment epithelium, and the like. About 3% to 5% of patients will have some transient nausea, and occasional vomiting 30 to 60 seconds following intravenous injection. Fluorescein absorbs blue light with maximum absorption at 480nm to 550nm and emits light and fluorescence from 500nm to 600nm with a maximum intensity at 520nm to 530nm.

fluorescence Property of a substance that, when illuminated, absorbs light of a given wavelength and re-emits it as radiations of another wavelength.

Fluoresoft Trade name for a form of fluorescent dye used to evaluate soft contact lenses, without staining or damaging the lens.

fluorine A non-metallic gaseous element of the halogen group; chemical symbol F, atomic number 9; a highly reactive poisonous gas; in the binary compound fluoride, is incorporated into bone and teeth, protecting against caries; used in contact lens material and commonly added to drinking water supplies. Discovered in 1886 by French chemist Ferdinand F.H. Moissan (1852–1907), who received a Nobel Prize in chemistry in 1906.

fluoro-silicone acrylate A silicone, rigid, gas-permeable (RGP) contact lens material; the addition of fluorine monomers improves oxygen permeability, wetting characteristics, deposit resistance and dimensional stability.

flux The rate of flow of fluid or energy.

flux, luminous The amount of light power leaving a source.

focal length See *length, focal.*

focal point See *point, focal.*

focal power See *power, vergence.*

foci (fō'sī) The plural of focus.

foci, conjugate A pair of object and image points in an optical system that are interchangeable. Light diverging from either point focuses at the other.

foci, cylinder A line or linear array of focal points generated by light emerging from a cylindrical power element which produces two principal line foci each at right angles to one another separated by a distance equal to the reciprocal of the cylindrical dioptric power component.

focimeter (fō-sim'i-ter) An optical instrument for determining vertex power, axis location, optical center, error-free point, and prism power at a given point on an ophthalmic lens; may be manual or automated. Trade names, Lensometer and Vertometer. First instrument of this type attributed to Troppmann in 1912, but based on awkward phakometer designed as a bench instrument, lensmeter, in 1876 by Hermann Snellen (1834–1908), ophthalmologist of Utrecht.

-focon Combining suffix for hydrophobic (non-hydrogel) contact lens polymers; terminology established by U.S. Adopted Names Council, Chicago, Illinois.

focus

1. A point at which rays of light converge or from which rays of light appear to diverge when entering or emerging from an optical system.
2. To adjust the elements of an optical system to achieve sharp imagery. See *point, focal.*

focus, back Distance between the rear surface of a lens and its focal point.

focusing, automatic Instrumental system used with cameras in self-adjusting focal length of the lens system to the object distance; sometimes based on ultrasound emitted from the camera and converting the time required for ultrasound to travel to the object and back into linear object distance.

fogging The deliberate overcorrection of hyperopia or the undercorrection of myopia for various purposes in refractive examination of the eye. It is used during subjective testing for astigmatism to reduce the tendency of the eye to accommodate during the test. Technique elaborated in the 1920s by U.S. ocular physiologist Charles Sheard, Ph.D.

follicular conjunctivitis See *conjunctivitis, follicular.*

Food and Drug Administration, U.S. (F.D.A.) A government agency (instituted in 1906), now within the Department of Health and Human Services, that sets standards and approves the use of foods, drugs, cosmetics and, since 1976, medical devices. It concerns itself with ophthalmic products, such as impact-resistant lenses, flammability of frame materials, and ultraviolet transmission of lenses; also operates the "Ophthalmic Device Panel" under F.D.A. device amendments of 1976 overseeing contact lenses, lens implants and about 1300 other devices, through its Center for Devices and Radiological Health, Rockville, Maryland 20857.

footcandle (fc) A psychophysical unit of illuminance of one lumen per square foot. Superseded by the metric lux (q.v.), one lumen per square meter.

foramen, optic (fo-ra'men) The opening of the optic canal into the bony orbit that transmits the optic nerve and the ophthalmic artery; located in the lesser wing of the spheroid bone.

foreign body See *body, foreign.*

form, face The curve in a spectacle front that follows the contours of the human face as viewed from above; also called head curve; parabolic curve frame.

former See *pattern, lens.*

fornix of the conjunctiva (for'niks, kon"junk-tī'vah) Loose fold of tissue which joins the bulbar and palpebral (tarsal) portions of the conjunctiva.

fossa (fos'ah) A cavity; depression; pit.

Foundation, Opticians Association of America Corporation established in 1990 to promote and further education, research, and scientific development in the field of optics, optical dispensing, and related subjects; established Muth Museum and Library, Fairfax, Virginia, in honor of master optician Eric P. Muth, Ph.D.

fovea (fō've-ah) Small glistening depression in the retina; the part of the macula adapted for most acute vision and color discrimination. It consists largely of specialized cone receptors and contains no blood vessels. (fovea centralis)

foveola (fō-ve-ō'lah) Base or bottom of the fovea centralis. The image of the point of fixation is formed on the foveola in the normal eye. Contains cone cells only.

fracture, fatigue (chronic stress fracture) A seemingly spontaneous breakup of poorly annealed or unevenly heat-tempered glass or other glass under stress or tension; may be precipitated by a minor impact or by heating when the glass is in a tight mounting.

fracture, lens A crack in an ophthalmic lens through its entire thickness and across a complete diameter creating two or more separate pieces, or when any piece of lens material, visible to the naked eye, becomes detached from the lens surface if a test ball or other object impacts a lens.

fracture, percussion cone A characteristic round indentation or conical excavation with many small spalls of glass, seen often following impact on glass with a BB shot or bird shot.

frame (ophthalmic or spectacle) A device for holding ophthalmic lenses in proper position on the head in front of the eyes. A frame typically consists of a front that holds the lenses and a pair of temples or earpieces to secure the unit to the head.

frame center distance See *distance, frame center.*

frame, combination A spectacle frame in which the front consists of a metal chassis with attached trim parts, sometimes known as top-rims. The trim parts are typically plastic, aluminum, or other metal, and are attached to the upper portion of the chassis. Top-rims may serve functional or cosmetic purposes, or both.

frame, doublet See *frame, flip up.*

frame, dress ophthalmic A frame for prescription corrective lenses, intended for use in correcting or improving vision (A.N.S.I. Z80.5). Such a frame is not intended for occupational, active sport, or safety use (A.N.S.I. Z87).

frame, flip up A spectacle with an auxiliary frame front glazed with prescription or absorptive lenses and hinged from the top of the primary frame front so that they may be easily lowered over or lifted away from the primary lenses; flip-front frames, flip-down spectacles, or doublet frame.

frame, gold-filled An ophthalmic frame constructed primarily of gold-clad metal. The term gold-filled indicates a layer of 10K gold or better, bonded by heat and pressure to one or more surfaces of a supporting metal. The karat gold layer must be at least 1/20th by weight of the total metal content.

frame, make-up A spectacle frame in which either lens may be flipped up or down singly to facilitate application of cosmetics to either eye for a presbyopic patient.

frame, metal An ophthalmic frame constructed primarily from a class of chemical elements, as aluminum, gold, nickel, silver, graphite, titanium, and the like.

frame, Oxford An eyeglass mounting, usually with metal eyewires connected by a flat spring across the top of the eyewires; the whole usually retained by a ribbon about the wearer's neck.

frame pantoscopic angle See *angle, frame pantoscopic.*

frame, parabolic curve An ophthalmic frame whose front top rim follows the contour of the forehead in a smoothly curving manner. (cf. *form, face.*)

frame, plastic An ophthalmic frame constructed primarily of synthetic material produced by chemical condensation or polymerization, frequently cellulose acetate or cellulose butyrate.

frame pupillary distance See *distance, frame center.*

frame, Titan 10 The trade name for a combination plastic metal frame made by Bausch & Lomb, in which the difference between the A and B dimensions is 10 mm.

frame, trial An adjustable spectacle-like device used to hold multiple trial lenses during subjective refraction.

frame, wraparound An ophthalmic frame, usually goggle-type, extending over the temporal orbital rim to provide lateral protection. See *frame, parabolic curve.*

frequency The number of waves passing a fixed point in one second; cycles per second or Hertz.

frequency, spatial In the design of grating targets to test visual acuity (or resolving power) of the eye, the number of cycles (test line plus equal space) per millimeter of target dimension.

Fresnel lens See *lens, Fresnel.*

Fresnel prism See *prism, Fresnel.*

fringes, Newton See *rings, Newton.*

front In spectacle optics, a component of an ophthalmic frame typically consisting of a bridge, rims and usually endpieces; function is to retain the ophthalmic lenses.

front vertex power See *power, front vertex.*

frontal angle See *angle, frontal.*

Fuchs dystrophy See *dystrophy, Fuchs.*

Ful-vue (Hibo) A spectacle frame design with the earpieces (temples) hinged high or 30° above the horizontal lens bisector (180° line of the lenses).

function, optical transfer A mathematical expression of the relationship between the light distribution received to form an optical image and that transmitted by an object for a given frequency; often expressed as a ratio of output contrast to input contrast; modulation transfer function.

fundus, ocular Concave interior of the eye, consisting of the retina, choroid, optic disc, and blood vessels; generally visible on ophthalmoscopic examination.

fused bifocal contact lens See *lens, contact, fused bifocal.*

fused segments See *segments, fused.*

fusion, binocular The cortical integration of the images received simultaneously by the two eyes. The function of merging simultaneous bilateral retinal images into a single perceptual image; sensory fusion. Divided in 1921 into first-, second- and third-degree fusion (the latter is true stereopsis) by London ophthalmologist Claud Worth (1869–1936).

fusional convergence See *convergence, fusional.*

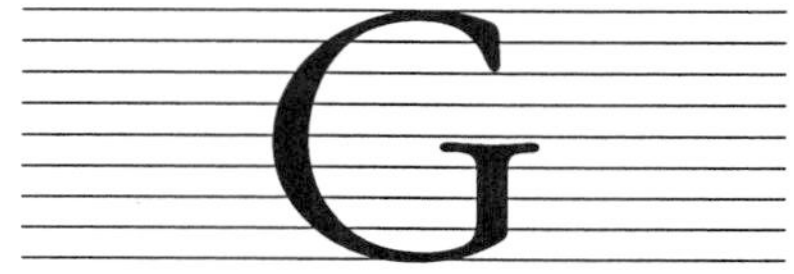

g The symbol for gram (S.I. unit). The basic unit of mass or weight in the metric system. Also abbreviated gm.

G The symbol for Gauss; q.v.

gain, optical In the human eye, the ratio of corneal to retinal increase of irradiance from focusing of incident light; normally in the magnitude of 100,000 times.

Galilean telescope See *telescope, Galilean.*

gamma, Γ, γ Third letter of the Greek alphabet; the third in a series of units or compounds.

ganglion cells See *cells, ganglion.*

garnet A crystalline, hard silicate mineral (generally $A_3B_2(SiO_4)_3$ of deep red color); Mohs hardness 6.5 to 7.5; used as a lasing medium; available in both natural and synthetic form; also used as an abrasive.

gas-permeable lens See *lens, gas-permeable.*

gauge A measuring instrument or device calibrated to a previously established standard, or system of units (e.g., thickness gauge).

gauge, Boley A mechanical caliper designed to measure inside or outside diameter; usually fitted with a lock and vernier scale.

gauge master A hand-held device containing standard lenses, curvatures, and thickness plates, all of known value, used to calibrate ophthalmic instruments.

gauge, segment A mechanical measuring device which may be inserted into an unglazed spectacle rim to determine height of bifocal or trifocal add; usually made in heights from 20mm to 30mm.

gauge, thickness See *caliper, lens.*

gauss An S.I. unit of magnetic energy or flux density. Superseded by the more convenient Tesla (T = 10,000 gauss); in 1934, superseded the unit Oersted; named for Croatian-born electrical engineer Nikola Tesla (1856–1943), and naturalized (1884) American citizen.

Gaussian optics See *optics, Gaussian.*

gc **1.** Abbreviation for the bacterium gonococcus, which causes potentially blinding keratoconjunctivitis.
2. In uppercase, abbreviation for geometric center; q.v.

Ge The symbol for the chemical element germanium; q.v.

gel Contracture for the word gelatin, a semi-solid material such as jelly or a colloid; q.v.. See *hydrogel.*

Geneva lens measure See *clock, lens.*

geometric center line See *line, geometric center.*

geometric center thickness See *thickness, geometric center.*

geometric center See *center, geometric.*

geometric optics See *optics, geometric.*

germanium A rare element of bluish-grey metallic appearance; chemical symbol Ge, atomic number 32; used in construction of lasers and diodes. Isolated in 1886 by Clements Alexander Winkler (1838–1904), German chemist; named for his nation.

ghost image See *image, ghost.*

ghost vessels See *vessels, ghost.*

giant papillary conjunctivitis (GPC) See *conjunctivitis, giant papillary (GPC).*

glabella In gross anatomy, the smooth and prominent area between the eyebrows and immediately above the depression of the nasal crest.

gland, lacrimal An exocrine secretory gland located at the upper outer area of the orbit that forms the aqueous or watery portion of the tears; almost identical histology to salivary glands.

glands, Krause Small accessory lacrimal glands that contribute to the production of the pre-corneal tear film, located deep in the upper and lower conjunctival fornices; structurally identical to the lacrimal gland. First described in 1854 by Karl Friedrich Theodore Krause (1797-1868), German anatomist.

glands, Meibomian (mī-bō′me-an) Series of sebaceous glands located in the tarsal plates whose ducts empty through the lid margin; produce the oily layer of the tear film; named for Heinrich Meibom, anatomist (1638–1700) of Helmstadt, Germany, who published first exact description of these tarsal glands in 1666.

glands of Moll Accessory sweat glands found at the base of the eyelashes along the upper and lower lid margins; first described in 1857 by Jacob Anton Moll (1833–1914), physician of Utrecht.

glands, tarsal See *glands, Meibomian.*

glands, Zeis Acinous, sebaceous glands found at the base of the eyelashes along the upper and lower lid margins; discharge a fatty sebaceous material, first described in 1835 by Dresden ophthalmologist Edourd Zeis (1807-1868).

glare Relatively bright light entering the eye creating dazzle, discomfort, or visual impairment. Within the visual field, a brighter light or greater illumination level than that to which the eyes are adapted; the contrast-lowering effect of stray light; may cause temporary loss of visual performance or acuity, annoyance, or blindness. Glare can be classified as direct or reflected.

glare, diffuse Reflected light that does not produce a clearly discernible image, i.e., a hazy, bright area.

glare, direct Relatively bright light that is not reflected, but emanates from a source such as the sun, oncoming automobile headlights, or other light source.

glare intensity See *intensity, glare.*

glare, reflected Relatively bright light that does not enter the eye directly from the light source, but after it has been deflected by a surface which the direct light has illuminated. It can be either diffuse or specular.

glare, specular Relatively bright light deflected off a mirror-like surface that produces a clearly identifiable image; creates dazzle, discomfort, or visual incapacity.

glare, veiling Excess light distributed over the visual field, creating reduction of contrast and visual acuity.

glass A hard, brittle, amorphous substance made from heat-fused (approximately 900°C) silicates with soda or potash, lime, metallic oxides, and similar elements of transparent quality and used in lens manufacture; developed as a commercial product about 1500–2000 B.C.

glass, barium crown A spectacle lens material of index 1.523 to approximately 1.610, containing 25% to 40% barium oxide (as barium carbonate) and having low dispersive power (i.e., Abbé number or Nu value 58).

glass beads See *beads, glass.*

glass, crown A highly uniform, isotropic, transparent, alkali-lime glass. An exceptionally stable glass of refractive index 1.523 at the sodium D line, wavelength 589.3nm, and low dispersive power (i.e., high Abbé number or Nu value, e.g:, 58), ophthalmic crown glass; spectacle crown glass; named for round, or crown-like shape given to a hot parison of glass as it is rotated in air by the glassmaker. Developed between 1807 and 1814 in France.

glass, flint Highly refractive index glass in which calcium has largely been replaced by lead; has a high dispersion relative to its refractive index; has higher surface reflection than crown glass, refractive index of 1.61 to 1.89. Trade names, High-Lite; Thinlite; Schott SFG.

glass, index 1.60 A relatively high-index optical glass; also available in phototropic composition (trade names PhotoGray, PhotoBrown); can be chemically tempered.

glass, index 1.70 An ophthalmic glass of high refractive index which is thinner but lighter than flint glass, and can be chemically hardened; contains titanium rather than lead oxide; has relatively high surface reflectivity (6.7% at each surface); Abbé value 38. Schott trade name High-Lite L; also called Hi Lite, Philtex, High-Lite.

glass, index 1.80 A glass of very high index of refraction having characteristics of softness of surface and a high dispersion; used to produce thinner lens configuration in high dioptric power. Trade names for lenses of this material, High-Lite; Auralite 1.80; Hidex.

glass, lead Generic name for high refractive index glass containing lead oxide (e.g., flint glass, Thinlite).

glass, natural Glass derived from the high heat of volcanic activity mainly from silicate melts; varies widely in composition over the range of common igneous rock; may be colorless to dark brown or opaque.

glass, ophthalmic crown See *glass, crown.*

glass, Pfund's A radiation protective lens for occupational use; made by placing a very thin layer of gold between a layer of ordinary crown glass and one of Crookes' "A" glass, an efficient UV absorber; gold reflects 98% of incident infrared wavelength light, but in thin layers is highly transparent to visible light.

glass, silica A very clear, strong glass produced by fusing pure SiO_2 at high temperature; used in high precision optical instruments; quartz glass; gives relatively high transmission of ultraviolet light.

glass, spectacle crown See *glass, crown.*

glasses A pair of lenses arranged in a holding device to keep them in proper position before the eyes as an aid to vision or for protection of the eye.

glasses, safety Pairs of ophthalmic lenses of special construction and mounting to protect the eyes from injury as by impact, heat, excessive irradiation, or liquid chemicals, meeting the requirements of A.N.S.I. Standard Z87; available as either corrective or non-corrective lenses.

glasses, scissors Eye glasses mounted as a pair on a downward-extending handle to be held with the hand before the user's chin.

glaucoma (glaw-kō′mah) A group of ocular diseases usually marked by abnormally high intraocular pressure, resulting in damage to the optic nerve and loss of visual field. Many types are classified. The existence of the disease in a first-order relative is a strong predisposing factor.

glaucoma, acute angle closure Sudden and painful elevation of intraocular pressure due to dilatation of the pupil or forward displacement of the iris obstructing aqueous drainage from the anterior chamber of the eye.

glazed

1. Furnished or fit with glass.
2. Assembled with appropriate ophthalmic lenses; used with respect to ophthalmic frames.

glazing

1. The process of inserting lenses into frames or mountings.
2. The work of a glazer fitting windows with glass.

globe of the eye Eyeball; bulbus oculi; the organ of vision.

glossy (adjective) Polished surfaces possessing a mirror-like or shiny finish.

gm Abbreviation for gram; q.v.

goggle An ocular protective device designed to fit the orbital area of the face to shield the eyes from a variety of hazards; may be ventilated or non-ventilated.

goggles, alpine skiing Special-purpose lenses to protect against high intensity visible and ultraviolet light at high altitudes on bright snow. (A.S.T.M. F 659-80.)

goggles, chipping Mechanical safety device worn in tight configuration over each eye or both orbits to protect the eyes from mechanical injury by flying particles or flakes during the act of chipping or hacking a surface to remove debris; may be designed to incorporate a refractive prescription or as coverall or over spectacles worn over prescription glasses.

goggles, cup Industrial or safety optical devices with individual components for each eye closely fitted to the orbital configuration of the face.

goggles, night vision A developing optical device to enhance vision in low light, frequently by means of infrared wavelengths; the light assistance used primarily by police and military personnel.

goggles, stack-trap Snug fitting safety goggles with anti-splash guards vented through shielded posts to prevent fluid entry.

goggles, swimmer's Individual cup goggles with plastic lenses; tight adaptation to orbital contours to seal water away from lids and eyes; held by tight elastic headbands. Usually allow insertion of plano or prescription lenses.

goggles, welding Protective eye shields worn to prevent eye injury, by reflection or absorption of excessive ultraviolet light and infrared light. Classified by U.S. Dept. of Commerce, National Bureau of Standards, 1928, No. 369 (N.B.S. shade numbers 1 to 14 which are logarithmic notations of visual transmission; the higher the number, the lower the transmission); more commonly, helmets or face shields are used to avoid burns of the skin.

gold A ductile, malleable, hypo-allergenic precious metal element, yellow in color; chemical symbol Au, atomic number 79; used as money, jewelry, spectacle frames, and to coat the surface of welders' goggles and face shields for astronauts while on the surface of the moon; has very high reflective value for infrared; absorbs UV; in thin layers has high transmittance for visible light.

gold-filled frame See *frame, gold-filled.*

gonio- Prefix meaning angle.

goniolens (gō′ne-o-lenz″) Contact lens to view the filtration angle of the anterior chamber, the iris root, ciliary body, and ora serrata; used with a slit lamp or gonioscope.

gonioprism A modification based on a contact lens having a greater index of refraction than does the cornea and incorporating a prism to bend forward the emerging rays of light, thus enhancing inspection of the anterior chamber angle.

gonioscope (gō′ne-o-skōp″) An instrument consisting of a biomicroscope in conjunction with a prismatic contact lens used to observe the angle of the anterior chamber of the eye; facilitates the diagnosis of open from closed or narrow-angle glaucoma; term and practical technique introduced in 1925 by M. Uribe Troncoso (1867–1959), ophthalmologist of Mexico City and New York.

gonioscopy (gō″ne-os′ko-pe) Observation of the angle of the anterior chamber of the eye; term coined by Alexis Trantis (1867–1961), a Greek ophthalmologist, who made various refinements between 1901 and 1907.

GPC Mnemonic for conjunctivitis, giant papillary; q.v.

gradient density lenses See *lens, gradient density.*

graft, corneal A disc or button of corneal tissue excised under sterile conditions from a donor eye, and placed in a prepared site of a host or recipient eye; corneal transplant.

gram The basic unit of weight or mass in the metric system; 1/1000 of the S.I. base unit, the kilogram; the weight of one cubic centimeter of distilled water at 4°C; approximately 1/28 of an ounce.

-graph Suffix meaning drawn, written.

graphite A form of native minearlized carbon, steel gray to black in color; a hexagonal crystal of high strength, used in spectacle frame construction.

graticule A grid or scale incorporated in transparent material in a focal plane of an optical instrument as an aid in localizing or measuring other objects.

grating, diffraction A plate of glass or polished metal ruled with a series of very close, equidistant, parallel lines to produce a spectrum by the diffraction of light. See *diffraction.*

gravity, specific The weight or mass of a substance compared to that of an equivalent volume of another substance taken as a standard, usually water, for measurements of solids or liquids; physical density.

gray A unit of Roentgen-absorbed radiation dose equal to 100 rads. Named in honor of Louis Harold Gray, Ph.D. (1905–1965), English medical physicist and radiobiologist.

grayness (or short finish) A surface defect in a finished or uncut lens caused by incomplete or incorrect fining or polishing that results in fine surface pits; sometimes referred to as short finish.

grid, Amsler's A chart of horizontal and vertically intersecting straight lines numbering about 5 squares to the inch used to evaluate macular alterations; devised 1947–1949 by Professor Marc Amsler (1891–1968), Swiss ophthalmologist.

grid, Esterman scoring A graphic plotting process used to establish a percentage value of the visual field, giving higher values to areas close to and immediately below fixation; introduced in 1967–1968 by Benjamin Esterman (b. 1906), New York ophthalmologist.

grid, optical An arrangement of parallel lines, grooves, etchings, or the like, constituting a graph or test chart, usually used to measure resolving power in an optical system. See *Z80.7.*

GRIN Acronym for gradient index lens. See *lens, gradient index.*

grinding, bicentric A process of surfacing or molding an ophthalmic lens to reduce vertical prismatic effect in the reading portion of an ophthalmic lens without affecting the error-free point of the distance portion of the lens. Used to balance vertical prismatic effects induced by anisometropic correcting lenses. Also called slab-off.

groove angle See *angle, groove.*

groove, eyewire See *groove, rim.*

groove, lens A narrow, shallow indentation on the edge of a lens for a rimless mounting designed to accept a cord or wire to retain the lens in the mounting.

groove, rim The recessed area of a spectacle front in which a beveled lens edge is seated.

groove, safety See *lip, posterior.*

guard The part of a spectacle front or mounting designed to support the spectacles by resting against either side of the nose; a nosepad.

guttata, cornea See *cornea guttata.*

Gy Abbreviation for unit of radiation energy, gray; q.v.

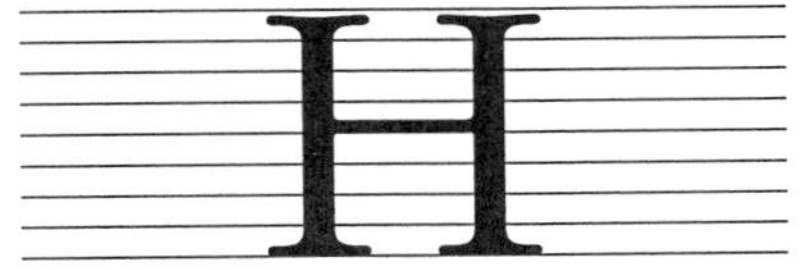

H Abbreviation for hardness; q.v.

H-R-R plates Abbreviation for Hardy-Rand-Rittler plates. See *plates, H-R-R.*

half-round pliers See *pliers, half-round.*

halides Binary chemical compounds of one of the halogens (usually fluorine, chlorine, bromine, or iodine) as a salt formed by direct union with a metal. Silver halides are the photosensitive compounds in phototropic or photosensitive lenses.

hallucinations, visual The subjective impression of visual sensations in the absence of appropriate stimuli and generally without impairment of consciousness.

halogen One of 4 or 5 closely related non-metallic elements (group VIIA of the periodic table) which form similar and salt-like compounds in combination with sodium and many other metals (including chlorine, fluorine, iodine, and bromine); used in high-efficiency light bulbs.

haptic Supporting component without refractive power. The part of a contact lens that touches the bulbar conjunctiva, or the part of an intraocular lens implant that touches the capsule or scleral sulcus; from the Greek "hapt(o)," to touch.

hard contact lens (HCL) See *lens, contact, hard.*

hard resin (plastic) See *CR-39.*

hardness (H) The ability of a substance to withstand indentation, penetration or deformation; often divided into macrohardness and microhardness; related to, but a variant of, scratch resistance.

hardness number See *number, hardness.*

hardware

1. Fittings or trimmings made of metal.
2. Metal components typically used to fasten together or strengthen portions of a spectacle frame.

haze In ophthalmic lenses, the presence of slight scratches, mars, coating delamination, or similar surface imperfections that interfere with light transmission by creating light scatter. (cf., *U.S. Federal Test Method 406, Method 3022.*)

HCL Mnemonic for lens, hard contact; q.v.

head curve See *form, face.*

heat-treated lens See *lens, heat-treated.*

height, apical See *depth, sagitta.*

height, fitting cross The vertical position of intersecting reference lines used to position a progressive-power lens in front of the eye, based on the manufacturer's design in relation to its horizontal lens bisector (HLB) (geometric center line). When specifying fitting cross height, it is not necessary to specify MRP height, because the MRP is a fixed position below the fitting cross, as designed by the manufacturer.

height (level), major reference point (MRP) The vertical distance in millimeters from the horizontal tangent at the lower lens bevel to the MRP. To avoid vertical prismatic imbalance or improper location of the MRP (especially in single lens replacement), it is good practice to specify the MRP height or level in relation to the horizontal lens bisector (HLB), similar to vertical segment position (VSP)—i.e., 4B, 2A, etc.

Commonly, if a bifocal is set at a usual position, such as 4mm below the HLB, the lab grinds the MRP on the HLB. With progressive-addition lenses, when the fitting cross height is specified, there is no need to specify the MRP height, because it is a fixed distance below the fitting cross.

In trifocal lenses, unusual positioning of bifocals, or the fitting of high-power or high-index lenses, the MRP height should be specified (e.g., VSP of trifocal segment = 2mm above (2A) the HLB). If no MRP level is specified, the lab may grind the MRP on the segment line or on the HLB. If the desirable position for the MRP is 2mm above the segment line, it must be specified as 4mm above (4A) the HLB.

height, optical center See *height, major reference point.*

height, segment (SH) The vertical distance in millimeters from the horizontal tangent at the lower finished lens edge to the horizontal tangent at the top of the segment in a multifocal spectacle lens. The top of the trifocal segment is specified in locating trifocal segment height. See Figure 20; see also *position, vertical segment (VSP).*

hema- Prefix meaning blood.

HEMA Acronym for **h**ydroxy**e**thyl **m**eth**a**crylate, the pioneer hydrophilic plastic polymer used in manufacture of some soft contact lenses; q.v.; Hydrogel.

hematoma (hē″mah-tō′mah) A tumor-like swelling due to hemorrhage of blood into soft tissues; this may occur in the eyelids (i.e., black eye), after a blunt blow.

hemeralopia (hem″er-ah-lō′pe-ah) Day blindness; defective vision in bright light. A turn of the century term describing a rare congenital and usually autosomal recessive cone dysfunction with color blindness, photophobia, and nystagmus; in last 30 years, commonly described as rod monochromatism, complete or incomplete.

hemi- Prefix meaning half.

hemianopsia (hemianopia) (hem″i-an-op′se-ah) Blindness of half the visual field of one or both eyes.

hemimeridian Half of a great circle of the cornea passing through the corneal apex; usually indicated in topographical analysis of the cornea for contact lens design or surgical intervention.

hemorrhage An extravasation of blood from arteries or veins.

hemorrhage, subconjunctival Blood loss from a small vessel beneath the conjunctiva; caused by high blood pressure, minor trauma, coughing, or sneezing. The blood is trapped between the conjunctiva and sclera, causing the eye to take on a blood-red color, with the blood being absorbed into the surrounding tissue over the course of about one week.

hemorrhage, vitreous Extravasation of blood into the large cavity of the eye (vitreous chamber); frequently associated with diabetes mellitus or trauma to the eye.

Herapathite A salt of quinine made by treating the sulfate with iodine utilizing its rhomboid crystals to polarize light. Technique developed in 1927–1928 by Edwin H. Land (1910–1991), American light science inventor. Named in honor of the English physician William Bird Herapath who initiated the concept in 1852, but did not bring it to a practical level. Crystals may be embedded in thin sheets of polyvinyl alcohol.

Hertz The expression of frequency in cycles per second (Hz). Named in honor of Heinrich Rudolf Hertz (1857–1894), German physicist who discovered radio waves.

hetero- Prefix meaning different.

heterochromia (het″er-o-krō′me-ah) Difference in the color of the two irides; sometimes associated with uveitis in the lighter colored eye (Fuchs heterochromia).

heterophoria (het″er-o-fō′re-ah) Tendency of the eye to deviate from normal alignment generally in the absence of adequate fusional stimuli. Esophoria: inward; exophoria, outward; hyperphoria, upward; hypophoria, downward; cyclophoria, rotational on front to back axis.

heterotropia (het″er-o-trō′pe-ah) Deviation of an eye not held in alignment by the fusion mechanism. Esotropia, eye turned in (cross-eyed); exotropia, eye turned out (wall-eyed); hypertropia, eye turned upward; hypotropia, eye turned downward; cyclotropia, eye rotation on its front to back axis.

heterotropic Pertaining to or having heterotropia.

Hg Chemical symbol for the metallic element mercury; q.v.

hidden hinge See *hinge, hidden.*

hide-a-bevel A special type of spectacle lens edge contour used for cosmetic effect; a flatter bevel generally used on strong minus lenses to minimize bevel appearance from frontal view. See *coating, edge.*

Hidex Trade name for a high-index glass containing lead oxide; refractive index 1.806.

high velocity impact test See *test, high velocity impact.*

High-Lite Trade name for glass lens, index 1.70.

hinge An interlocking, pivotal device that joins a spectacle front and temple while facilitating a swinging motion between them; made of a variable number of barrels or leaves (commonly three barrels, five barrels, or seven barrels).

hinge, English A type of hinge construction on early 1900 zylonite-type frames that embody metal-to-metal contact of the temple butt end to the front endpiece hinge.

hinge, hidden In a spectacle endpiece, an embedded hinge-anchoring device that is not visible from the front surface.

hinge screw See *screw, hinge.*

hippus Abnormally exaggerated rhythmic dilation and constriction of the pupil.

HLB Mnemonic for bisector, horizontal lens; q.v.

Ho Chemical symbol for the metallic element holmium; q.v.

holmium A metallic element of the rare earth group; chemical symbol Ho, atomic number 67; sometimes called neoholmium because original preparations were impure. Approved for ophthalmic laser use in 1990 in combination with YAG; particularly useful in glaucoma control; named for the city of Stockholm near where it was discovered in 1878 by J.L. Soret and M. Delafontaine, Swedish chemists.

holography The recording of images in a hologram or three-dimensional form on photographic film by exposing it to a laser beam reflected from the object under study; may be projected into three-dimensional space. Theoretical basis developed in 1947 and practical technique produced in 1965 by Hungarian-born physicist Dennis Gabor (1908–1979), working in London and Connecticut; received 1971 Nobel Prize in physics.

homocentric In optics, the condition in which more than one optical beam or pencil share the same ray path, as in the ophthalmoscope where the path of illumination and observation follow the same principal axis.

honey bee lens See *lens, honey bee.*

hordeolum (hor-de'o-lum) A localized purulent infection of one or more glands of the eyelid, usually due to staphylococcus. An external hordeolum points through the skin surface; an internal hordeolum points through the tarsal conjunctival surface; stye. A contraindication to fitting or wearing contact lenses.

horizontal segment position (HSP) See *position, horizontal segment.*

horopter (ho-rop'ter) The location of all object points in three-dimensional space simultaneously stimulating corresponding points on the retina from a given distance. The contour of the horopter depends on the distance from the eyes to the fixation point. The concept and name were introduced in 1613 by Franciscus Aguilonius (1567–1617), a Jesuit priest of Belgium.

horopter, Nonius longitudinal An experimental measuring device, forerunner of the vernier, to establish the horizontal field of corresponding retinal points. Nonius is the Latinized form of (Pedro) Nunes (1502–1578), Portugese professor of mathematics and cartographer, who established the graduating device.

horopter, Vieth-Müller A theoretical circle passing through the fixation point and entrance pupils of the two eyes; any point on such circle stimulates corresponding retinal elements. Described in 1818–1826 primarily by the German ocular physiologist Johannes Müller (1801–1858).

housing, lamp See *lamphouse.*

Hruby lens See *lens, Hruby.*

hue The particular aspect of color or wavelength that enables it to be assigned a position in the visible spectrum; distinct from saturation and brightness; chroma.

humor, aqueous The normally clear, watery fluid that fills the anterior and posterior chambers of the eye. It is formed by secretion from the ciliary body and drains out of the eye through the Canal of Schlemm. It has a refractive index (1.33) lower than the crystalline lens (variably 1.38 to 1.40); it surrounds the crystalline lens and is involved in the metabolism of the cornea and the lens.

humor, vitreous The gelatinous, colorless, transparent substance (refractive index 1.336) filling the vitreous chamber of the eye, i.e., the space between the crystalline lens, the ciliary body, and the retina. It contains mucoid, collagen fibers and hyaluronic acid, but is mostly water.

hyaline plaque See *plaque, hyaline.*

hydration The absorption or combination of water with a tissue or substance; water of hydration.

hydro- Prefix meaning water.

hydrogel A colloid made from various polymers that absorbs and binds with water; used as a material for contact lenses.

hydrogel lens See *lens, hydrogel; lens, contact, soft.*

hydrophilic Having an affinity toward water; water-loving. A class of soft contact lenses that absorb and retain water; trade names, Permalens; Hydrocurve; Silsoft; Aquaflex; AO Soft; Soflens; Softcon; CibaSoft; Gel Flex; SofForm; Tresoft; etc.

hydrophobic Having little or no affinity for water; as in contact lenses with a poor wetting angle.

hydrops (hī'drops) An abnormal accumulation of fluid in the tissues or a body cavity.

hydrops, corneal An abnormal accumulation of watery fluid, presumably aqueous humor, in the stroma and usually the epithelium of the normally clear cornea.

hydroxyapatite (hī-drok"se-ap'a-tīt) An inorganic compound found in coral and in the matrix of bone and teeth ($Ca_{10}(PO_4)_6(OH)_2$) that provides rigidity to those structures; as coralline hydroxyapatite, a chemical derivative of coral skeletal corbomate is used in porous spheres as volume-replacing implants after enucleation; blood vessels and fibrous tissue grow into its structure creating firm adhesions. Released by F.D.A. in September 1989.

hydroxyethyl methacrylate (HEMA) In contact lens materials, one of several similar synthetic hydrogel polymers which absorbs and binds water into its molecular structure; developed in late 1950s by Otto Wichterle and Drahoslav Lim, Prague (Czechoslovakian) chemists; first HEMA contact lenses were manufactured in 1960 and released as an investigative new drug in the United States in 1964 with full F.D.A. clearance in 1971.

hypaesthesia Alternate spelling for hypesthesia; q.v.

hyper- Prefix meaning above, higher, excessive.

hyperemia (hī"per-ē'me-ah) Congestion of the blood vessels, characterized by their fullness of excessive blood; seen in all infections and inflammations of the eye (engorgement).

hyperflange A special thinned area at the edge of a high minus contact lens to reduce edge awareness and lens movement. A hyperflange is configured to the edge thickness of a plus (+) lens and allows a lens of high minus power to center better.

hyperlacrimation (hī"per-lak"ri-mā'shun) An excess flow of tears, usually from the lacrimal gland, and containing primarily the aqueous portion of the tears. (cf. *epiphora.*)

hypermature cataract See *cataract, hypermature.*

hypermetropia (hī"per-me-trōp'e-ah) Refractive error or optical defect of the eye in which parallel rays of light, as from a distant light source, strike the retina before coming to a focus. Term proposed, clarifying difference between presbyopia and farsightedness, in

1859 by the Dutch ophthalmologist and physiologist Franciscus Cornelis Donders (1818–1889) of Utrecht. Synonym, *hyperopia.*

hypermetropic (hī″per-me-trop′ik) Pertaining to or having insufficient refractive power for the length of the eye; farsightedness; correctable by plus lenses; hyperopia.

hyperopia (hī″per-ō′pe-ah) Refractive error or optical defect of the eye in which parallel rays of light, as from a distant light source, strike the retina before coming to a focus; correctable by plus lenses; farsightedness. Term proposed in 1859 by the German physiologist and physicist Hermann von Helmholtz (1821–1894). Synonym, *hypermetropia.*

hyperopia, axial Refractive error of farsightedness due to abnormal shortness of the eye as measured from front to back; confirmed by ultrasound examination.

hyperopia, curvature Optically underpowered eye caused by curvature of the cornea or lens that is too flat for the axial length of the eye, confirmed by keratometer reading, or Purkinje images from the lens.

hyperopia, latent Portion of total farsightedness not apparent to a patient because of compensation by accommodation.

hyperopia, total Entire amount of farsightedness present in an eye from any and all mechanisms.

hyperphoria (hī″per-fō′re-ah) A tendency for an eye to deviate upward; occurs on interruption of binocular fusion as when an eye is covered and is detectable on uncovering the eye, at which time it returns to its normal position.

hypersensitivity A marked or exaggerated tissue response to a foreign substance in amounts which are innocuous to most individuals; may be immediate or delayed response.

hypersensitivity, contact A delayed type of inflammatory reaction to direct contact of skin or other epithelium (e.g., cornea or conjunctiva) to any of a variety of chemicals or chemical compounds (e.g., contact lens material); may be lymphocyte mediated.

hypertelorism (hī″per-te′lor-izm) Abnormally wide distance between the two eyes; usually congenital defect affecting both sides symmetrically; may be reduced by major facial surgery.

hypertonic Any solution with a higher osmotic pressure in reference to another.

hypertropia (hī″per-trō′pe-ah) An upward deviation of one eye while the other remains straight and fixates normally.

hypesthesia (hīp″es-thē′ze-ah) Reduction in sensitivity; when occurring in the cornea, contraindicates the wearing of contact lenses; older spelling, hypaesthesia; optional spelling hypoesthesia.

hyphema (hyphemia) (hī-fē′mah) Blood within the anterior chamber of the eye; commonly follows blunt injury to the eye; a serious problem because of tendency to rebleed in 4 or 5 days, and development of secondary glaucoma.

hypo- Prefix meaning below, lower, deficient.

hypophoria (hī″po-fō′re-ah) The tendency for one eye to deviate downward; occurs on the interruption of binocular fusion, as when one eye is covered.

hypopyon (hī-pō′pe-on) Pus in the anterior chamber associated with inflammatory diseases of the cornea, the iris, or the ciliary body.

hypotonic Any solution with a lower osmotic pressure in reference to another.

hypotony (hī-pot′o-ne) Low pressure within the eye, often associated with wound leaks, retinal detachment, or cyclitis; the opposite of glaucoma.

hypotropia (hī″po-trō′pe-ah) Downward deviation of one eye.

hypoxia An inadequate supply of oxygen to tissues; may occur in the cornea under a tight contact lens. Mountain climbers at high altitude commonly develop retinal hemorrhages from hypoxia. (cf. *anoxia.*)

Hz Abbreviation for Hertz; q.v.

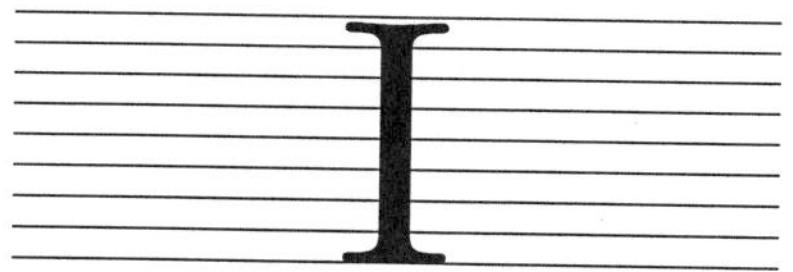

I.E.C. Abbreviation for the International Electrotechnical Commission; q.v.

I.S.E.T. Abbreviation for International Society of Eye Trauma.

I.S.O. Abbreviation for International Organization for Standardization; q.v.

I.S.O.T. Abbreviation for International Society of Ocular Trauma; q.v.

icon

1. From the Greek, a sacred image.
2. An image, figure or representation displayed on a microcomputer screen representing a variable function or resource.

illiterate E A simple optotype for testing visual acuity in non-readers or children who are mature enough to point with their hand or finger to indicate the direction of the three-stroke component of the figure; introduced in 1885 by Giuseppi Albini (1825–1911), ophthalmologist of Naples, Italy.

illuminance Psychophysical description of light falling on a surface; may be expressed in candela per square meter, lux, or the older foot candle (1 lumen per square foot) equal to slightly more than 10 lux. Illumination.

illumination, diffuse An ocular biomicroscopic examination technique with non-focal light directed broadly to the anterior structures of the eye to facilitate gross observation or details of contact lens fit.

illumination, direct focal An ocular biomicroscopic examination technique with light focused frontally or straightforward on an area of localization. Concept introduced in 1919 by Alfred Vogt (1879–1943), Swiss ophthalmologist.

illumination, indirect lateral An ocular examination technique with light focused closely (usually about a 60° angle) to one side or the other of an area under biomicroscopic localization; a variation of retroillumination, sometimes called "proximal" illumination. Technique introduced in 1919 by Alfred Vogt (1879–1943), Swiss ophthalmologist.

illumination, sclerotic scatter A biomicroscopic technique of ocular examination with high-intensity light to assess corneal relucency, degree of corneal edema, corneal abrasion, or tear interchange. A beam 1mm to 3mm wide is brought to focus on the temporal corneoscleral limbus creating a perilimbal or circumcorneal illumination which reveals minute or faint pathologic changes in the cornea. This illumination causes light to be carried across the cornea by reflecting off both the anterior and posterior corneal surfaces. May be performed with or without fluorescein. Originally described in 1923 by Basil Graves, London ophthalmologist.

Illuminator, True Daylight Trade name for a C.I.E. illuminant source of "C" characteristics; delivers approximately 100 lux; supersedes the discontinued Macbeth lamp. Manufactured by Richmond Products, Boca Raton, Florida 33307. See also *Vitalite* (fluorescent tube illuminant of Duratest Corp., North Bergen, New Jersey.)

image That which is formed as a counterpart or likeness of something else. Visual impression of an object formed by a lens or mirror; may be real (projectable on a screen) or virtual (located mathematically by ray tracing).

image, catoptric The image formed by regularly reflected light.

image, dioptric The image formed by regularly refracted light.

image displacement See *displacement, image.*

image, entopic Image formed on the retina by objects inside the eye or on the surface of the eye, i.e., shadows of vitreous floaters (muscae volitantes), mucus on the cornea, retinal vessels, and the like.

image, ghost In spectacle optics, an unwanted secondary image formed by internal reflections from the rear, i.e., ocular surface of an ophthalmic lens, or by reflection from the anterior surface of the cornea and a second reflection from the ocular (eye) surface of a spectacle lens.

image, inverted Visual impression of an object as formed by a lens or mirror, in which the upper and lower portions of the image appear as exchanged.

image jump See *jump, image.*

image polarity See *polarity, image.*

image, real An optical image that actually exists, formed by the convergence of refracted or reflected light rays that can be projected on a screen and viewed without looking into the optical system.

image, reversed Visual impression of an object as formed by a lens or mirror in which the right and left portions of the image appear as exchanged.

image size compensation See *compensation, image size.*

image, virtual An optical image that has no real existence and cannot be projected on a screen; apparent; created by emanating rays diverging from an optical system.

imbalance A state or condition when something is out of equilibrium or unequal.

imbalance, muscular In visual physiology, a generic description for heterophoria or heterotropia. A dissimilarity in the position of one eye in relation to the other.

imbalance, prismatic The difference in prism power in a pair of ophthalmic lenses at corresponding specified reference points.

imbalance, vertical A generic description for unequal vertical positioning of one eye in reference to the other. See *imbalance, prismatic.* See also *hyperphoria, hypertropia, hypophoria, hypotropia* in relation to extraocular muscles.

immature cataract See *cataract, immature.*

impact resistance See *resistance, impact.*

impact-resistant lens See *lens, impact resistant lenses for dress eyewear; lens, impact-resistant lenses for occupational and educational protection.*

implant, orbital

1. Volume-replacing devices to place within the extraocular muscle cone after surgical enucleation of an eye, or within the scleral shell after evisceration of an eye. Implant within Tenons capsule introduced in 1877 by London ophthalmologist William Lang (1863–1937) using a glass ball; scleral implant introduced in 1885 by Philip Henry Mules (1843–1905), ophthalmologist of Liverpool.
2. Plastic material, usually silicone, sutured on or into the sclera to compress a retinal break.

incidence, angle of See *angle of incidence.*

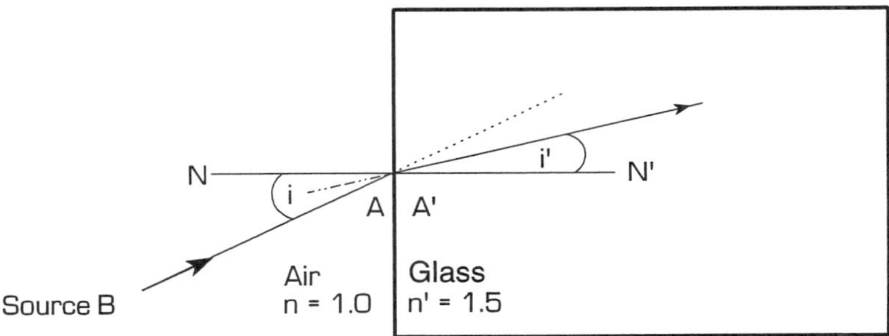

Figure 23 Snell's (Descartes') law of refraction. n(SIN i) = n'(SIN i').

incident light See *light, incident.*

incident ray See *ray, incident.*

incipient cataract See *cataract, incipient.*

Inconel Trade name for a reflective metal coating used on the front surface of some sunglasses; comprised of approximately 80% nickel, 14% chromium, and 6% iron; also Inconel-X, a metal alloy used in surface coating of rocket space craft which can withstand frictional heating to 1,200°F.

index 1.70 glass See *glass, index 1.70.*

index 1.80 glass See *glass, index 1.80.*

index of refraction The ratio of the velocity of light in air to the velocity in a given medium. This ratio expresses the ability of a lens material to refract or bend a ray of light of given wavelength. It is usually stated for the wavelength of the first sodium D lines (587.56 nanometers [nm]); the higher the index, the more the refractive power. For the ophthalmic glass most commonly in use, n = 1.523, ±0.0015. Allyl resin and polycarbonate plastic materials used in the manufacture of ophthalmic lenses have typical indices of refraction of 1.4975 and 1.586, respectively. Diamonds have an index of refraction of 2.417; *Snell's law of refraction* (Figure 23). See also *Table I, Index of Refraction* in the Appendix.

indium A soft malleable low melting point (c. 120°F), metallic element, chemical symbol In, atomic number 49, which resists tarnishing; named for its two indigo blue lines in the visible spectrum; used in metallic alloys as a bonding agent between lens blanks and blocking bodies for lens surfacing or edging operations. Discovered in 1863 by the color-blind Ferdinand Reich (1799–1882), German mineralogist.

indocyanine green A fluorescent dye administered intravenously to demonstrate deep structure of the retina and choroid with a maximum light absorption at 805nm and peak fluorescence at 835nm—a near infrared level that penetrates the retinal pigment epithelium.

induced prism See *prism, induced.*

industrial "safety" lenses See *lens, impact resistant for occupational and educational protection. (A.N.S.I. Z87)*

infection Swelling and inflammatory reaction in an organ due to invasion of bacteria, fungi, viruses, and the like.

inferior Lower or downward direction.

inferior oblique muscle See *muscle, inferior oblique.*

inferior punctum See *punctum, inferior.*

inferior rectus muscle See *muscle, inferior rectus.*

infinity In optical science, a distance great enough so that rays of light from that distance may be regarded as parallel; 20 feet or 6m or greater.

infrared Electromagnetic radiation with wavelengths longer than visible light, but shorter than microwave radiation (i.e., 700nm to 10M); divided (approximately) into near infrared (IR-A), 700nm to 1,000nm; middle infrared (IR-B), 1,400nm to 3,000nm; and far infrared (IR-C), 3,000nm to 10,000nm; creates heat in substances that absorb such wavelengths.

injection

1. Tissues rendered red and swollen from dilated blood vessels.
2. A technique of molding by inserting material into a form; used in preparation of most plastic lenses.
3. The technique of forcing a liquid into a part of the body, commonly done with a needle and syringe.

injection, conjunctival Redness caused by congestion of the capillaries within the mucus membrane covering the eye; usually caused by irritation or mechanical manipulation.

innervation The distribution or supply of nerves to a body part; motor innervation, conducting a stimulus to a muscle; sensory innervation, conducting a reaction of sensation centrally or to the brain.

inset See *inset, segment (SI).*

inset, bridge A configuration of a spectacle bridge with the nasal contact area located behind the plane of the lenses (nearer the face).

inset, segment (SI) The horizontal distance in millimeters between the vertical major reference point bisector and the vertical segment bisector; based on the formula (see Figure 20):

$$\text{segment inset, SI} = \frac{(\text{DIOD} - \text{NIOD})}{2}$$

where
DIOD = distant interocular distance in millimeters.
NIOD = near interocular distance in millimeters.

inset, total segment (TSI)

1. The sum of the segment inset and distance decentration for each lens.
2. The horizontal distance between the vertical lens bisector and the vertical segment bisector;.based on the formula (see Figure 20):

$$\text{total (segment) inset, TSI} = \frac{(\text{FCD} - \text{NIOD})}{2}$$

where
FCD = frame center distance, A + DBL.
NIOD = near interocular distance.

instrument compensation See *compensation, instrument.*

insufficiency, convergence Inability to adduct the eyes to the average or normal near point of convergence; may be alleviated by base in prism in the reading portions of a pair of spectacle lenses.

intensity, glare The amount or concentration of light energy per unit area of source; inversely proportional to the square of the distance from the eye and the cosine of the angle of incidence.

intensity, luminous The amount of light leaving a point source through a given sector (measured in steradians) of space; luminous flux; radiance.

inter- Prefix meaning between, among.

interference In physical optics, the process in which two or more electromagnetic waves of the same frequency combine to reinforce or cancel each other; also occurs with sound waves.

interferometer In ophthalmic optics, a diagnostic instrument which projects a series of progressively finer black and white sine wave gratings onto the macula to evaluate macular function.

interferometry (in″ter-fer-om′i-tre) The measurement of the process in which two or more electromagnetic waves of the same frequency combine to reinforce or cancel each other; particularly used with twin laser beam potential acuity meters to estimate visual resolving power (acuity) through a partial cataract.

intermediate

1. Being or happening between two things, places, stages, or the like.
2. The area in a trifocal lens or blank which has been designed to correct vision at ranges between distant and near objects.

intermediate interpupillary distance See *distance, intermediate interocular (IIOD).*

intermediate peripheral curve (IPC) See *curve, intermediate peripheral.*

internal rectus muscle Incorrect term; see *muscle, medial rectus.*

International Academy of Sports Vision (I.A.S.V.) A voluntary organization promoting public education concerning eye safety and performance in sports; approximately 1000 members; since 1953, publishes the *Journal of the International Academy of Sports Vision,* and since 1984, the quarterly Journal *Sportsvision.* Office: 200 S. Progress, Harrisburg, Pennsylvania 17109.

International Electrotechnical Commission (I.E.C.) Voluntary agency which develops light, electrical, and laser standards; established in 1913. Abbreviated I.E.C. (Technical Committee 76, Radiation Safety and Laser Products and Equipment 1979). Office: Geneva, Switzerland.

International Eye Foundation (I.E.F.) A voluntary, professional association of ophthalmologists and related specialists promoting and providing care of ocular disease in underdeveloped nations. Established in 1961 by John Harry King (1911–1986), Washington ophthalmologist. Office: Bethesda, Maryland 20814.

International Ophthalmological Congress (I.O.C.) A series of worldwide scientific meetings of ophthalmologists occurring every 4 to 5 years since 1857 and held in various world capital cities. The 1994 meeting was in Toronto, Canada, and the 1998 meeting will be in Amsterdam, the Netherlands. Publishes transactions or *Acta* of each Congress.

International Organization for Standardization (I.S.O.) Treaty agency which supervises international standards; established in 1947 in Geneva, Switzerland; evaluates recommendations by Technical Advisory Groups (T.A.G.) from each participating nation. Standards become binding on each of approximately 85 signatory nations through General Agreement on Tariffs and Trade, G.A.T.T. (established 1947). Office: Geneva, Switzerland.

International Society of Ocular Trauma (I.S.O.T.) A voluntary professional organization of individuals interested in prevention and repair of ocular injuries; established in 1989; conducts triannual international symposia; approximately 2,000 members from 34 countries; publishes quarterly *Journal of Eye Trauma.* Office: Tel Hashomer, Israel.

interocular distance (IOD) See *distance, interocular (IOD).*

interocular Between the eyes.

interpalpebral (in-ter″pal-pē′bral) Located within the space defined between the margins of the upper and lower eyelids. See *fissure, palpebral; fissure, interpalpebral.*

interpupillary distance See *distance, interocular (IOD).*

interval, astigmatic (interval of Sturm) The linear distance between the two focal lines or ellipses of an astigmatic eye or toric optical system. A component within the conoid of Sturm; q.v. (See Figures 6 through 11.)

intra- Prefix meaning within.

intracapsular cataract extraction See *extraction, cataract, intracapsular.*

intraocular pressure See *pressure, intraocular.*

intraocular Within the eye.

intrinsic Belonging to the real nature of a thing; inside; pertaining exclusively to a part.

intumescence (in″tyu-mes′ens) A swelling up, as with congestion; commonly in reference to the lens of the eye as it develops cataractous changes and induces a myopic shift in refractive correction.

invariant Having no degree of freedom or change; constant; said of certain linear optical functions.

iodopsin (ī″o-dop′sin) A photosensitive violet pigment in retinal cones which subserves photopic vision and is important in color vision.

IOL Mnemonic for **i**ntra**o**cular **l**ens (pseudophakos) implant; lens is introduced surgically after removal of a cataract; initially achieved in 1949 by Harold Lloyd Ridley (b. 1906), London ophthalmologist.

ionic

1. Pertaining to ions—atoms or radicals having a charge of positive (cation) or negative (anion) electricity.
2. A type of Greek or Ionic architecture characterized by ornamental scrolls.
3. Commonly used in relation to contact and spectacle lens material, designating its ability to attract minute particular debris.

IPC Mnemonic for curve, intermediate posterior; q.v.

ipsilateral Located on the same side; homolateral; opposite of contralateral.

iridectomy (ir″i-dek′to-me) Surgical removal of part of the iris; usually peripheral in location or sector in radial configuration; often done with cataract extraction or to remove a tumor of the iris.

irideremia (ir″id-er-ē′me-ah) Congenital absence of part of the iris; in contrast to aniridia, or total absence of the iris.

irides (i′ri-dēz) The plural of iris.

iridocyclitis (ir′i-do-si-klī″tis) Inflammation of both the iris and the ciliary body; may be due to systemic inflammatory disease, autoimmune disease, or local injury.

iridodonesis (ir″i-dō-don-ē′sis) An abnormal tremulousness or shaking of the iris on movement of the eye; seen in posterior dislocation or subluxation of the crystalline lens; also seen after uncomplicated intracapsular cataract extraction.

iridotomy (ir″i-dot′o-me) The making of a hole or slit through the iris; this may be done with surgical instruments or by laser application.

iris The pigmented or variously colored anterior component of the uvea, which surrounds a central opening (pupil); it controls the amount of light reaching the lens by altering the pupillary diameter; separates anterior chamber from posterior chamber of the eye. Named in 1721 by J.B. Winslow (1669–1760), Parisian anatomist, but described in its diverse colors by Greek philosopher Aristotle (384–322 B.C.).

iris dilator muscle See *muscle, iris dilator.*

iris sphincter muscle See *muscle, iris sphincter.*

iritis (ī-rī′tis) Inflammation of the iris due to infection, trauma or autoimmune processes; term introduced in 1801 by Johann Adam Schmidt (1759–1809), anatomist and ophthalmologist of Vienna, Austria.

iron A metallic element found in certain minerals and nearly all soils; chemical symbol Fe, atomic number 26. Used in some green (Crookes') sunglasses.

irradiance A physical or radiometric term for light or other electromagnetic energy falling on a surface per unit area; commonly expressed in watts per square meter or watts per square centimeter.

irradiation

1. General term for incident electromagnetic energy (photons, electrons, and the like) reaching a substance or surface.
2. The visual phenomenon in which objects having brighter illumination than their surround, appear to be larger than they are.

irregular astigmatism See *astigmatism, irregular.*

iseikonic lens See *lens, iseikonic.*

Ishihara test See *test, Ishihara.*

-ism Suffix meaning condition, action.

iso- Prefix meaning equal.

isochromatic (ī″so-kro-mat′ik) Possessing the same color throughout.

isocoria (ī′so-kō′re-ah) Equality in size of the two pupils.

isopter A line depicting or connecting locations of equal characteristics or power; in visual-field testing, a line connecting loci of equal sensitivity to light; analogous to contour lines indicating equal elevations on a geographic map.

isotonic The state of a solution having the same osmolar tonicity (effective osmotic pressure equivalent) as another solution with which it is compared; e.g., physiologic saline solution and blood serum; normal tears and properly constituted artificial tears.

isotropic (ī″so-trop′ik)

1. Having equal refractive power (index of refraction) in all directions; being singly refractive. This is a basic characteristic of high-quality ophthalmic glass, ophthalmic plastics and ophthalmic lenses; optical homogeneity.
2. Exhibiting properties (as velocity of light transmission, compression, or strain) with the same value when measured along a contour.

-itis Suffix meaning inflammation.

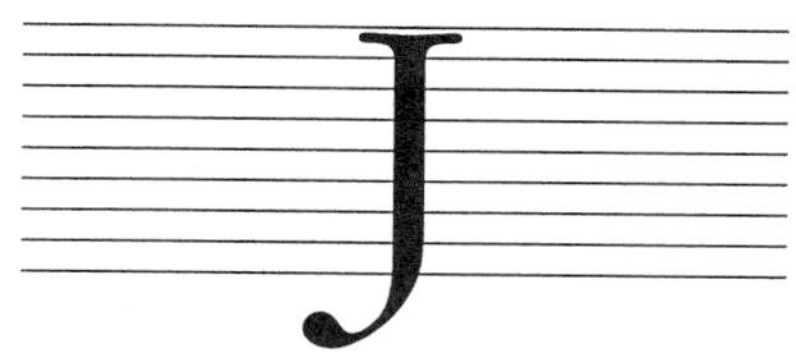

J Symbol for S.I.-derived unit of energy or work, joule.

J.C.A.H.P.O. Abbreviation for Joint Commission on Allied Health Personnel in Ophthalmology; q.v.

Jackson cross cylinder See *cylinder, cross.*

Jaeger test type See *type, Jaeger test.*

jelly bumps Informal designation of muco-lipid polysaccharide deposits that form lumps on the surfaces of a hydrophilic contact lens. See *lipoproteins.*

jitter Unwanted movements or vibration of an image as seen on a CRT display or through an optical instrument (binoculars or telescope) when viewing during motion of the instrument or the observer.

joint, butt A flat juncture between a spectacle front and temple with no miter cut on the endpiece of the front or temple.

joint, miter (mī'ter) A juncture between a spectacle front and temple wherein both mating surfaces are angularly machined.

Joint Commission on Allied Health Personnel in Ophthalmology (J.C.A.H.P.O.) Voluntary certifying agency in ophthalmology, established in 1969; approximately 15,000 certificants, at the entry level of assistants, intermediate level of technician, or highest level of technologist. Prepares and gives certifying examinations each year, both practical and written. Office: 2025 Woodlane Dr., St. Paul, Minnesota 55125-2995.

Jones test See *test, Jones.*

joule (jool) A derived S.I. physical unit of radiant energy or quantity of heat-expressing work done by a force (one newton acting over a distance of one meter); more suitable for objective measurement and generally preferred to the many psychophysical units sometimes used in quantitative photobiology. Symbol, J; used to designate laser energy; one joule = 10^7ergs, or 0.239 calories. Named in honor of James P. Joule (1818–1889), English physicist.

jump, image

1. The apparent sudden displacement of an object that occurs when the fixation axis passes abruptly from one viewing area of a non-progressive multifocal lens to another (i.e., looking back and forth from the distance to near areas). This can be disturbing in high-power lenses, but can be minimized by proper segment choice.
2. A rocking motion of the images of keratometer mires, frequently seen during keratometric examination of a keratoconic cornea, which interferes with aligning the two optical images.

junction, corneo-scleral The transition zone in which the edges of both the sclera and cornea join; also referred to as the limbus; q.v.

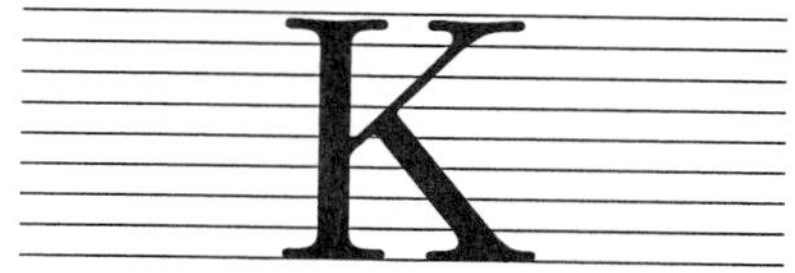

k 1. Symbol for kilo (1,000), in the metric system.
2. Symbol for mathematical constant, may be written in both capital or non-capital (small) type.

K 1. Chemical symbol for the metallic element potassium; q.v.
2. Abbreviation for keratometer reading of the curvature of the anterior corneal surface, usually expressed in diopters for each of the two principal axes.
3. Symbol for Kelvin, the S.I. unit of measurement on the absolute zero temperature scale; q.v.

Kalichrome lens See *lens, Kalichrome.*

Kelvin scale See *scale, Kelvin.*

keratic precipitates See *precipitates, keratic.*

keratitis (ker″ah-tī′tis) Inflammation of the cornea. Term introduced in early 1800s by James Wardrop (1782–1869), British ophthalmologist and pathologist.

keratitis, actinic Painful inflammation of the cornea due to excessive ultraviolet light exposure; welder's flash; snow blindness. A temporary destruction of the epithelial cells of the cornea.

keratitis, exposure Inflammation of the cornea secondary to incomplete lid closure, or corneal coverage by the upper eyelid, creating tear evaporation which leads in turn to dehydration of the corneal epithelium, and exposure of Bowman's membrane.

keratitis, punctate Inflammation of the cornea with clinical features of microscopic white or gray dots (punctates) located in the corneal epithelium that tend to coalesce into larger oval opacities that are arranged in groups; may be generalized or localized in the cornea.

keratitis sicca Irritation of the cornea due to deficiency of tears; usually keratoconjunctivitis sicca indicating inflammation of the cornea and conjunctiva; may be associated with dry mouth and dry joints; generally a contraindication to fitting contact lenses, unless specifically prescribed as a therapeutic or bandage lens.

keratitis, superficial punctate (SPK) Generic term for corneal inflammation of multiple etiologies characterized by epithelial irritation, photophobia, and foreign body sensation; may have a tendency to periodically recur. Thygeson's superficial punctate keratitis; particularly affects the central cornea with round to oval conglomerates of discrete white-gray intraepithelial dots. First described in 1950 by Phillips Thygeson (b. 1903), ophthalmologist of California.

keratitis, superior limbic Hyperemia and papillary hypertrophy of the cornea and conjunctiva in the area of the upper corneo-scleral junction; usually is bilateral and more common in females; superior limbic keratoconjunctivitis.

kerato- A prefix that indicates a condition involving the cornea.

keratoconjunctivitis sicca (ker″ah-to-kon-junk″ti-vī′tis) The ocular component of a triad of dry eyes, dry mouth, and rheumatoid arthritis; the lacrimal, parotid, and other salivary glands show infiltrative destruction of their secretory cells, and the tear film becomes slowly and progressively desiccated; disease predominantly occurs in postmenopausal women, and affects both eyes. Immune studies show multiple autoantibodies including antinuclear antibodies, and antibodies to two specific antigens, Ro (SSA), La (SSB). A relative contraindication to wearing contact lenses. Term introduced and extensive descriptions published by Henrik Samuel Conrad Sjogren (1899–1972?), ophthalmologist of Sweden. Includes earlier (1888) concepts of Mikulicz Syndrome and Mikulicz disease, described by Romanian surgeon, Johann Mikulicz (1850–1905), working in Germany.

keratoconus (ker″ah-to-kō′nus) Conical protrusion and thinning of central cornea (conical cornea); usually bilateral and progressive through early adult life. First described in 1747 by French ophthalmologist Pierre Demours (1702–1795); sometimes confused with his son, Parisian ophthalmologist Antoine Pierre Demours (1762–1836).

keratoglobus (ker″ah-to-glo′bus) A congenital enlargement of the cornea, usually bilateral and hereditary; megalocornea; macrocornea.

keratograph A diagrammatic scheme plot, or color display of the various isopters of anterior corneal curvature (topographic map).

keratometer (ker"ah-tom'i-ter) Optical instrument for measuring curvature of anterior corneal surface by double reflected images of mires; incorrectly called ophthalmometer. Actually determines radius of curvature in millimeters, but expressed by conversion values in diopters; Alcon Electronic Portable Automated Keratometer (1992) uses liquid crystal display of measurement in diopters and millimeters. Initial description published in 1856 by Hermann Von Helmholtz (1821–1893), German physiologist;

keratomileusis (ker"ah-to-mi-loo'sis) A surgical technique for altering the refractive status of the cornea by removing a trephined disc from its anterior surface, freezing it, reshaping it on a lathe to a desired front curvature, then suturing it back to the remaining cornea; introduced in 1958 by José I. Barraquer, ophthalmologist of Bogota, Columbia. Generally superseded by more recent laser surgical procedures.

keratomileusis in situ A technical modification of keratomileusis in which an automatic corneal shaper or excimer laser is used to sculpture the anterior cornea in place for surgical correction of a broad range of refractive errors.

keratopathy, bullous (bul"us ker"ah-top-ah'the) A chronic and painful corneal pathology characterized by small fluid-filled blisters or pockets in the corneal epithelium; may represent advanced stage of Fuchs corneal dystrophy developed from preceding endothelial cell loss; commonly is bilateral; at times treated provisionally with therapeutic soft bandage contact lenses.

keratophakia (ker"ah-to-fā'ke-ah) A surgical technique for altering the refractive status of the cornea by inserting an appropriately shaped button of donor cornea between layers of the recipient's cornea; developed in mid-1960s by José I. Barraquer, ophthalmologist of Bogota, Columbia.

keratoplasty (ker'ah-to-plas"te) Corneal grafting or plastic surgery of the cornea, commonly divided into penetrating or full thickness corneal transplant, versus lamellar or partial thickness (superficial) transplant.

keratoplasty, penetrating A surgical procedure placing a full thickness disk, or button of donor corneal tissue, into a recipient cornea, usually to improve vision by excising diseased tissue in the host cornea; full thickness keratoplasty.

keratoprosthesis An optical device, artificial corneal segment, sometimes of nut and bolt design, a few millimeters in diameter and usually made of methyl methacrylate; surgically implanted through the central cornea in the presence of extensive corneal opacification; Cordona implant. Developed in the late 1950s and reported in 1962 by Hernando Cordona, ophthalmologist working in New York City.

keratoscope (ker'ah-to-skōp) A reflecting optical instrument for examining the curvature of the cornea for irregularities or distortion by alternating black and white concentric circles; Placido's discs. Primarily developed in 1880–1882 by Antonio Placido (1848–1916), Portuguese ophthalmologist; battery handle, Kline keratoscope (1958), photo-keratoscope by several workers in the 1930s, video keratoscope, or video recording keratograph. Varidot Surgical Keratometer, a hand-held surgical keratoscope; disposable cylindrical keratoscope developed by William F. Maloney and Van Loenen, California ophthalmologists.

keratotomy, radial (ker"ah-tot'o-me) An ophthalmic surgical procedure in which multiple radially arranged incisions are made deep into the corneal stroma in an effort to flatten the cornea and reduce myopic or astigmatic error.

Kestenbaum's rule See *rule, Kestenbaum's.*

keyhole bridge See *bridge, keyhole.*

kg Symbol for kilogram, the S.I. unit of mass or weight in the metric system.

kinetic perimetry See *perimetry, kinetic.*

knife edge See *edge, knife.*

Kr Chemical symbol for the inert gaseous chemical element Krypton; q.v.

Krause glands See *glands, Krause.*

Krukenberg's spindle See *spindle, Krukenberg's.*

Kryptok Trade name for a fused bifocal lens having a 22mm round flint (i.e., lead oxide) segment, patented in 1908 by John Borsch, Jr. Name is taken from an earlier cemented flint-segment bifocal patented in 1899 by John Borsch, Sr.

krypton An inert, heavy gaseous chemical element found in the atmosphere; chemical symbol Kr, atomic number 36; used in lasers and as reference light spectrum. Discovered in 1898 by William Ramsay (1852–1919), Scottish chemist who received Nobel Prize in chemistry in 1904.

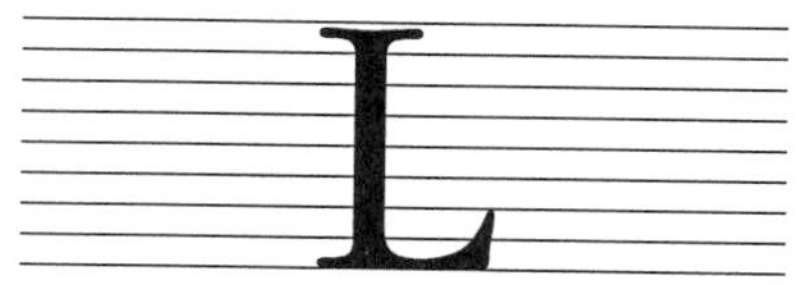

l Symbol for liter, a unit of volume equal to 1000 cubic centimeters (slightly more than 1 quart); a division of the S.I.-derived unit for volume, the cubic meter.

L Symbol for Lambert, a psychophysical unit of brightness diffusely emitting one lumen per square centimeter; named for Johann Heinrich Lambert (1728–1777), German mathematician and physicist.

LVES Abbreviation for Low Vision Enhancement System; q.v.

lacerate To tear or cut jaggedly.

lacrimal canal See *canal, lacrimal.*

lacrimal canaliculus See *canaliculus, lacrimal.*

lacrimal caruncle See *caruncle, lacrimal.*

lacrimal fluid See *fluid, lacrimal.*

lacrimal gland See *gland, lacrimal.*

lacrimal lens See *lens, lacrimal.*

lacrimation (lak″ri-mā′shun) The secretion and flow of tears, largely from the lacrimal gland, bathing the front surface of the eye; common connotation being excessive secretion or hypersecretion. (cf. *hyperlacrimation.*)

lagophthalmos (lag″of-thal′mos) A functional eyelid defect, particularly of the upper lid, in which the lid does not follow the globe when it is rotated downward; may be caused by thyroid exophthalmos, congenital defect, or facial nerve (VII) impairment.

lambda, λ Symbol for wavelength; eleventh letter of the Greek alphabet.

laminated Composed of layers of firmly united materials. See *lens, laminated.*

laminated lens See *lens, laminated.*

lamp, Dazor Trade name for a large series of high-intensity lamps with magnifying devices and patented floating arms. Introduced in 1938 by St. Louis, Missouri, lighting engineer Harry Dazey.

lamp, Macbeth (New London Easel Lamp) See *illuminator, true daylight.*

lamp, Nernst (Nernst rod) An early intense light source obtained by passing electric current through oxide of magnesium and rare earths; used in early slit lamps, but soon superseded by tungsten, wound filament nitra, and later halogen and neodymium bulbs; Nernst glower. Developed by Walther Hermann Nernst (1864–1941), German physical chemist and inventor who received the Nobel Prize in chemistry in 1920.

lamphouse

1. That portion of an optical instrument (e.g., focimeter, keratometer, slit lamp) that houses the source of illumination needed for proper operation of the instrument.
2. A protective encasement for potentially hazardous radiation, as from arc lamps and UV generators.

Landolt C (broken ring) test chart See Figure 17; see also *optotype.*

Lantern, Farnsworth The final validating test for color perception of U.S. Navy personnel simulating "lights at sea"; consists of 9 pairs of color-specific lights mounted in a rotating drum and viewed from a distance of 8 feet; abbreviation FaLant. Developed by Dean Farnsworth (1902–1959), U.S. Navy Commander and experimental visual scientist, New London, Connecticut.

lap (n) A tool used in the manufacture of precision or ophthalmic spectacle and contact lenses, made from cast iron, aluminum, or brass and occasionally from specially adapted plastic forms, with surfaces as portions of a spherical shell, flat cylinder, or torus and available in plus (convex) and minus (concave) mated halves of the same numerical surface markings; used either as grinding or polishing platforms to produce refractive or reflective surface powers on lenses or mirrors. See *Appendix, Table 5.*

Present day spectacle lens surfacing tools were designed to be used on an early (now obsolete) crown glass of index 1.530. Current ophthalmic lens indices of refraction are different from the index for which laps were previously designed, requiring the knowledge of the true powers of the surfaces to be generated and the appropriate lap for the lens material used. Contact lens surfacing tools are commonly made for polymethyl methacrylate (PMMA) n = 1.490.

lap (v) To cut or to polish, as a lens or a gem.

lap cutter See *cutter, lap.*

LARS (left add, right subtract) Acronym for technique or procedure used to compensate for the misorientation of a toric soft contact lens. If the lens in situ rotates to the fitter's left, add the amount of angular displacement in degrees to the spectacle axis; if it rotates to the fitter's right, subtract the amount in degrees; general rule is to add/subtract 15° for every unit or increment (i.e., 1/2 hour) of misorientation of the lens based on the face of a clock.

laser (**L**ight **A**mplification by **S**timulated **E**mission of **R**adiation) Acronym for an electro-optical device which transforms light of various wavelengths into an extremely intense, small and nearly non-divergent monochromatic beam with all waves in phase; focuses high-energy levels into very small areas; active medium may be chemical, solid state, dye, gas, or semiconductor. Developed in 1960 by Theodore Harold Maiman (b. 1927), American physicist. See *resonance, optical.*

laser refractometry See *refractometry, laser.*

laser, ruby Laser with active medium of ruby and wavelength 173.6nm. Developed in the early 1960s by Charles Hard Townes, Ph.D. (b. 1915), U.S. physicist; awarded Nobel Prize in physics in 1964 for initial invention of the laser from work done between 1953 and 1960.

laser, YAG An electro-optical instrument producing an intense monochromatic and coherent light beam whose active medium is a crystal of yttrium, aluminum, and garnet; wavelength 1060nm; used for capsulotomy after artificial lens implant surgery. Usually "doped" with neodymium.

latent hyperopia See *hyperopia, latent.*

latent nystagmus See *nystagmus, latent.*

lateral canthus See *canthus, lateral.*

lateral geniculate body See *body, lateral geniculate.*

lateral rectus muscle See *muscle, lateral rectus.*

lateral Of or pertaining to, situated at, proceeding from, or directed toward a side.

lathe-cut lens See *lens, contact, lathe cut.*

law, Lambert's The amount of light which passes through a clear or colored optical medium diminishes in geometric proportion as the thickness of the medium increases in arithmetic progression; described by Johann Heinrich Lambert (1728–1777), German physicist and mathematician; author of *Photometria*, 1760.

law, Prentice's An equation for prismatic effect induced in a lens; prismatic deviation, expressed in prism diopters ($^{\Delta}$), at a point on a lens is equal to the product of its refractive dioptric power (F_V) multiplied by the distance in centimeters of the point from the optical center of the lens; named for New York optician Charles F. Prentice (1854–1946). The formula to find how much to decenter a lens to obtain a given prism value is

$$\frac{10 \times \text{prism diopters } (^{\Delta})}{F_V} = \text{decentration in millimeters}$$

To find the prism when the decentration and power are given

$$\frac{F_V \times \text{decentration in millimeters}}{10} = \text{prism diopters } (^{\Delta})$$

where

F_V = lens diopter power in meridian of decentration.

law of refraction, Snell's (Descartes' Law of Sines) The sine of the angle of incident light bears a constant relation to the sine of the angle of refracted light for a given transparent substance (for a refracting medium in air, the sine of the angle of incidence divided by the sine of the angle of refraction is the index of refraction for that medium). Angles are measured to a perpendicular erected at the point of incidence. Originally described, but not published, in 1621 by Willebrord van R. Snell—also spelled Snel—(1591–1626), Dutch astronomer and mathematician; published independently by René Descartes, (1596–1650), French philosopher and mathematician (see Figure 23).

layer, depth of compression The linear distance from the surface of a heat-tempered or chemtempered glass lens where there is increased glass density of compaction, and no stress.

layout

1. The art or process of arranging.
2. The process of marking a blank or lens for positioning in surfacing or edging equipment.

lazy eye See *amblyopia*.

lead A soft, grayish-blue metal with poisonous salts; chemical symbol Pb, atomic number 82; used in glass lenses to increase the index of refraction (and concurrently, to increase chromatic dispersion).

lead glass See *glass, lead. (flint)*

LEAP (system) Trademark and acronym for Lens Edging Adhesive Pad, a lens layout blocking system developed by 3M company (Minnesota Mining and Manufacturing), utilizing a metallic (originally) block, to which the lens to be worked on is joined by a double adhesive-backed pad to establish centration or decentration of ophthalmic lens blanks for edging operations of simple or complex corrective lens prescriptions; blocks now emulated in plastic or metal form and distributed by numerous other suppliers.

LED Mnemonic for light emitting diode, a solid state semiconductor that provides light when voltage is applied to it; presents very little ocular hazard except at very close viewing distance where green, red, and infrared have a limited potential for retinal thermal risk.

left eye See *eye, left.*

legal blindness See *blindness, legal.*

legibility The degree to which individual symbols such as letters, digits, punctuation and specific symbols can be read (cf. *letters, test, equal difficulty,* a series of 10 non-serif letters of similar difficulty to resolve C, D, H, K, N, O, R, S, V, Z); described in 1959 by Louise L. Sloan, Ph.D., visual physiologist of the Wilmer Ophthalmological Institute, Baltimore, Maryland.

lehr A large, specially adapted type of annealing oven providing control of the reduction of heat to a continuous transit of newly formed glass objects or lens blanks, usually requiring 8 to 15 hours until room temperature is reached. Lehr is a spelling variant appearing in 1908 from the original, "leer" of 1662, for an annealing furnace; in nineteenth centry, appears at times as "lear." Current spelling is preferred.

length, axial Linear measure of the eyeball from the anterior pole (apex) of the cornea to the posterior pole of the sclera; commonly done with A-scan ultrasound and used in calculation of dioptric power for lens implants to be placed within the eye following surgical removal of cataracts.

length, chord Straight line measurement in millimeters across curved components, as in a contact lens; usually specified to two places beyond the decimal point.

length, focal (f) The distance from the back vertex of a lens to its focal point, strictly called the back vertex focal length. See *power, vertex.*

length, overall In ophthalmic optics, the total length of a spectacle earpiece or temple measured from the center of the center barrel screw hole to the tip with the temple in a straight position; measured either in millimeters or inches.

lens A piece of isotropic, transparent material having two opposite surfaces used to alter the characteristics of light rays incident to it.

lens aberration See *aberration, lens.*

lens, absorptive Lens which converts a portion of incident light to other forms of energy (usually heat) based on chemical ingredients or coatings.

lens, achromatic (āk″ro-mat′ik) A lens corrected by surface design to reduce chromatic aberration, often a combination of a plus lens and a minus lens of differing refractive indices. Invented in 1758 by John Dolland (1706–1761), London optician who became a Fellow of the Royal Society in 1761 and was appointed optician to the king.

lens, aphakic (a-fā′kik) (cataract lens). A high plus-power lens for optical correction of absence of the crystalline lens, usually following cataract extraction.

lens aplanatic (ap′lah-nat′ik) A lens designed with greater curvature on the anterior than the posterior surface to reduce off-axis and coma aberration.

lens, assembled A lens or lenses that have been combined with a frame or mounting to form a pair of spectacles.

lens, astigmatic Toric lens used to correct ametropia of the eye with differing refractive powers in the principal meridians; introduced in 1827 by Sir George B. Airy (1801–1892), British astronomer, who suffered from high, compound-myopic astigmatism and had lenses ground for himself by the optician Fuller of Ipswich, England.

lens, Bagolini A non-colored, diagnostic ophthalmic lens, very fine and lightly streaked, which permits the eye to be seen, but creates a streaked image, perpendicular to the axis of striation from a point light source; devised in 1958 by Bruno Bagolini (b. 1924), Italian ophthalmologist.

lens, bandage A soft, hydrophillic contact lens with no refractive power; used therapeutically to protect a damaged or chronically diseased cornea and promote healing; trade name, Softcon; planolens. (cf. *shield collagen.*)

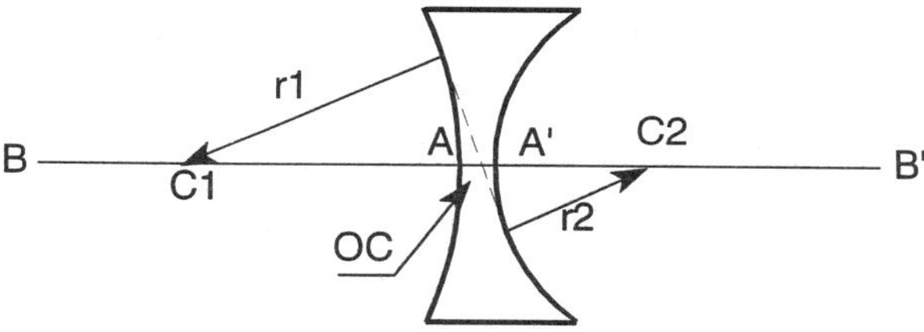

$AC_1 = r_1$; $A'C_2 = r_2$; $r_1 > r_2$; $r_1 \mid\mid r_2$; OC = optical center.

Figure 24 Biconcave lens—unequal radii of curvature.

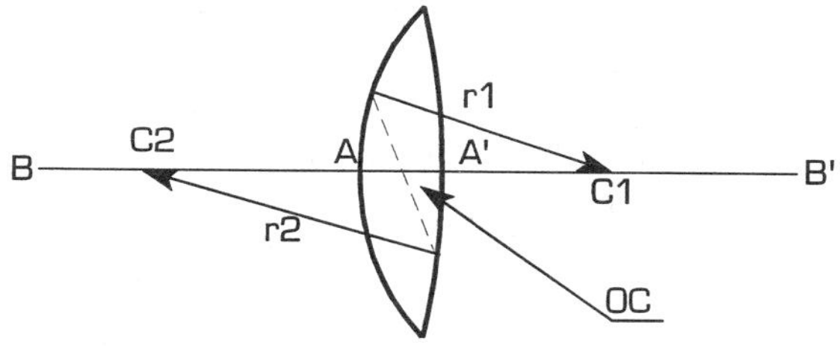

$AC_1 = r_1$; $A'C_2 = r_2$; $r_1 < r_2$; $r_1 \mid\mid r_2$; OC = optical center.

Figure 25 Biconvex lens—unequal radii of curvature.

lens, bent An early designation of ophthalmic lens form having both of its surfaces curved, one convex the other concave. (cf. *lens, flat; lens, meniscus.*)

lens, best form A series of spectacle lenses calculated on the basis of surface power to minimize optical aberrations by placing a circle of least confusion within a macular diameter of 0.002mm., the diameter of a macular cone cell, designed 1914–1926 by Archibald Stanley Percival (1862–1935), British ophthalmologist.

lens bevel See *bevel, lens.*

lens bevel angle See *angle, lens bevel.*

lens, biconcave A lens with hollow surfaces of unequal radii on each side; thinnest at its optical center (Figure 24); see also *lens, double concave.*

lens, biconvex A lens with bulging surfaces on both sides, usually of unequal radii; thickest at its optical center (Figure 25); see also *lens, double convex.*

lens, bifocal An ophthalmic lens designed to provide correction for two viewing ranges; introduced in 1784 by inventor and statesman Benjamin Franklin (1706–1790) of Philadelphia.

lens, bifocal, cement An early ophthalmic lens designed and patented by August Morck in 1888 (also attributed to the optician Samuel Gregg in 1866) with a spherical power wafer of crown glass cemented on the inferior (usually front) surface of the distance correction. Now used as a 22mm round aspheric acrylic (scratch-resistant-coated) adhesive-mounted add on the front surface of a single-vision lens; a low-vision aid (+8 to +24D); trade name, Univision.

lens, bifocal, cemented Kryptok An ophthalmic lens manufactured with a depression countersunk into the lower front surface of the crown glass lens in which a disc of flint glass was placed for near focusing. A cover glass was then cemented over the entire front of the lens; although less noticeable than previous bifocals, the placement of the flint segment in front of the crown glass carrier led to greater chromatic aberration; designed in 1899 by John L. Borsch, Sr. of Philadelphia; called cemented Kryptok.

lens, bifocal, flat-top (FT) A popular multifocal lens with a straight, horizontal dividing line delimiting the upper edge of the segment. Introduced in 1926 as fused construction by the Univis Lens Co. (U.S.).

lens, bifocal, Franklin The initial multifocal lens made by uniting the upper half of a distance power lens and the lower half of a near power lens in an eyewire; the two half lenses are independent of each other. Developed in 1784 by Benjamin Franklin.

lens, bifocal, fused A crown glass ophthalmic lens with a segment of flint glass (later, barium crown glass) heat-blended into position. Invented in 1908 by John L. Borsch, Jr. of Philadelphia; called fused Kryptok, to distinguish it from the cemented Kryptok earlier invented by his father. The fusion process was patented in 1915 by Henry Courmettes.

lens, bifocal, one-piece See *Ultex; lens, one-piece multifocal.*

lens, bifocal, prism A special construction of the near focal portion of a spectacle lens where prism power (commonly base-in) is incorporated in the bifocal only, to assist near-point convergence.

lens, bifocal, solid upcurve A multifocal lens ground from one solid glass blank without a dirt-collecting edge; manufactured by grinding off the top portion of a single-vision reading glass; has a strong base-down effect in the distance correction. Invented in 1837 by Isaac Schnaitmann of Philadelphia.

lens, bifocal, Younger seamless A heat-blended multifocal ophthalmic lens with its distance and near curvatures rendered inconspicuous; developed in mid-1950s by Irving Rips, Los Angeles optician; manufactured by Younger Lens Co. (est. 1954) using its name to suggest youthfulness.

lens, bitoric Most commonly a type of contact lens having a toric surface on each side of the lens; occasionally found as an ophthalmic lens used to correct aniseikonia; trade name, Troptic. See *iseikonic.*

lens, blended See *lens, bifocal, Younger seamless.*

lens caliper See *caliper, lens.*

lens, Calobar Trade name for a green-colored lens, highly absorptive of ultraviolet and infrared light; generally manufactured in three densities.

lens cap See *cap, lens.*

lens capsule See *capsule, lens.*

lens, carrier The major portion of a lens that has a differing power component cemented or fused to it, creating the combined lens power, e.g., fused segment multifocal.

lens, Cartesian A lens shaped so there is no spherical aberration; calculated and proposed by René Descartes (1596–1650), French philosopher and mathematician.

lens, case-hardened Glass lens which has been toughened by heating to the near-viscosity range (1330°F) and then rapidly chilled in cold air to create a surface compression layer and radial tension forces in the slowly cooling core. Initially developed and granted U.S. patent in 1874 by Francois B.A. Royer de la Bastie of Paris, France.

lens, cataract See *lens, aphakic.*

lens, Chavasse An occluder lens that reduces acuity of the emmetropic eye to about 20/200. Posterior surface has pebble finish and lens appears clear to the observer looking at the wearer's eye. Developed by F. Bernard Chavasse (1889–1941), ophthalmologist of Liverpool, England.

lens, chem-hardened See *lens, chem-tempered.*

lens, chem-tempered Glass lenses that have been made more impact-resistant by timed treatment in a hot, ion-exchange bath chemically replacing, from each surface of the lens, small ions with larger ions into a thin, toughened, surface layer. Chem-hardened; introduced by Corning Glass Works in 1962 under the trade name, Chemcor.

lens clock See *clock, lens.*

lens, cobalt blue Tinted industrial lenses of deep blue color, particularly used by workers on steel melts or open hearth furnaces; the lenses help to evaluate the ore melt, but offer little ultraviolet and infrared protection; incorporates cobalt oxide and alumina into the glass melt.

lens, collimating An optical lens which renders light rays parallel.

lens, compensated base curve Semi-finished ophthalmic lens blank with its base curve ground and polished to a curvature different from that stated on the box or envelope housing the lens. The actual base curve is greater or less than that nominally stated to allow for the difference in the refractive index of the lens material being ground, i.e., ophthalmic crown n = 1.523; CR-39 = 1.498; polycarbonate n = 1.586; high index n = 1.80, etc.; the lens index for which grinding and polishing equipment were designed to produce curves, i.e., glass of index 1.530. See *lap (n).*

lens compensation See *compensation, lens.*

lens, complex A homocentric optical system composed of multiple groups of lens elements, usually including linear separation of some of the elements.

lens, compound

1. A lens that functions as a combination of a spherical lens and a cylindrical lens; spherocylinder.
2. A homocentric system of multiple refracting surfaces or lenses that may be in direct contact or separated by a calculated distance in air; generally a single group of two or more lenses. (cf. *lens, doublet.*)

lens, concave A lens that diverges light rays, said to have minus power.

lens, confocal A system precisely coordinating a very narrow beam of laser light with the focal plane of a high-power magnification system or microscope; permits visualization of very thin, subcellular planes.

lens, conoid High dioptric power, aspheric lens providing major correction of spherical abberation by utilizing surfaces described by rotation of a conic section about its axis. The two basic types of conoid surfaces are closed curves or ellipses; and open curves or hyperbolas; separating these two is the parabola. Used as spectacle-mounted or hand-held low-vision aids (c. 1954); condensing lenses for indirect ophthalmoscopy, and smaller diameter hand-held lenses for fundus examination at the slit lamp. Developed by David Volk (1917–1987), ophthalmologist of Cleveland, Ohio.

lens, contact

1. Scleral. A form of contact lens designed to cover both the cornea and a contiguous segment of the bulbar conjunctiva; divided into an optical zone (optic), and a scleral zone (haptic), of differing curvatures; now used primarily for theatrical and cosmetic purposes. Early scleral lenses were pioneered by Zurich ophthalmologist Adolph Eugen Fick (1829–1901) in the late 1880s and in 1937 by New York City optometrist William Feinbloom (1904–1985). The Feinbloom lens had a glass optic and a plastic haptic. The all-methyl methacrylate-molded scleral lens developed in 1938 by New York optician Theodore E. Obrig (1895-1967) is the most satisfactory scleral flange lens. Such lenses are fitted by making an impression of the surface of the cornea and anterior bulbar conjunctiva.
2. Corneal, A reduced-diameter, polymethyl methacrylate contact lens approximating the standard corneal diameter, or less. Introduced in 1948 by California optician Kevin M. Tuohy, leading to many modifications and further reduction in diameter—the "microlenses" of the mid–1950s. *Note:* A small-diameter glass contact lens was unsuccessfully tried in 1888 by August Müller in Kiel, a 14-diopter myopic medical student.

lens, contact, annular design A design form of multifocal contact lens with distant powers confined to the central zone and near-range powers in concentric-ring configuration toward the lens edge. (cf. *lens, contact, simultaneous vision.*)

lens, contact, bicurve An early-design corneal contact lens with a posterior surface curvature composed of two different and concentric zones, the central zone, called the optical zone, and the outer zone, called the bearing surface.

lens, contact, bitoric A contact lens designed for astigmatic corneas, the lens having two perpendicular radii of curvature on both its posterior and anterior surfaces. The posterior radii determine the fitting curves of the lens to the cornea, and the anterior radii complete the prescription power requirements.

lens, contact, color changing (cosmetic) Large corneal contact lens with embedded or layered hue over the patient's iris to provide major hue alteration, as from brown to blue; diameter essentially equals visible iris diameter, and the pupillary zone of approximately 5mm diameter is clear.

lens, contact, color enhancing (color altering) Large corneal contact lens tinted in the area overlying the iris, but clear in the approximately 5mm diameter pupillary zone; intended to alter or intensify hue of light irides; diameter essentially equals visible iris diameter.

lens, contact, daily wear A designation for contact lenses that need to be removed on a daily basis.

lens, contact, diffractive bifocal A simultaneous vision design having bifocal or multifocal optical powers created by a series of concentric rings engraved in the periphery of the lens with small facets which diffract about 50% of incident light into a separate focus. The faceted rings are generally on the posterior surface, and are located progressively closer to one another as near-addition power is increased.

lens, contact, double slab-off A modification of toric soft contact lens design using superiorly and inferiorly thinned zones to limit lens movement and rotation on the cornea.

lens, contact, extended wear A contact lens that is designed to be worn on a continuous, 24-hour basis, following approval by the U.S. Food and Drug Administration. Current policy limits this to 7 days of continuous wear.

lens, contact, flat A contact lens that has a longer posterior radius of curvature than does the anterior surface of the cornea that it is placed on; causes central corneal touch or bearing. (cf. *lens, contact, loose.*)

lens, contact, flexible wear A hydrophilic soft contact lens containing about 45% water, capable of extended (overnight) wear, but generally removed daily; may be used beneath a hard contact lens (piggyback configuration); trade name, Flexlens.

lens, contact, fused bifocal A one-piece rigid bifocal contact lens that has a molded anterior surface, and a lathe-cut posterior surface.

lens, contact, hard (HCL) A class of inflexible lenses which may be surfaced to high optical precision and will retain their configuration under usual wearing conditions; first satisfactory material used for this purpose was polymethyl methacrylate (PMMA) introduced in 1938; subsequently, cellulose acetate butyrate (CAB) was adapted to contact lens manufacture in 1974; later introduction of silicone, or copolymers, such as silicone-acrylic have led to many modifications of hard or rigid lens materials.

lens, contact, lathe-cut A contact lens with the posterior radius of curvature generated by a micro-cutting machine on which the semi-finished plastic disk is spun on a horizontal axis and shaped by a fixed cutting tool.

lens, contact, loose A contact lens that has a longer posterior radius of curvature than that of the front surface of the cornea for which it is prescribed; a contact lens in which the sagittal value produces a flat lens/corneal-fitting relationship. Such lenses tend to move excessively over the anterior corneal surface. (cf. *lens, contact, flat.*)

lens, contact, minus lenticular modification Special anterior-edge treatment of a high plus (+) contact lens which produces edge configuration similar to a minus lens, providing centration of the otherwise low-riding plus (+) lens.

lens, contact, multifocal Any contact lens having more than one optical power zone.

lens, contact, piggyback A contact lens fitting mode employing a rigid contact lens overriding a soft contact lens; particularly used to fit highly astigmatic or keratoconic corneas.

lens, contact, prism ballast A contact lens having an increased thickness along one edge, designed to reduce the tendency of the lens to rotate. The increased edge thickness causes the lens to orient with the ballasted area inferiorly. The weight causes the lens to ride lower and is generally applied to toric, high-riding, or multifocal contact lenses.

lens, contact, rigid gas permeable (RGP) A firm or hard contact lens constructed of material with high-oxygen permeability, originally (1974) cellulose acetate butyrate made into contact lenses; more recently of silicone acrylate, fluoropolymers, and the like.

lens, contact, semiscleral A soft contact lens of sufficient diameter to overlie the limbus or adjacent bulbar conjunctiva.

lens, contact, simultaneous vision A multifocal contact lens which provides two or more focal points on the retina at the same time. The wearer learns to ignore all but one image and concentrates on the specific focal length desired. (cf. *lens, contact, annular design*).

lens, contact, single-cut Corneal contact lens designed with a single curvature on the posterior surface, instead of the usual multicurve design.

lens, contact, soft A contact lens made from a hydrophilic (water-loving) organic polymer or copolymer; lens may be manufactured by lathe cutting, spin-casting, or molding. Generally the diameter is larger than that of rigid corneal lenses. The lenses have a general water content ("water of hydration") of 30% to 75%; when left to dry in the open air, they become small and brittle; used primarily for correcting refractive errors, particularly irregular errors which cannot be corrected by spectacle lenses; also used as bandage lenses and for cosmetic purposes; generally more easily accepted by patients, and easier to fit than hard contact lenses. Introduced in 1960 by Otto Wichterle and Drahoslav Lim, polymer chemists of Prague, Czechoslovakia.

lens, contact, spin-cast A soft contact lens manufactured by injecting a predetermined amount of the appropriate polymer into a spinning metal mold of elected radius of curvature for a predetermined time; this avoids the use of cutting tools as in lathe-cut lenses.

lens, contact, steep A contact lens that has a central posterior curve of a shorter radius of curvature than the cornea to which it is fitted, creating a potential interruption of the normal tear interchange and resultant hypoxia.

lens, contact, Tangent Streak Bifocal Trade name of Fused Kontacts, Inc., for a truncated, prism-ballasted, RGP, anterior surface, one-piece bifocal contact lens of translating design—employs a horizontally split distant and reading field through the usable optical zone; derives its name from the juncture of the distant and near fields and somewhat resembles an executive bifocal. Developed in 1985 by Chicago optometrist George Tsuetaki (d. 1990).

lens, contact, therapeutic A contact lens designed to promote healing and/or to provide a smooth refracting surface for the cornea. Soft therapeutic lenses may be used as a delivery system for ocular medication. May also be used to protect the corneal surface from mechanical injury from certain lid deformities.

lens, contact, translating bifocal Imprecise term used to describe the combination of vertical ocular rotations and movement of a multifocal contact lens in situ; when the eye rotates downward for near viewing, the multifocal contact lens generally shifts upward to allow the use of the lower (i.e., near) correction of the contact lens.

lens, contact, tri-curve An early-design corneal contact lens with a posterior surface curvature composed of three different concentric zones, the central zone called the optical zone and the two outer zones called the bearing surface.

lens, contact, truncated A corneal contact lens that has had a section of its edge squared or flattened to create a stabilizing effect on the orientation of the lens, and minimize rotation.

lens, contact, X-Chrom Trade name for a monocular contact lens, best worn on the non-dominant eye of red-green color-deficient persons, designed to assist in color discrimination; controversial. Other trade name, Rhodalux.

lens, convex A lens that converges light rays, said to have plus power. (See Figures 31, 32, 34.)

lens, Corlon (C-lite) Trade name of Corning Glass Co. for a single-vision ophthalmic glass lens employing a layer of pliable plastic over the rear surface of the lens to act as a deterrent to eye damage caused by lens fracture or disintegration under impact. Obsolete.

lens, corrected curve A lens designed to reduce peripheral power errors (aberrations) for the conditions of intended use over a specified portion of the field of view. The use of different performance criteria establishes different curvatures for different prescription powers. A group of such lenses covering a range of prescription powers and based on the same performance criteria is referred to as a corrected curve series; for example, Wm. H. Wollaston, deep periscopic (1804–1812); M. Tscherning, M.D., orthoscopic (1908); Zeiss, Punktal (1908–1911); F. Oswalt shallow curve periscopic (1898); Percival Best-Form (1914–1926); E.D. Tillyer, (1917); Shuron, Widesite (1917); W.B. Rayton, B&L Orthogon (1928); Continental, Kurova (1920); Titmus, Normalsite (1950); Univis, Uni-Form (1964); Davis, J.K., Fernald and Rayner, A.O. Tillyer Masterpiece (1964); Shuron/Continental (i.e., S/C Shursite, 1966), now Textron.

lens corridor See *corridor, lens.*

lens, cover A disposable pane or film of optically clear material (e.g., cellulose acetate) to protect an ophthalmic lens from damage; e.g., used in welding.

lens, CR-39 See *CR-39.*

lens, Crookes Glass lens developed from extensive research in 1913 by Sir William Crookes (1832–1919), brilliant physicist of England; blocks UV and infrared by incorporating cerium and ferrous oxide into the glass. Introduced as Crookes Sage Green, then later another glass, not as opaque to infrared, Crookes "A."

lens, Cruxite (Cruxite Ax) Trade name for lenses of pink tint which absorb UV wavelength light by incorporation of cerium, iron, and similar compounds.

lens, crystalline The variably biconvex, normally transparent, and resilient lenticular body suspended directly behind the pupil in a normal phakic eye by zonule fibers from the ciliary body, having high refractive power and altering its convexity by action of the ciliary muscle.

lens, cylinder Ophthalmic lens in which one of the principal meridians has zero refractive power; first ground in America in 1829 by the optical firm of McAllister of Philadelphia, Pennsylvania.

lens deposits See *jelly bumps.*

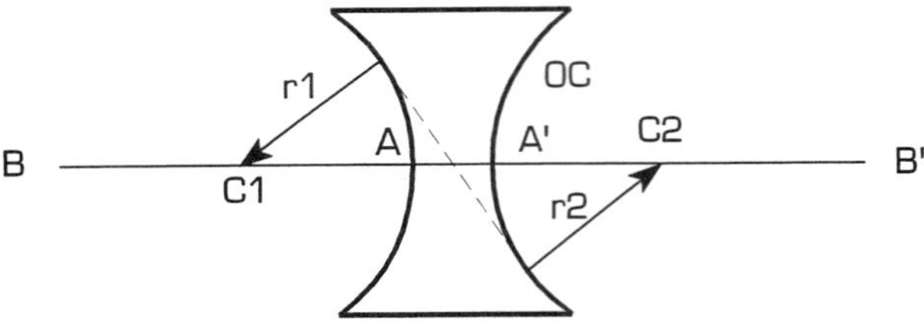

$AC_1 = r_1$; $A'C_2 = r_2$; $r_1 = r_2$; $r_1 \mid\mid r_2$; OC = optical center.

Figure 26 Double concave lens—equal radii of curvature.

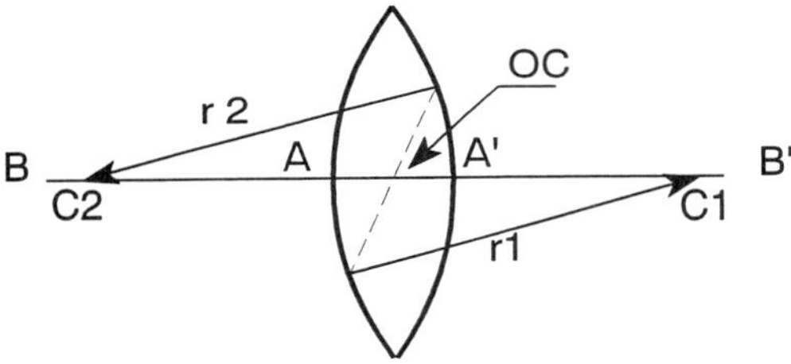

$AC_1 = r_1$; $A'C_2 = r_2$; $r_1 = r_2$; $r_1 \mid\mid r_2$; OC = optical center.

Figure 27 Double convex lens—equal radii of curvature.

lens, didymium Protective filter lens containing neodymium and praseodymium which are particularly effective in absorbing high sodium or yellow light as in silver soldering; has a light-pinkish tint.

lens difference See *difference, lens.*

lens, dislocated Crystalline lens out of its normal position; luxated (totally dislocated) or subluxated (partially dislocated); may be congenital or following injury to the eye.

lens, double concave A biconcave lens of special form having hollow surfaces of equal radii on either side (Figure 26).

lens, double convex A biconvex lens of special form having bulging surfaces of equal radii on either side (Figure 27).

lens, double D A multifocal spectacle lens with a flat, edged segment both at the upper and lower extremities of the lens; helpful in overhead near work.

lens, doublet A pair of lenses, usually of differing refractive index and curvature, designed and ground to eliminate aberrations; may be cemented in direct contact, or separated by an air space determined by the dioptric powers.

lens, dress-hardened See *lens, impact resistant for dress eyewear (A.N.S.I. Z80.1)*

lens, edged An ophthalmic lens whose periphery has been ground (flat, rimless, grooved, or beveled) to a specified size and shape.

lens, Executive A one-piece multifocal lens with the near and intermediate power segments extending over the full width of the lens, characterized by an inverted (dirt-catching) ledge at the juncture of the foci; also referred to as "E" or "M" style.

lens, filter An ophthalmic lens that absorbs or attenuates specific wavelengths of light.

lens, finished An ophthalmic lens that has been ground and polished on both sides to a specific prescription power and thickness; has been edged, rendered impact-resistant, if necessary, and prepared for insertion or mounting into eyeglasses.

lens, flat An early form of lens having both surfaces convex, both surfaces concave, or one surface flat and the other curved (either convex or concave) to provide the desired lens power (cf. *lens, bent; lens, meniscus; lens, corrected curve.*)

lens fracture See *fracture, lens.*

lens, Fresnel (frā'nel) A lens surface of narrow concentric rings or prism sections of a specified power that gives the effect of a continuous lens surface with the same power, but without the usual thickness and weight. Introduced in 1822 by Jean Augustin Fresnel (1788–1827), a French military engineer. Fresnel lenses may be made of a pliable plastic that can be cut and applied to existing lenses, making them a valuable diagnostic tool.

lens, gas-permeable Contact lens made of (hard) plastic material, such as cellulose acetate butyrate (CAB), silicone, or (soft) hydroxy methyl methacrylate that transmits oxygen through it with relative ease. See *lens, contact, rigid gas-permeable.*

lens, gold-coated An industrial or aerospace lens, particularly used for protection in welding, because gold reflects almost all infrared wavelengths and in thin layers is highly transmittant to visual wavelengths. Trade name, Uvex.

lens, gradient density An ophthalmic lens whose luminous transmittance varies significantly from one area of the lens to another; commonly with greatest density in the upper portion of the lens; trade name, Gradutint.

lens, gradient index Lenses which vary in refractive index from a maximum on the optical axis to a minimum at the outer extremity of the lens; the lens material is usually glass and the decrease of refractive index is usually parabolic from the center to the periphery; commonly used in small (1mm–3mm) diameters to couple laser beams or fibre optics. The human lens has a gradient index. Acronym, GRIN.

lens, heat-treated Lenses that have been rendered impact-resistant by hot-oven treatment (to 1330°F), just below the viscosity range, and chilled by forced air to create a compressed surface layer; lens, case hardened; q.v.

lens, honey bee A compound magnifying lens design consisting of three to six small telescopes mounted in the upper portion of a spectacle lens, including prisms, to reduce visual interruption on shifting from one to another telescope; proposed as a low-visual aid for distance use.

lens, Hruby (roo"be) A –55.00 Diopter lens attached to the biomicroscope used to neutralize the refractive power of the eye, as an aid to binocular examination of the fundus; placed very close to corneal surface; introduced in 1941 by Karl Hruby, Austrian ophthalmologist; refined from 1923 lens of Lemoine and Valois of France.

lens, impact-resistant for dress eyewear Ophthalmic lens that conforms to the detailed requirements for impact resistance in the American National Standard Recommendations for Prescription Ophthalmic Lenses, Z80.1, section 4.6. For dress (or street wear); not to be confused with special-purpose occupational and educational or recreational protective lenses which must meet or exceed A.N.S.I. Z87 standards.

lens, impact-resistant for occupational and educational protection Lens that conforms to the requirements of American National Standard Practice for Occupational and Educational Eye and Face Protection, A.N.S.I. Z87.1–1989 (or the latest version).

lens, industrial "safety" See *lens, impact resistant, for occupational and educational protection, meeting or exceeding A.N.S.I. Z87 standards.*

lens, intraocular implant (IOL) See *pseudophakos.*

lens, ion-exchange See *lens, chem-tempered.*

lens, iseikonic (īs-i-kon′ik) A lens made with special thickness, surface curvatures, and bevel-edge location to control the magnification of an image while maintaining the prescribed refractive power; used to compensate for aniseikonia.

lens, Kalichrome Trade name for an absorptive lens of yellow color, often containing silver oxides, absorbing large amounts of ultraviolet and blue light, while transmitting most of the remainder of the spectrum; used for image definition in haze and fog. Sometimes promoted as a "shooting" lens; Wratten K1 or K2 filter equivalents. Other trade names, Noviol, Hazemaster, Rifilite.

lens, lacrimal The optical component created by the pre-corneal tear film between the posterior surface of a contact lens and the anterior surface of the cornea; may be varied in its dioptric power by changes in the posterior contact lens curve.

lens, laminated A lens formed by two or more layers of refracting material firmly joined together for special optical or safety purposes; developed in 1903 by Eduard Benedictus (1879–1930), Parisian chemist; trade names, Triplex; Salvoc; Scutoid; Motex; Willson-Triplex; I-Safe; Schott KG3.

lens, lenticular A lens, usually of strong refractive power, in which the prescribed power is provided over only a limited central region of the lens called the lenticular portion. The remainder of the lens is called the carrier and provides lesser or no refractive correction, but gives increased dimensions to the lens for mounting. See *lens, Myo-Disc.*

lens, liquid See *lens, lacrimal.*

lens measure See *clock, lens.*

lens, melanin A proprietary optical material promoted for ultraviolet light absorption, particularly in polycarbonate lenses. U.S. patent issued to James M. Gallas of Texas in 1987.

lens, meniscus (me-nis′kus) Meniscus (i.e., little or crescent moon). An ophthalmic lens having base curves of plus (+) or minus (–) 6 diopters; may be plano or of a specified refractive power; having a convex configuration on one side and a concave configuration on the other. Introduced in 1611 by Johann Kepler (1571–1630), German astronomer and mathematician, in his book *Dioptrice.*

lens, minus A lens having negative dioptric power; thinner at the center than at the edge (concave).

lens, mounted Ophthalmic lens that has been inserted into a spectacle frame front or secured in a rimless mounting.

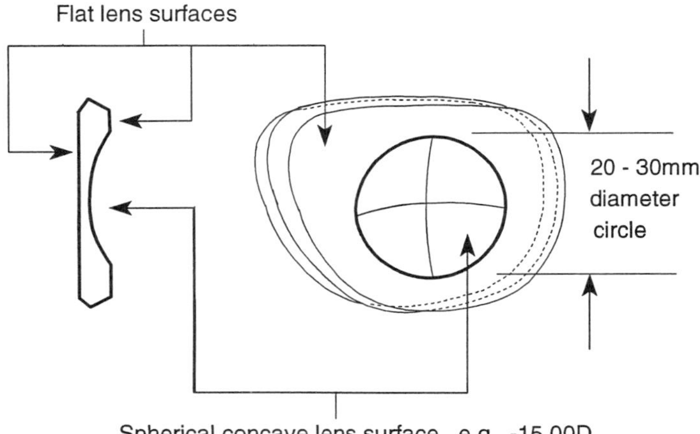

Figure 28 Myo-Disc lens.

lens, multifocal An ophthalmic lens designed to provide correction for two or more viewing ranges; for example, bifocal, trifocal, etc.

lens, multifocal flat-top See *lens, straight-top multifocal.*

lens, Myo-Disc In the correction of high myopia, a lenticular lens, having a concave, central corrective area 20mm to 30mm in diameter and a flat peripheral or carrier area; was also made in bifocal form (Figure 28). Introduced in 1933 by New York City optician Theodore E. Obrig (1895–1967).

lens, neodymium See *lens, didymium.*

lens, neutral gray An ophthalmic lens designed for ocular protection against high light intensities by generally even reduction of light transmission across the visible spectrum; does not distort color values. Introduced as G-15 by Bausch & Lomb in 1953.

lens, Noir Trade name for a series of ophthalmic filter lenses in a broad range of colors and levels of absorption; originally an acronym for **No i**nfra**r**ed.

lens, non-removable A unitized lens and ophthalmic front constructed of one piece of optical plastic; particularly used for safety and protective products.

lens, Noviol Trade name for a yellow-colored absorptive lens with a sharp cut-off in the 490nm to 510nm wavelength (i.e., **No viol**et).

lens, Omnifocal Trade name for a progressive power lens designed in 1962 by David Volk and J.W. Weinberg; vision progressed gradually from distance into the bifocal area with no lens channel; produced distortion to either side.

lens, one-piece multifocal A multifocal ophthalmic lens or blank fabricated from a single piece of optical glass or plastic; trade names, Ultex; Philtex. See *Ultex.*

lens opening See *opening, lens.*

lens, ophthalmic A piece of transparent and homogeneous substance having two highly polished, opposing, refracting surfaces for use close to the eye to assist the functions of the eye.

lens, orthoscopic See *lens, Tscherning.*

lens pattern See *pattern, lens.*

lens, periscopic A shallow, base curve, spherical correcting lens series in which the minus-powered lenses have base curves of +1.25D and the plus-powered lenses have base curves of –1.25D. The initial deep curve design of lenses (i.e., periscope, to see all around) was developed in 1801 and patented in 1804 by Wm. H. Wollaston (1766–1828), English physicist and physician. Originally manufactured by a London optician, Dolland, and about 1818 by London optician Charles West.

lens, photochromic See *lens, phototropic.*

lens, phototropic (fō-to-tro'-pik) Glass ophthalmic lenses of special chemical composition containing silver halides (Cl, Fl, Br) that darken on exposure to ultraviolet light and lighten with reduced exposure; photosensitive lenses; photochemical lenses. Developed in early 1960s by W.H. Armistead and S.D. Stookey, Corning Glass Co. research chemists. Recently available in plastic lenses by addition of phototropic films to the lens surface.

lens, plano (plā'no) A lens having zero refractive power (afocal); lens surfaces may both be flat or equally meniscus in shape.

lens, plano concave A lens having one flat and one concave surface.

lens, plano convex A lens having one flat and one convex surface.

lens, plus A lens having positive dioptric power; thicker at the center than at the edge (convex).

lens, polarizing A lens which includes a layer of parallel-oriented crystals or material (Herapathite, calcite, stressed polyvinyl alcohol, or the like) that transmits light waves vibrating in one direction, but not at right angles to this; not to be used for laser protection. Trade names, Photopolar; Polar-Ray; Polarlite; Polarex; Polarguard; SpecPol; Vergopol.

lens, Polaroid Trade name. Word coined by Clarence Kennedy, a Smith College professor, and commercialized by Edwin H. Land (1910–1991). See *lens, polarizing.*

lens power See *power, refractive.*

lens, prescription An ophthalmic lens manufactured to the wearer's individual refractive needs; refractive power is specified in diopters.

lens, prism ballast In contact lens design, a lens that has a thicker cross-section, and hence is heavier on one edge than the opposite; the thicker edge orients downward.

lens, progressive An ophthalmic lens, introduced in 1959, designed and developed by Bernard Maitenaz (b. 1926), optical engineer of Paris, France, in which the power changes continuously rather than discretely in order to provide correction for more than one viewing range; also referred to as progressive-addition or progressive-power lens (Figure 29). Trade names, Adaptar; Omnifocal; Omnivarilux; Prima; Progressive Power; Progressor; Progressive R; Technica; Ultraview; Varilux; Varilux Infinity; Varilux Comfort; Younger 10/30.

lens, progressive addition See *lens, progressive.*

lens, progressive power See *lens, progressive.*

lens protractor See *protractor, optical.*

lens, Punktal A highly precise, early German toric lens series corrected for astigmatic aberrations over the entire lens surface; designed by Dr. Moritz von Rohr, and manufactured by Carl Zeiss (1913-) as the first corrected-curve toric lenses to be introduced commercially.

lens, quadrifocal A multifocal ophthalmic lens having four finite focal distances, usually a typical trifocal with one additional segment at the top for above-eye-level viewing.

lens, RedeRite A bifocal ophthalmic lens with the major area for near viewing and having a small negative segment at the top for distance viewing; introduced about 1836 by the Philadelphia optician Isaac Schnaitmann, who ground off an upper portion of the reading lens to give distant vision.

lens, reflective A lens that has been coated, usually with a metallic layer 10–15u thick to return specific wavelengths of incident light (e.g., gold-coated lenses to reflect infrared); silver- and copper-coated lenses of personal choice.

lens retention See *retention, lens.*

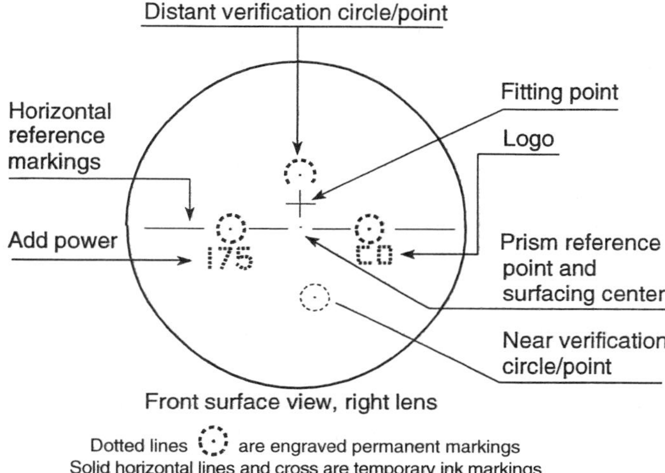

Figure 29 Progressive lens markings.

lens, rimless An ophthalmic lens with a flat or faceted edge for use in mountings without rims or eyewires.

lens, safety A generic term for various ophthalmic lenses designed to protect the eye from injury.

lens, sapphire An extremely durable lens of high transmittance made in the single hexagonal-crystal form of alumina Al_2O_3; extremely hard; birefringent.

lens, semi-finished A lens having only one finished surface.

lens, shooting A yellow filter lens (similar to Wratten K1 or K2) promoted to reduce apparent haze; absorbs most wavelengths below 500nm and reduces scotopic sensitivity by about 50%; not indicated for night driving. Trade names, Acutone; Hazemaster; Night Hawk; Noviol; Nupro; Orgalux; Rifilite; Roadmaster; Starlight. See lens, *Kalichrome.*

lens, single-cut In contact lenses, a hard contact lens, the anterior surface of which is of a single radius of curvature.

lens, single-vision An ophthalmic lens designed to provide correction for only one viewing distance.

lens size See *size, lens.*

lens speed See *number, f.*

lens, spherical A lens that has the same refractive power in all meridians. Such a lens may have rotationally symmetrical aspheric surfaces; Cartesian lens.

lens, spherical plus A convex lens having the same refractive powers in all meridians to make incident light more convergent or increase its vergence.

lens, spherocylinder A lens having different refractive powers in its two principal meridians. It is sometimes referred to as a toric lens or, incorrectly, as a cylinder lens. See *lens, cylinder.*

lens, stock or factory-finished uncut An ophthalmic lens with both surfaces finished to specific back vertex power(s) supplied by a manufacturer. Such a lens has yet to be edged to a specific shape.

lens, Stokes A rotating combination of a plano convex and a plano concave cylinder of equal power; used to check power and axis in cylindrical refractive examination. Introduced in 1849 by Sir George Gabriel Stokes (1819–1903), Irish physicist and mathematician, while working at Cambridge.

lens stop See *stop, lens.*

lens, straight-top multifocal A multifocal ophthalmic lens with a straight line of transition from distance to near power which is aligned parallel with the horizontal lens bisector (0° to 180° line); commonly referred to as "D" style multifocal because of the segment's shape.

lens, telescopic In ophthalmic lenses, a compound lens system, usually Galilean, with plus objective and minus ocular components for magnification of image size, usually from 2X to 4X in magnifying power. As low-vision aids, mounted for one or both eyes; first produced in 1907 by the Carl Zeiss Works of Jena, Germany.

lens, tempered See *lens, impact resistant for dress eyewear.*

lens, Therminon (ther′mi-non) Trade name for a Corning glass of pale greenish-blue color that absorbs both ultraviolet and infrared light.

lens, Thinlite Trade name for a high-index flint (lead oxide) glass lens; suffers from significant chromatic aberration and weight.

lens, tinted See *lens, absorptive.*

lens, toric A lens to correct astigmatic ametropia with one or both surfaces having different power meridians of least and greatest curvature located at right angles to each other (usually a meniscus-type lens). First developed in America about 1830 by Philadelphia optician, Zentmayer. Also, a contact lens design, usually toric on the posterior surface, but may be toric on both surfaces (bitoric).

lens, trial

1. A loose lens in a series used in patient examination to determine the desired refractive power for ophthalmic lenses or contact lenses. First produced as a set of lenses in 1778 by Paul Hirn, "Electoral Spectacle and Lens Maker"; contained 17 lenses.
2. An individual spherical, cylindrical, or prism lens in an examination set or case. (cf. *phoropter.*)

lens, trifocal A multifocal, ophthalmic lens designed to provide correction for three viewing distances. Introduced in 1826 by John Isaac Hawkins (1772–1855), inventor, musician, and engineer of London and Philadelphia.

lens, trifocal, standard Imprecise designation of trifocal dioptric power as 50% of the near-vision addition. (Actual amount should be specified from available manufacturer's inventory, ordinarily from 40% to 75% of the near add).

lens, triplet, A high-powered hand-held magnifier, composed of two concave meniscus lenses cemented to a double convex lens; Hasting's triplet; outer lenses are usually high index and center lens is low-index glass; very little aberration.

lens, Triplex Trade name for a pioneering British and French impact-resistant lens made of two layers of optical glass with a plastic interlayer. Developed in 1903–1905 and patented in 1906 by Parisian chemist Edouard Benedictus (1879–1930). See *lens, laminated.*

lens, Tscherning's orthoscopic (chern'ingz or'tho-skop"ik) A corrected curve series of lenses to reduce distortion and peripheral aberration; designed in early 1900s by the Danish ophthalmologist Marius Hans Eric Tscherning (1854–1939) during 26 years at the Sorbonne in Paris; design published in 1904.

lens, Ultex Trade name for a multifocal ophthalmic lens made of a solid piece of lens material (uniform optical density throughout) with add power(s) created by a difference in surface curvature. Developed and patented in 1910 by Indianapolis, Indiana, optician Charles W. Conner.

lens, Ultex A Trade name for a one-piece bifocal lens with a semicircular segment shape and near-vision image with base-down prism effect.

lens, ultraviolet absorbing A lens in which the average transmittance between 280nm and 315nm (UVB) is zero (0), and the average transmittance between 315nm and 380nm (UVA) is reduced and specified; trade names, Hallauer's glass; Cruxite Ax; Crookes; Photochromic; Noviol. (cf. *A.N.S.I. Z80.3.*)

lens, uncut An ophthalmic lens that has been ground and polished on both sides to a specific prescription power and thickness, but not yet sized, edged to shape, or, if specified, made impact-resistant.

lens, uniform density A lens with luminous transmittance which does not vary significantly over the entire area of the lens.

lens, universal Informal designation of the pinhole effect through an opaque disc, reducing the blur circles and improving acuity in ametropia.

lens, verant A meniscus or corrected-curve ophthalmic lens adapted to range of movement of the eye; forerunner of the Zeiss punctal lens. Designed in 1902 by Swedish ophthalmologist Dr. Allvar Gullstrand (1862–1930. From the Latin, "verus," true.

lens, Volk A series of aspheric double convex lens for indirect ophthalmoscopy in powers of +14 to +40 diopters, and for panretinal (slit lamp) examination in powers of +60 to +90 diopters; Conoid lens. Developed by David Volk (1917–1987), ophthalmologist of Cleveland, Ohio.

lens, yellow See *lens, Kalichrome*; *lens, Noviol.*

lens, zoom A compound lens system usually of three or more elements with continuous mechanical alteration of power rather than in discrete steps or units; classified as uncompensated or compensated (mechanically or optically). In the latter, the image is always at the same position relative to the front element.

Lenscorometer Trade name for a hand-held mechanical screw gauge with a guard ring used to determine linear distance between the back surface of trial lenses in a phoropter and the front surface of the eye. See *distance, vertex.*

lensectomy (lenz-ek'to-me) Surgical removal of a lens with or without cataract formation within it; lentectomy.

lensmeter Instrument for determining optical characteristics of a lens; may be mechanical/optical, projection, electronically displayed, or fully automated with printout findings; focimeter; trade names, Lensometer; Vertometer.

Lensometer (lenz-om'i-ter) Trade name for a lensmeter (focimeter) used for verification of ophthalmic lens characteristics and their preparation for assembly into spectacles; manufactured by American Optical Corporation.

lenticular (len-tik'yu-lar) Pertaining to the lens; lens shape. See *lens, lenticular.*

lenticular astigmatism See *astigmatism, lenticular.*

lenticular lens See *lens, lenticular.*

lenticular, minus See *lens, Myo-Disc.*

-less Suffix meaning without.

letter, Snellen A standard visual acuity test letter (optotype) that subtends an angle of 5 minutes of arc at specified distances, each portion of the letter subtends an angle of 1 minute of arc. Developed in 1862 by Utrecht professor of ophthalmology Hermann Snellen (1834–1908).

letters, test (test types) Specifically sized letters for measuring visual acuity at a given distance from the eye; generally based on 1 minute of arc resolution as the minimal separation which the average human eye can resolve; optotypes.

letters, test, equal difficulty A series of letters (D, K, R, H, V, C, N, Z, S, O) presenting similar construction and optical loading of the letter space, introduced in 1959 by Louise L. Sloan, Ph.D. (1898–1982), visual scientist of Baltimore, Maryland.

leukoma (loo-kō"mah) A dense white opacification of the cornea.

lexigram A symbol, device, geometric form, or the like, standing for a word, phrase, simple description, or simple direction.

library temple See *temple, library.*

licensed optician See *optician, licensed.*

lid edema See *edema, lid.*

LIDAR Acronym for **Li**ght **D**etection **a**nd **R**anging; q.v.

lifestyle dispensing An opticianry analysis of exposure, work, and recreation relative to suggesting appropriate ophthalmic lenses and frames for a patient.

lift-front spectacles See *spectacles, lift-front.*

ligaments, suspensory See *zonule of Zinn.*

light Electromagnetic radiations visible to the human eye, approximately 380nm to 760nm in wavelength; gives rise to the sensation of vision by stimulating the rod and cone cells of the retina; absence of darkness. See *spectrum, visible.*

light, actinic Rays of light shorter than those in the violet spectrum and capable of producing photochemical effects; e.g., a component of light from a welding torch causing painful destruction of the corneal epithelium.

light, coherent Electromagnetic radiations in the visible spectrum traveling in strictly spherical wavefronts (spatially coherent) and in phase (temporally coherent); particularly said of tightly collimated light as in laser emissions.

light emitting diode (LED) display See *display, light emitting diode.*

light, incident Light falling on a surface.

light perception See *perception, light.*

light pipe See *optics, fibre.*

light, polarized See *polarization.*

light scatter, Rayleigh See *light, scattered.*

light, scattered Random, radiating electromagnetic fields to all directions (oscillating acceleration of electrons moving from their usual orbits about a heavier nucleus) appearing as light traveling in all directions; loosely, diffusion of light in passing through a medium having turbidity or random particles, as smoke or moisture. Irregular reflection of light from a matt surface; light scatter, Rayleigh. The amount of light scatter varies as the inverse of the 4th power of the incident light wavelength; accounts for blueness of the sky. Calculated (c. 1870) by Lord John Wm S. Rayleigh (1842–1919), English physicist, who received a Nobel Prize in 1904 for work on wave motion.

light, ultraviolet A component of the electromagnetic energy spectrum of wavelengths from 10nm to 400nm; Finsen light; Minen light; Wood's light. Subdivided since 1932 into three main categories:

UVC – Radiation from 100nm to 280nm; normally filtered out by the atmospheric ozone layer surrounding the earth;

UVB – Radiation between 280nm and 320nm; causes sunburn and destroys bacteria;

UVA – Radiation between 320nm and 400nm; may cause suntanning. (Wood's light). Subdivided since 1986 into UVA I (340nm–400nm) which may cause tanning, and UVA II (320nm–340nm) which produces erythema and pigmentation.

light, visible The portion of the electromagnetic energy spectrum between 380nm to 400nm and 760nm to 780nm. Values established by C.I.E.

light, Wood's A low-intensity diagnostic light source of mercury-vapor origin in the near ultraviolet, peak emission 365nm to 375nm., usually passed through cobalt-blue glass tubes with a nickel-oxide filter and fitted with a magnifying lens, used to evaluate corneal surface abnormalities and contact lens in situ in the presence of sodium fluorescein; black light; also available with white fluorescent tubes in tandem with above; developed and named by Robert Williams Wood (1868–1958), American physicist; manufactured by Burton Medical Products of Van Nuys, California (i.e., Burton lamp).

Light Detection and Ranging A laser light modification of RADAR (Radio Detection and Ranging) generally used in outdoor environments, as in astronomy and tactical military needs; of concern to eye safety or retinal safety.

Lighthouse, The Voluntary, nonprofit agency, based in New York City, involved in direct services to the blind and visually handicapped, established in 1906; has research division engaged in fundamentals of visual reception and guidance.

limbus A border, edge, or junction often distinguished by color.

limbus, corneal The transitional ring 1nm to 2mm wide where the cornea and sclera unite; the corneo-scleral junction of the eye.

limen The threshold or beginning point; plural is limina.

line, 180 See *bisector, horizontal lens; 180° line.*

line, center See *bisector, horizontal lens.*

line, cutting See *line, geometric center.*

line, datum (British term) See *line, geometric center.*

line, dividing See *line, segment.*

line, geometric center A horizontal line, passing through the intersection of diagonal lines joining opposite corners of a box, that circumscribes the lens shape; previously called normal mounting line. See Figure 22; see also *bisector, horizontal lens (HLB).*

line, normal mounting See *bisector, horizontal lens (HLB).*

line of sight See *axis, fixation; axis, visual.*

line, reference A long, thin mark that constitutes a beginning or mark of comparison.

line, segment In spectacle optics, the horizontal boundary that indicates the uppermost edge of a multifocal addition in an ophthalmic lens.

linear

1. Extended or arranged in a row.
2. Involving measurement in only one dimension.

linear magnification See *magnification, linear.*

linear magnifying power See *power, linear magnifying.*

lip, posterior A slightly extended retaining edge in the inner side of the rim groove (eyewire groove) in a safety spectacle front; aids in retaining an ophthalmic lens in its frame when impacted frontally; is generally 0.2mm to 0.6mm higher than the outer edge of the rim groove; safety flange; safety groove.

lipoprotein deposits See *jelly bumps.*

lipoproteins Combination of fat (lipid) and organic complexes usually containing sulphur and nitrogen (protein) possessing the general properties and solubility of proteins that are the principal constituents of all the protoplasm of cells. In response to an individual patient's biocompatibility with various contact lens materials, there may be such deposits formed on both surfaces of contact lenses. These tend to be roundish in configuration, and slightly yellowish or brown in color; informally designated "jelly bumps."

liquid lens See *lens, liquid.*

loading, rate of A major variable in the mechanical characteristics of impact resistance. Slow loading over minutes or hours may result in chronic-fatigue (static fatigue) fracture, whereas rapid loading over milliseconds creates an entirely different (shock) fracture mechanism and possible percussion-cone fracture or explosive fracture patterns.

locus A system of points, lines or the like that satisfies one or more set of conditions.

logMAR (logarithmic Minimal Angle of Resolution) A proposed (1972) visual acuity test system and notation based on 0.1 log unit, chart-line size progression, but utilizing the 1-minute Snellen minimal angle of resolution; introduced by Australian optometrists I.L. Bailey and J.E. Lovie.

logo Shortened form of logogram or logotype. A distinctive mark, letter, symbol or character used as a trademark or colophon.

-logy Suffix meaning science.

longest diagonal See *diagonal, longest.*

longest dimension See *dimension, longest.*

lorgnette (lorn-yet′) Eyeglasses, either folding or non-folding, mounted on a handle or slide.

lorgnon (lorn-yon′) Eyeglasses of delicate folding construction, generally of nose-glass design rather than hand-held.

loupe (loop) A magnifying optical system based on a Galilean telescope with additional plus power in the objective lens designed for near-visual use; jewelers loupe. (*Note:* Terminology differs in Great Britain.)

loupe, jewelers A single or double lens magnifying system which clips to a spectacle front, or endpiece, and may be moved in or out of the ipsilateral line of sight; also called spectacle loupe.

Low Vision Enhancement System (LVES or VEH) Trade name for a spectacle top rim or brow-bar mounted miniaturized pair of telescopes (3, 4, or 6X) giving flip-front construction which may be changed to different pairs of spectacles; available in focusing or reading cap design.

lubricants, ocular Pharmaceutical agents used to moisten the surface of the eye to promote healing and prevent corneal/ocular dehydration.

lumen (loo′men)

1. Psychophysical optics. In the S.I. system, a derived unit of luminous flux emitted in a unit-solid angle by a uniform point source of one candela.
2. Anatomy. The internal cavity or hollow portion of a structure, as the passage way within a blood vessel, or the lacrimal duct.

luminance Psychophysical term for the amount of light emitted by a source; flux or intensity per unit solid angle.

luminous flux See *flux, luminous.*

luminous intensity See *intensity, luminous.*

luminous transmittance properties See *transmittance properties, luminous.*

lux (meter-candle) In the Système International (S.I.), a derived unit of illuminance expressed as lumen per square meter (formerly called meter-candle), or 0.0001 phot. Division by 10 gives the approximate footcandles, the corresponding English unit. Slit lamps provide 200,000 lux to 400,000 lux.

luxation In ocular pathology, complete dislocation of the crystalline lens relative to the pupil; may be anterior (in front of the iris) or posterior (behind the iris). (cf. *subluxation.*)

lysozyme (lī'so-zīm) An enzyme of the hydrolase class naturally occurring in tears, saliva, and egg white which breaks down some bacterial cell walls and thereby destroys bacteria; contributes to maintaining a bacteria-free tear film; first discovered and named in 1922 by London bacteriologist Alexander Fleming (1881–1955), who was later knighted (1944) and received a Nobel Prize (1945).

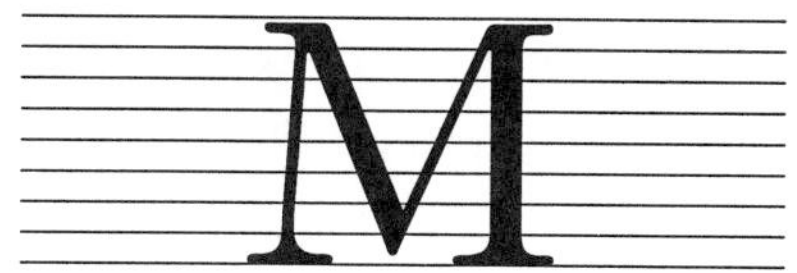

m **1.** Symbol for meter, in the Système International (S.I.); the unit of linear measurement, one of seven base units.
2. Symbol for linear magnification in a lens or lens system.

M Roman numeral for one thousand (1,000).

ma Abbreviation for milliampere (1/1000 of an ampere).

M.C.E. Abbreviation for the term mandatory continuing education; q.v.

MLC Abbreviation for **m**inimum **l**ash **c**learance; a convenient notation of trial lens position at refraction and after fabrication and fitting of spectacle lenses.

M.P.H. Abbreviation for the academic degree Master of Public Health, a sequential degree to a bachelor's degree, and before the terminal degree D.P.H. (Doctor of Public Health).

macro- Prefix meaning large, long, great.

macrocornea An abnormally large cornea. See *megalocornea; keratoglobus.*

macula (mak'yu-lah)
1. An oval area in the posterior polar retina, 3mm to 5mm in diameter, usually located temporal to and slightly below the level of the optic disc; characterized by the presence of a yellow pigment (leaf xanthophyll) diffusely permeating the inner layers; contains the fovea centralis in its center, and provides color detection and the best photopic visual acuity.
2. A moderately dense scar of the cornea that can usually be seen without optical aids.

macula, ectopic A macular area located away from or eccentric to its usual position.

macular degeneration See *degeneration, macular.*

madarosis (mad″ah-rō′sis) Loss of lashes or eyebrows. (cf. *alopecia.*)

Maddox rod See *rod, Maddox.*

Magnatel Trade name for a lightweight (2.5 oz) inexpensive, British magnifying spectacle with distant refractive correction in the near lenses (ocular) and plus spherical lenses in the objective lenses. Distant magnification to 3X by adjusting the distance between the objective and ocular lenses.

magnesium A light, silvery, metallic element, chemical symbol Mg, atomic number 12; as a fluoride, it is an effective anti-reflective lens coating; its salts are essential in nutrition; other compounds are used orally as antacids and laxatives. First isolated in 1808 by English chemist Humphry Davy (1778–1829).

magnesium fluoride (coating) See *coating, anti-reflective.*

magnification The increase in the apparent or perceived size or subtended angle of an image in relation to actual size of object. See *power, magnifying.*

magnification, angular The mathematical ratio of the angle subtended by the image to that subtended by the object with respect to a viewing point of reference, such as the entrance pupil of the eye. More specifically expressed as a ratio of the tangents of the angles. By convention, expressed for the near-focusing distance of 25cm or 10 inches (M).

magnification, approach Increase in image size by coming closer to an object.

magnification, linear Mathematical ratio of image size to object size (M). Not an absolute value in case of direct visual observation because of accommodative range in the human eye.

magnification or magnifying power See *power, magnifying.*

magnifier An optical or electronic device that produces an enlarged image of an object.

magnifier, Coddington A spherical or nearly spherical single glass lens with a deep V-shaped equatorial groove covered or filled with opaque material. Image quality is improved by the groove acting as a diaphragm. Developed about 1810 by Henry Coddington (d. 1845), English mathematician and optical scientist.

magnifier, line A near-reading aid of plus cylinder design with fixed distance supports to enlarge one or two lines of type at a time.

magnifier, measuring An optical device used to view and evaluate the surface or parameters of a contact lens. A magnifying device used to measure the diameter and posterior optical zone of a contact lens. (cf. *graticule.*)

magnifier, paperweight A fixed-focus, plano-convex lens of about 4X magnification, used in direct contact with a printed page, and of light-gathering design; usually housed in an opaque ring. (cf. *Visolett.*)

magnifier, pendant A chain-supported, single-piece spherical lens of intermediate power; often styled as a dressing accessory.

magnifying power See *power, magnifying.*

major blank See *blank, major.*

major reference point (MRP) See *point, major reference.*

major reference point height See *height, major reference point.*

Mandatory Continuing Education (M.C.E.)

1. A grass-roots voluntary effort by numerous state organizations and some licensing boards to promote the concept of obligatory continuing education as a requirement to recertification or relicensure within that state.
2. Similar principle as adopted by several state boards of medical licensure.

mandrel A metal spindle, either tapered or cylindrical, designed to be fitted with a choice of selected tool bits for removal of broken screws, pressing holes in plastic ophthalmic frames, and the like.

manufacturing optician See *optician, manufacturing.*

marginal

1. Occurring at or near the edge.
2. At or near a tolerance.

mark Any letter, figure, numeral, symbol, sign, word, or device, or any combination thereof, applied to an article.

marked surface power See *power, marked surface.*

marking, alignment reference Location points, inked or etched on the surface of an ophthalmic lens, provided by designers and manufacturers to establish the proper rotational alignment of a progressive-addition ophthalmic lens blank or re-establish other reference points.

marking pins See *pins, marking.*

MASER Acronym for **M**icrowave **A**mplification by **S**timulated **E**mission of **R**adiation; the conceptual and working forerunner of LASERs as conceived in 1954 by Charles Hard Townes, Ph.D., (b. 1915), American physicist, who received a Nobel Prize in 1964.

master optician See *optician, master.*

mastoid bend See *bend, mastoid.*

material, non-ionic A contact lens polymer which has little electronic activity, and does not tend to attract airborne debris.

matte (mat) A finish or surface that scatters reflected light in all directions; a dull finish.

mature cataract See *cataract, mature.*

McCullough effect A perceptual sensation following 2 to 4 minutes of alternate gazing at vertical and horizontal gratings of complementary color (i.e., orange and blue-green in the normal color vision subject) in which aftereffects are of opposite color and linked to the direction of the grating even in 90° rotation; this edge effect will persist for many hours; conceptualized in 1965 by Celeste McCullough.

mcg Abbreviation for microgram, one millionth of one gram (i.e., 10^{-6}).

measurements, binocular PD See *distance, interpupillary.*

measuring magnifier See *magnifier, measuring.*

media, ocular Transparent substances of the eye through which light passes prior to stimulation of the retina. These include the tears, cornea, aqueous humor, crystalline lens, and vitreous humor.

medial canthus See *canthus, medial.*

medium, optical Any material, substance, space or surface regarded in terms of its transmission of light.

mega- Prefix meaning large; great; million.

megalocornea (meg″ah-lo-kor′ne-ah) Abnormally large cornea; usually a bilateral and hereditary developmental enlargement of the cornea; macrocornea. See *keratoglobus.*

Meibomian gland See *gland, Meibomian.*

melanin (mel′ ah-nin) Dark, amorphous pigments of the skin, hair, and uvea of the eye; produced by polymerization of oxidation products of tyrosine and dihydrophenyl compounds; contains carbon, hydrogen, nitrogen, oxygen and often sulfur; synthesized in cells called melanoblasts; absorbs radiant energy; first described in an organized way by C.L. Pierre Masson (1880–1959), French physician and pathologist.

melanoma A dark-colored tumor consisting of cells containing the pigment melanin; may be benign or malignant; very common in Caucasian races, intermediate in Chinese races, and very rare in blacks. The most common tumor inside the adult Caucasian eye, where it is frequently malignant; in the iris, it is more often benign.

membrane A thin layer of tissue which lines a cavity or covers a surface, as the corneal epithelium.

membrane, Bowman's Second layer of the cornea; a glass-like layer between the corneal epithelium and the corneal stroma. Named for Sir William Bowman (1816–1892), English ophthalmologist and anatomist, who first described its histologic details in 1847.

membrane, Descemet's (des-eh-mā̄z') Fourth layer of the cornea; a glass-like layer between the corneal stroma and the corneal endothelium; can regenerate after injury. Named for Jean Descemet (1732–1810), Parisian physician and botanist who elaborated upon it in his 1758 dissertation, though it had been referred to by others several years earlier.

membrane, hyaloid The condensed gel at the anterior and posterior surfaces of the vitreous humor; structureless and optically homogeneous; a surface layer and not a true anatomical membrane.

meniscus (me-nis'kus) A crescent-shaped structure.

meniscus lens See *lens, meniscus.*

meniscus, tear The pre-corneal tear accumulation, roughly triangular in cross-section, which is normally formed between the border of the lower eyelid and the ocular surface with the lids open; also called river of Norn (after M.S. Norn, Copenhagen ophthalmologist), tear prism, inferior marginal tear strip (IMTS).

mercury A metallic element, liquid at ordinary temperature; silver colored; chemical symbol Hg, atomic number 80; quicksilver; used in contact lens disinfecting solutions (as Thimerosal); may cause allergic reaction on contact. Electrical discharge through mercury vapor yields bright bluish light rich in UV. Known to ancient Chinese and Egyptians as early as 1500 B.C.

meridian An imaginary line on the surface of a spherical body making intersection with a plane perpendicular to the surface at a specified point. When applied to a lens, it may also be defined as an imaginary line on its surface at the intersection of the surface with a plane that contains the optical axis. Also applies to the cornea and the eye as a whole.

meridians, principal The two mutually perpendicular meridians of a spherocylinder lens or toric optical surface with minimum and maximum power.

meridional power See *power, meridional.*

meshwork, trabecular (trah-bek′u-lar) A fine net of fibrillar tissue located at the angle of the anterior chamber of the eye and leading to the canal of Schlemm.

mesopic vision See *vision, mesopic.*

metal frame See *frame, metal.*

metall Seventeenth century term for glass in its molten state.

metamorphopsia (met″a-mor-fop′se-ah) A pathologic disturbance of vision in which objects appear to be distorted or twisted; frequently derives from pathologic changes in the macular area.

-meter Suffix meaning measured.

meter (m)

1. The basic unit of linear measurement in the metric (S.I.) system; now standardized in terms of the wavelength of a line in the Krypton spectrum.
2. A combining suffix indicating to measure.

meter-candle Psychophysical term for illumination produced on a flat surface by one candela of light one meter from the surface (lux).

meter, potential acuity Optical instrument used to estimate the resolving power of the macula and evaluate the likely level of improved acuity to be obtained following a cataract extraction. Uses a reduced Snellen acuity chart in very near range; developed by Johns Hopkins ophthalmologists David L. Guyton (b. 1944) and John S. Minkowski (b. 1951); abbreviated PAM. (cf. *Visometer, Lotmar.*)

metric system See *system, metric.*

-metry Suffix meaning the process of measuring.

MEVA Abbreviation for Miniaturized Electronic Visual Aid; q.v.

Mg Chemical symbol for the metallic element magnesium; q.v.

micro- Prefix meaning small; one millionth part of a ~.

microcoria (mī″kro-kō′re-ah) Abnormally small pupils, as from instilling the drug pilocarpine, or congenital developmental defect of the iris, or acquired disease as neurosyphilis.

microcornea Abnormally small cornea.

microlens

1. A general description for small diameter near (reading) lenses about 15mm in diameter; usually of high dioptric power for low-vision patients; microglasses.
2. A group of corneal contact lenses designed specifically smaller than the diameter of the cornea; introduced in 1948 by California contact lens technician Kevin M. Tuohy (d. 1990?).

micrometer An instrument, usually mechanical, used for measuring very small linear distances.

microphthalmos (mī″krof-thal′mus) Pathologically small size of the eye or eyes from birth; usually a static birth defect. In extreme cases may be cosmetically aided with orbital implant surgery and insertion of a reform prosthesis.

microscope A compound magnifying system whose elements are of high dioptric power and very short focal distances; the magnifying power is the product of the linear magnification of the objective multiplied by the angular magnification of the ocular.

microscope, specular (spek′yu-lar) Optical instrument for examining and photographing the size and regularity of corneal endothelial cells in specular-reflected light; endothelial microscope; scanning specular microscope.

microwatt A unit of power per unit of time; one millionth of a watt; the watt is an S.I.-derived unit.

milli- Prefix meaning one thousandth (1/1000) (i.e., 0.001, or 10^{-3}).

millijoule (mil′i-jool″) A unit of work; one thousandth of a joule; used to compare energies of laser burns. The joule is an S.I.-derived unit.

millimeter A subunit of linear measurement in the S.I. system; one thousandth of a meter; abbreviated mm.

millimeter rule See *rule, millimeter.*

milling A dry-cutting, lens-generating machine using a rotating cutter of 2-, 4-, or 12-flute design (in contrast to a single-point lathe), usually computer-controlled; particularly useful for edging polycarbonate and high-index plastic lenses.

mineralogy, optical The science of solid, homogeneous crystalline elements or compounds (minerals) that are non-opaque (e.g., quartz, ruby, diamond), and result from inorganic processes of nature; particularly, the study of their crystallography, physical and chemical compositions, and their effects on light). (cf. *optics, crystal.*)

Miniature Electronic Visual Aid (MEVA) Trade name for a self-contained, battery-powered, portable closed-circuit television system to afford magnified reading in any location; weight under 10 lbs; available magnification at 4X, 7X, and 11X; LED display. Current model is the MEVA II.

minification A decrease in the apparent size or perceived size of an object, by image size reduction in relation to object size; sometimes referred to as negative magnification.

minifier A lens system that reduces image-size in expectation of increasing visual field.

minimum separable angle See *angle, minimum separable.*

minus Algebraic term used to indicate a negative quantity or the vergence power of a concave lens surface; diverging power.

minus lens See *lens, minus.*

minus power See *power, minus.*

miosis (mī-o'sis) Contraction of the pupil or condition in which the pupil is very small, 2mm or less in diameter.

miotic drugs See *drugs, miotic.*

mire Focusing guide or target for an optical measuring instrument, commonly used in illuminated form on a keratometer; meridian mark.

mirror A surface capable of reflecting light rays and forming optical images. Such surface is smooth and made of highly polished metal or a thin film of metal on glass, quartz, or plastic.

mirror, cold A glass mirror designed to reflect most (90%) visible light and allow most infrared light (80%) to pass through.

mirror, first surface A highly polished, reflecting boundary where light is reflected without passing through any glass or optical medium.

mirror, parabolic A smoothly polished, aspheric reflecting surface in which the intersection of a perpendicular plane passing through its focal point creates a conic section; reflects parallel light rays to a point focus.

miter joint See *joint, miter.*

mixed astigmatism See *astigmatism, mixed.*

MLC Abbreviation for minimal lash clearance to indicate the position of the back surface of a spectacle lens as worn; q.v.

mm Abbreviation for millimeter; q.v.

modulation transfer function See *function, optical transfer.*

Mohs scale See *scale, Mohs.*

molded blank See *blank, molded.*

molding, corneal A change in corneal curvature due to the mechanical pressures of a contact lens. Alters refraction and may require corneal rehabilitation.

molding, impression The production of negative and positive casts of a patient's cornea and anterior bulbar curvatures for preparation of molded contact lens. Technique introduced in 1933 by Joseph Dallos (1905–1979), Hungarian ophthalmologist.

Moldite A trade name; see *alginate.*

Moll glands See *glands of Moll.*

Monel Trade name for a metal made by direct reduction of suitable ore; used in spectacle frames manufacturing; contains approximately 67% nickel, 28% copper, 5% other elements.

mono- Prefix meaning single; one.

monochromacy, cone (mon″o-krō′ma-se) Rare, total, congenital colorblindness, but with relatively normal visual acuity, normal electroretinogram and oculogram; may be complete or incomplete.

monochromacy, rod Rare, non-progressive, total, congenital color blindness, associated with poor vision, light sensitivity, and nystagmus.

monochromat A person with complete colorblindness; inability to discriminate hues; all colors appearing as shades of gray; also called achromat.

monochromatic Composed of light of one color or narrowly specified wavelength.

monochromatic radiation See *radiation, monochromatic.*

monocle A single eyeglass, designed to be worn or hand-held in front of one eye; usually provided with an attached cord or chain; introduced about 1800.

monocular (mo-nok'yu-lar) Pertaining to one eye or vision with one eye; uniocular.

monocular distance See *distance, monocular.*

monomer A simple molecule of a compound of relatively low molecular weight, capable of reaction by condensation or polymerization to form a dimer (2), trimer (3) or polymer (many).

monovision A contact lens fitting technique in which the dominant eye is corrected for distance vision and the non-dominant eye is corrected for near vision.

motile (mō'tīl) The capability of movement, generally spontaneous.

motility, ocular The science and study of extraocular muscles, their neural components, and the capability of spontaneous or induced movement of the eye or of its parts.

motion, against An optical phenomenon of retinoscopy in which the light image is displaced in a direction opposite to the movement of the light source, the retinoscope.

motion, with An optical phenomenon of retinoscopy in which the light image is displaced in the same direction as the movement of the light source, the retinoscope.

mounted See *lens, mounted.*

mounting In spectacle optics, the bridge, endpieces, and temples attached to rimless ophthalmic lenses to hold the lenses in position in front of the eyes.

mounting, finger-piece Pince-nez eyeglasses in which the pads that clasp the nasal bridge with spring tension are released or positioned by compression between the wearer's thumb and finger; patented and popularized by Charles H. Pixley of Chicago and Jules Cottet of France around 1900.

mounting, rimless In spectacle optics, the use of lens-holding devices located both temporally and nasally, the temporal piece holding a temple to either lens and the center piece holding both lenses together, the pieces being totally independent of each other (i.e., without a metallic or plastic rim to connect them together).

mounting, semi-rimless In spectacle optics, the use of lens-holding devices employing a center piece with metallic rims following the upper nasal to temporal edge of the lens and hinged there to the temples (i.e., two-hole mounting), or hinged through endpieces to appropriate temples (four-hole mounting).

MRP Abbreviation for major reference point; see *point, major reference.*

multi- Prefix meaning many.

multifocal See *lens, multifocal.*

multifocal contact lens See *lens, contact, multifocal.*

multifocal flat-top See *lens, straight-top multifocal.*

multifocal semi-finished blank See *blank, multifocal semi-finished.*

multifocal straight-top See *lens, straight-top multifocal; lens, bifocal flat-top.*

Multiframe Trade name for brow-bar suspension system for lenses. See *bar, brow.*

Munsell chromaticity (color diagram) See *color.*

Munson's sign See *sign, Munson's.*

muscae volitantes (mus'ā vol"i-tan'tez) Particles in the vitreous casting shadows on the retina, a visual sensation as of dark spots or specks floating before the eye. Their sudden appearance, particularly if associated with flashes of light, may be evidence of serious retinal detachment (vitreous floaters).

muscle, ciliary Smooth muscle portion of the ciliary body responsible for near-visual focusing. (cf. *ciliary body.*)

muscle, inferior oblique An extraocular muscle taking origin from the bony floor of the orbit nasally and passing laterally beneath the inferior rectus to insert, with no apparent tendon, variably between the lateral rectus muscle and the macular area into the sclera; innervated by the inferior division of the oculomotor nerve (Cranial Nerve III); in the primary position, this muscle rotates the eye upward and outward, as well as supplying excyclotorsion; its antagonist is the superior oblique of the same side.

muscle, inferior orbital A muscle of the lower eyelid taking origin from the inferior orbital periosteum, and inserting into the fascia of the lower eyelid and tarsal plate; innervated by sympathetic fibers; action is to retract the lower lid downward; its antagonist is the orbicularis oculi.

muscle, inferior rectus An extraocular muscle taking origin from the circumference of the optic foramen, and passing forward to insert on the under side of the sclera about 23° temporal to the median sagittal plane of the eye; innervated by the inferior division of the oculomotor nerve (Cranial Nerve III); in the primary position this muscle rotates the eye downward and secondarily adducts the eye; its antagonist is the superior rectus muscle of the same side.

muscle, iris dilator Within the iris, a radially arranged smooth muscle that is responsible for opening the pupil.

muscle, iris sphincter Within the iris, a circular smooth muscle that encircles the pupillary opening and is responsible for constriction when the eye is exposed to bright light; innervated by Cranial Nerve III, the oculomotor nerve.

muscle, lateral rectus An extraocular muscle which takes origin from the lateral margin of the optic foramen, and inserts on the lateral aspect of the sclera along the horizontal plane of the globe; rotates the eye outwardly; innervated by abducens nerve (Cranial Nerve VI); its antagonist is the medial rectus of the same side.

muscle, medial rectus An extraocular muscle taking origin from the circumference of the optic foramen, and inserting in the medial aspect of the sclera along the horizontal plane of the globe; innervated by the inferior division of the oculomotor nerve (Cranial Nerve III); rotates the eye medially; its antagonist is the lateral rectus muscle of the same side.

muscle, orbicularis oculi (or-bik″yu-lar′is ok′yu-lī) Thin, oval sheet of striated muscle which surrounds the interpalpebral fissure, covers the eyelids, and spreads out for some distance onto the temple, forehead and cheek; responsible for active eyelid closure.

muscle, superior levator An elevating muscle of the upper eyelid which takes origin from the upper border of the optic foramen, and has complex insertions on the top edge and lower front area of the tarsal plate of the upper eyelid with insertional horns extending medially and laterally to bony orbital tubercles; innervated by the superior division of the oculomotor nerve (Cranial Nerve III); elevates upper lid; its antagonist is the orbicularis oculi muscle of the same side.

muscle, superior oblique An extraocular muscle taking origin from the lesser wing of the sphenoid bone above the optic foramen; its long tendon passes through the trochlea (pulley), anchored to the bony medial orbital wall slightly anterior to the equator of the globe, and passes backward under the superior rectus muscle to insert into the lateral sclera variably between the insertion of the lateral rectus muscle and the optic nerve; in the primary position, this muscle rotates the eye down and outwardly, as well as supplying incyclotorsion. Innervated by the trochlear nerve (Cranial Nerve IV); its antagonist is the inferior oblique muscle of the same side.

muscle, superior rectus An extraocular muscle taking origin at the upper border of the optic foramen, and inserting into the upper lateral aspect of the sclera, about 23° temporal to the median sagittal plane of the eye; innervated by the superior division of the oculomotor nerve (Cranial Nerve III); in the primary position, this muscle rotates the eye upward, but secondarily adducts the eye; its antagonist is the inferior rectus of the same side.

muscular imbalance See *imbalance, muscular.*

mydriasis See *dilation.*

mydriatic drugs See *drugs, mydriatic.*

Myo-Disc lens See *lens, Myo-Disc.*

myoflange Anterior edge-shaping of a high plus contact lens creating an anterior configuration similar to a minus (–) power contact lens, providing centration of the commonly low-riding plus (+) lens.

myopia (mī-ō'pe-ah) "Nearsightedness." A refractive error of the eye in which light rays from infinity focus in front of the retina of an uncorrected eye; generally corrected by minus (–) powered or concave lenses (hypometropia).

myopia, axial A nearsighted refractive error in which the eye is too long from front to back for its optical power.

myopia, curvature Optically overpowered eye caused by steeper than normal corneal curvature or a crystalline lens that is too convex for the eye's axial length.

myopia, total (overall) The sum of all the ocular refractive components creating a nearsighted refractive error.

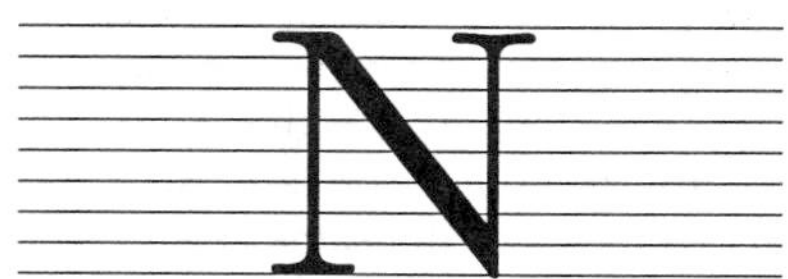

n The symbol for index of refraction; q.v. For example, crown glass, n = 1.523; hard resin; 1.498 polycarbonate, n = 1.586. See also *Table I* in the Appendix.

N **1.** Chemical symbol for nitrogen; q.v.
2. The S.I. symbol for the measure of force, a Newton, expressed in $kg/m/s^2$.

N.A. **1.** Abbreviation for numerical aperture, a measure of the optical efficiency of the objective lens of an optical system; the ratio of a lens diameter to its focal length.
2. Abbreviation for not applicable.

N.A.M.O. Abbreviation for National Association of Manufacturing Opticians; q.v.

N.A.O. Abbreviation for National Academy of Opticianry, Inc.; q.v.

N.A.O.O. Abbreviation for National Association of Optometrists and Opticians; q.v.

N.A.S.V. See *International Academy of Sports Vision.*

N.A.V.H. Abbreviation for the National Association for Visually Handicapped; q.v.

N.A.V.P.C. Abbreviation for National Association of Vision Program Consultants. Now known as National Association of Vision Professionals (N.A.V.P.); q.v.

N.B.S. Abbreviation for the U.S. National Bureau of Standards (name no longer used). See *National Institute for Standards and Technology* (name changed in 1989).

N.B.S. density number See *number, N.B.S. density.*

N.C.L.E. Abbreviation for the National Contact Lens Examiners; q.v.

N.C.S.O.L.B. Abbreviation for National Committee of State Opticianry Licensing Boards; q.v.

N.E.B.O. Abbreviation for the National Examining Board of Ocularists; q.v.

N.E.I. Abbreviation for the National Eye Institute; q.v.

N.E.I.S.S. Abbreviation for the National Electronic Injury Surveillance System; q.v.

N.I.O.S.H. Abbreviation for National Institute for Occupational Safety and Health; q.v.

N.I.S.T. Abbreviation for National Institute for Standards and Technology; q.v.

N.O.A. Abbreviation for the National Optometric Association; q.v.

N.S.P.B. Abbreviation for the National Society to Prevent Blindness; q.v. (Renamed Prevent Blindness America in 1994.)

Na Chemical symbol for the soft, alkaline, metallic element sodium, atomic number 11; a major cation in drugs; also used as an oxide in phototropic glass.

nanometer (nan-om′i-ter) Abbreviation nm. A unit of length equal to one-millionth of one millimeter or 10 Ångström units; used to measure the wavelengths of light; 10^{-9} meters. Replaces obsolete unit millimicron (mu).

nasal crest See *nasion.*

nasal edge See *edge, nasal.*

nasion Depression across the root of the external nose just below the level of the eyebrow; commonly called crest of the nose or nasal crest.

nasolacrimal duct See *duct, nasolacrimal.*

National Academy of Opticianry, Inc. (N.A.O.) A voluntary national organization whose primary function is the education of opticians; 6,000 + individual members, established in 1973. Office: 10111 M.L. King, Jr., Hwy. 112, Bowie, Maryland 20720-4299.

National Academy of Sports Vision (N.A.S.V.) See *International Academy of Sports Vision.*

National Association for Visually Handicapped (N.A.V.H.) A voluntary service organization established in 1954 in New York and San Francisco to help low-vision patients requiring special attention.

Provides large assortment of low-vision aids, trial and practice facilities.

National Association of Manufacturing Opticians (N.A.M.O.) A trade association incorporated in 1977; former office in Dallas, Texas, but phased out of operation in mid–1980s.

National Association of Optometrists and Opticians (N.A.O.O.) A voluntary organization established in 1960 to promote activities between optometrists and opticians; 13,500 members. Office: Cleveland, Ohio 44128.

National Association of Vision Professionals (N.A.V.P.) (Formerly National Association of Visual Program Consultants, 1976–1986.) Professional association primarily of program administrators in various aspects of preventing blindness; established 1976; 200 members. Office: Washington, D.C. 20036.

National Bureau of Standards, (U.S.) (N.B.S.) A federal agency located in Washington, D.C.; established in 1901 as a part of the U.S. Department of Commerce; maintains a major division in optics and established density filter numbers for eye protection in various types of welding. The name of this organization was changed in 1989 to the National Institute of Standards and Technology.

National Committee of State Opticianry Licensing Boards (N.C.S.O.L.B.) A voluntary organization of executive officers and members of state opticianry licensing boards and/or authorized agencies established in 1979 and organized for the purpose of improving the stature and conduct of opticianry licensing nationwide. Office: 10341 Democracy Lane, P.O. Box 10110, Fairfax Virginia 22030-8010.

National Contact Lens Examiners (N.C.L.E.) An examining and credentialing agency established to develop requirements and examinations for voluntary credentialing of contact-lens fitters and opticians designing and fabricating contact lenses. Established c. 1975 (originally as National Committee of Contact Lens Examiners); 7,710 credentialed individuals. Office: 10341 Democracy Lane, P.O. Box 10110, Fairfax, Virginia 22030-8010.

National Electronic Injury Surveillance System (N.E.I.S.S.) A division of the Consumer Product Safety Commission which maintains hospital emergency room census of injuries related to products, including spectacles and contact lenses.

National Examining Board of Ocularists (N.E.B.O.) A voluntary, U.S. examining and credentialing board established in 1980 for individuals devoting their professional activities to ocular prosthetics.

Formalized from earlier A.S.O. Education and Training Program for Ocularists.

National Eye Institute (N.E.I.) A division of the federally funded National Institutes of Health and part of the U.S. Public Health Service; established in 1970. Office: Bethesda, Maryland.

National Institute for Occupational Safety and Health (N.I.O.S.H.) A federal agency established by the U.S. Congress in 1970 to conduct research and promote worker protection: within the U.S. Department of Health and Human Services. Principal office: Atlanta, Georgia.

National Institute for Standards and Technology (N.I.S.T.) Federal agency, established in 1901 as National Bureau of Standards within the U.S. Department of Commerce; charged with the supervision of all units of weight and measure; name changed in 1989.

National Optometric Association (N.O.A.) A professional association primarily of minority ethnic members, founded by black optometrists in 1969; 350 members; devoted to increasing minority optometric manpower. Office: Columbus, Ohio 43205.

National Society to Prevent Blindness (N.S.P.B.) A voluntary charitable organization established in New York in 1908; 27 state affiliates. Renamed in 1994, Prevent Blindness America. Office: 500 Remington Rd., Suite 800, Schaumburg, Illinois 60173-4557.

Nd Chemical symbol for neodymium; q.v.

near interocular distance (NIOD) See *distance, near interocular.*

near intersection point (NIP) See *point, near intersection.*

near-point vision See *vision, near point.*

near point See *point, near.*

near reference point (NRP) See *point, near reference.*

nearsightedness See *myopia, hypometropia.*

nebula

1. A slight clouding of the cornea due to pathologic changes.
2. A liquid preparation used as a spray.

negative accommodation See *accommodation, negative.*

Negocoll Trade name for a hydrocolloid formulated by Dr. Alphonse Poller of Vienna for impression molding of the cornea or the enucleation socket. Adapted in 1933 as molding for contact lens manufacture by Josef Dallos (1905–1979) of Budapest.

neodymium A rare metallic element of yellowish tinge. Chemical symbol Nd, atomic number 60. Used in Nd-YAG laser providing the charged ions which "dope" the YAG crystal providing effective laser cutting of transparent membranes at the lens capsule. A successor to tungsten lamp filaments giving more light and longer life. Isolated in the early 1840s by Carl Gustav Mosander (1797–1858), Swedish physician and chemist.

neoprene Originally a trade name for the first widely successful synthetic rubber; developed in 1929 by Belgian-born, U.S. chemist Julius Arthur Nieuwland (1878–1936); made by polymerization of chloroprene; has greater stability than rubber; used in gasket on top of supporting tube for drop-ball impact test (A.S.T.M. methods D1415, D412); polychloroprene.

neovascularization (nē″o-vas-kyu-lar-i-zā′shun) An abnormal growth of blood vessels into an area generally without such vessels. In the cornea this occurs particularly from the limbal area spreading into the clear or avascular cornea. Generally a contraindication to the wearing of contact lenses.

Nernst lamp See *lamp, Nernst.*

nerve, optic Second cranial nerve; connects the ganglion cell layer of the retina to the optic chiasma and thence by the optic tract to the lateral geniculate ganglion, connecting the retina to the visual cortex; contains over 1,000,000 afferent fibers from the retina and some efferent fibers that end in the retina. Classified as a nerve of special sense, its length is divided into intraocular, intraorbital, intracanalicular, and prechiasmal or intracranial portions. It leaves the orbit through the optic canal to enter the middle fossa of the cranial cavity where it forms the optic chiasma. First described about 500 B.C. by Alcmaeon of Crotona, physician and dissecting anatomist, pupil of Pythagoras.

neur-, neuro- Combining prefix indicating relationship to nerves or the nervous system.

neutralization

1. Utilizing a focimeter to determine the dioptric power of an ophthalmic lens.
2. The combining of plus with minus or minus with plus lenses so as to produce a combination without power, thus determining the power of the examined lens.

Ni Chemical symbol for nickel; q.v.

nickel A silver-white metallic element, chemical symbol Ni, atomic number 28. Used in metal spectacle frame manufacture; a cause of contact dermatitis.

nickel silver A silver-white-appearing alloy of copper, zinc, and nickel; resistant to oxidation and used in spectacle frame manufacture.

nit
1. A psychophysical unit of luminance recently adopted by the Commission Internationale de l'Eclairage (C.I.E.), expressed as one candela per square meter of light source, or 1/10,000 stilbs.
2. The egg of a louse.

nitrogen A gaseous element, chemical symbol N, atomic number 7; found free in the atmosphere.

nm Abbreviation for nanometer; q.v.

nodal points See *points, nodal.*

NOIR Trade name for large line of goggles and filters; many incorporate ultraviolet absorbers, blue blockers, and infrared absorbers; originally an acronym for **No i**nfra**r**ed.

nominal Pertaining to a name, or existing in name only; trifling or small amount.

nominal surface power See *power, nominal surface.*

nomogram
1. A figure consisting of multiple straight or curved lines, each graduated for differing variables and aligned so that intersections have specific mathematical relationships.
2. In contact lens fitting, a graphic figure or table relating the keratometric readings to the selection of the lens curvature, power and diameter.

nomogram, Dyer A table based on keratometric findings from which computations are derived to design a contact lens. Developed in 1968 by John Allen Dyer, M.D. (b. 1923), ophthalmologist of Mayo Clinic, Rochester, Minnesota.

non compos mentis (non kom'pos men'tis) Not of sound mind.

non-linear optics See *optics, non-linear.*

non-removable lens See *lens, non-removable.*

norm
1. Standard; model; pattern.
2. General level; average.

normal In optics, a perpendicular

1. To a tangent of a curve or surface at the point of tangency; preferably referred to as a perpendicular.
2. Through an interface at a point of incidence, refraction and/or reflection of a ray, labeled as N in the object medium and N' in the image medium.

normal blind spot See *blind spot, normal.*

normal mounting line See *bisector, horizontal lens (HLB).*

nosepad The nasal bearing surface member of a spectacle front, also called pad.

notch, Izod A small, specific surface defect in glass (or metal) created or accidentally developed that concentrates strain or focalizes rupture on impact testing; concept developed by twentieth century English mechanical engineer, E.G. Izod.

Nu value, ν See *number, Abbé.*

nuclear sclerosis See *cataract, nuclear sclerotic.*

number A figure, word, or group of figures or words graphically representing an arithmetic sum.

number, Abbé (ab'ā) Sometimes called Nu value (ν). An arithmetic value between 1 and 100, derived as the reciprocal of the relative dispersion of a refracting medium; the closer the Abbé number is to 100, the more efficient the refractive medium, i.e., the ability to keep white (polychromatic) light from being dispersed (e.g., spectacle crown glass—Nu value, ν = 59), indicates the least amount of chromatic dispersion, suggesting a desirable refractive efficiency. Thinlite, i.e., a lead oxide glass with a lower Nu value, ν = 30, reveals a greater amount of chromatic dispersion, recognized as color fringes around reading material. Described by Ernest K. Abbé (1840–1905), German optical physicist.

Algebraically defined by the following formula

$$\text{If } \delta = \frac{(n_F - n_C)}{(n_D - 1)} \quad \text{and Nu, } \nu = \frac{1}{\delta} \quad \text{then } \nu = \frac{1}{\dfrac{(n_F - n_C)}{(n_D - 1)}}$$

$$\text{or } \nu = \frac{(n_D - 1)}{(n_F - n_C)}$$

where:

ν = the reciprocal relative dispersion (i.e., Abbé number or Nu value)

δ = the relative dispersion (i.e., delta)

n_D = the index of refraction for radiation of wavelength ≈ 589nm yellow

n_F = the index of refraction for radiation of wavelength ≈ 486nm blue

n_C = the index of refraction for radiation of wavelength ≈ 656nm red

number, aperture An optical constant determined by the apical angle (from a point source of light) of the maximum diameter cone of light which can pass through a given lens; numerical aperture.

number, atomic The number of protons in the nucleus of an atom (Z number).

number, f The ratio of the focal length of the lens to the diameter of the effective aperture (i.e., entrance pupil of the lens system). For example, stated f/2, f/4, or f/8, where the effective aperture is 1/2, 1/4 or 1/8 the focal length respectively. Also known as "f" value, "f" stop; sometimes called lens speed.

number, hardness A reference number indicating the relative degree of indentation resistance on Brinell, Knoop, Mohs, Rockwell, Vickers, and similar scales.

number, N.B.S. density Log scale of visual transmission of welder's goggles or shields, developed empirically in 1928 and experimentally refined in the 1940s by National Bureau of Standards (now U.S. National Institute of Standards and Technology). Shade numbers 1 to 14 specified in N.B.S. Circular 471, published in 1948; revised by A.N.S.I. in 1959.

Numont arm See *arm, Numont.*

Numont arm pliers See *pliers, Numont arm.*

nyctalopia (nik″ta-lō′pe-ah) Night blindness; impaired vision under reduced light; may be congenital or acquired; originally referred to in the writings of Hippocrates (c. 460–375 B.C.) to describe day blindness or the ability to see beter at night. Term introduced in 1684 by William Briggs (1642–1704), English physician.

nylon Trade name for a synthetic long-chain polymeric amide used for sutures and spectacle frames; a long-lasting material of great strength and wide industrial use.

nystagmus (nis-tag'mus) Involuntary, repeated oscillation of one or both eyes in any or all fields of gaze (dancing eyes).

nystagmus, latent An oscillation of the eyes which occurs and reduces visual capability only when one eye is covered.

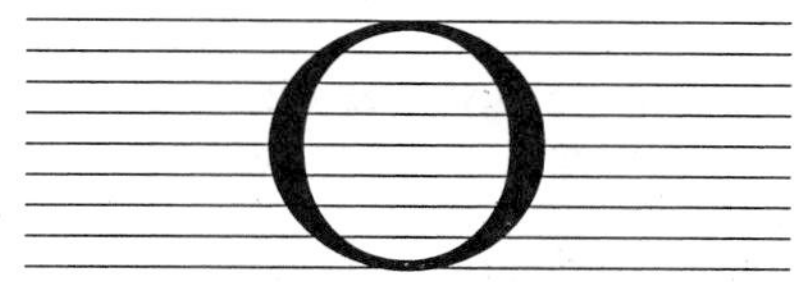

O **1.** Chemical symbol for oxygen; q.v.
2. Often used as the integer for zero; naught.

O_2 Symbol for molecular oxygen; the diatomic (two atoms) form of oxygen.

O.A.A. Abbreviation for Opticians Association of America; q.v.

O.D., OD Abbreviation for:
1. Oculus Dexter, Latin for right eye; see *oculus.*
2. Optical density; see *density.*
3. Doctor of optometry; see *optometrist.*
4. Popular term for overdose.

O.H.S.T. Abbreviation for Certified Occupational Health and Safety Technologist; q.v.; see *technologist, certified.*

O.L.A. Abbreviation for Optical Laboratories Association; q.v.

O.M.A. Abbreviation for Optical Manufacturers Association; q.v.

O.S. Oculus Sinister, Latin for left eye.

O.S.A. Abbreviation for Optical Society of America; q.v.

O.S.H.A. Abbreviation for the U.S. Occupational Safety and Health Administration; q.v.

O.U. Oculi Uterque; Latin for both eyes.

OWS Abbreviation for overwear syndrome; see *syndrome, overwear.*

O_2 flux The quantity of oxygen that will pass through a predetermined area of a contact lens material over a specified time when exposed to a pressure difference of oxygen.

ob- Prefix meaning toward; to; on; over; against.

objective refraction See *refraction, objective.*

oblique Slanting; not at right angles; other than perpendicular or parallel.

1. Ophthalmic terminology. The direction of any meridian other than 90° (vertical) and 180° (horizontal).
2. Ocular anatomy. Description of the two extraocular muscles, inferior oblique and superior oblique, that move the eye up and out or down and out, respectively.

oblique astigmatism See *astigmatism, oblique.*

obsidian A hard, usually dark-colored or black, volcanic glass yielding smooth convexities or concavities (conchoidal) when fractured; chemical composition is rich in silica, and similar to granite; very prevalent; sometimes used as a gemstone; named by Pliny (23–79 A.D.) for a Roman traveller, Obsius, whom Pliny credited with discovering the material in Ethiopia.

OC Abbreviation for center, optical; q.v.

occluder An opaque plastic device used to cover one eye; positioned during the evaluation of visual acuity or other ocular examination of one eye; worn therapeutically by young patients with strabismus to assist visual development in a deviating amblyopic eye by covering the preferred eye.

occlusion (o-kloo'zhun)

1. The act of blocking vision with a device placed before an eye; eye shield.
2. The obstruction or closing off of a structure, as in nasolacrimal occlusion or blockage of the tear duct.

Occupational Safety and Health Administration (O.S.H.A.) A U.S. federal agency established in 1971 by Congress, within the Department of Labor; enforces industrial safety and health standards, including those for workplace eye protection.

octo- Prefix meaning eight.

Octopus Trade name for a complex, computerized instrument for examination of the visual fields by static testing of visual thresholds in a programmed sequence over a given radius from fixation; manufactured by Interzeag of Switzerland.

ocul- A combining prefix denoting relationship to the eye; also oculo-.

ocular (ok'yu-lar)

1. Pertaining to the eye.
2. The eyepiece or proximal lens component of an optical system (e.g., Huygenian ocular); a negative eyepiece consisting of two

plano convex lenses, the convexities being directed toward the objective; developed by the Dutch physicist Christian Huygens (Huyghens) (1629–1695).

ocular albinism See *albinism, ocular.*

ocular decongestant See *decongestant, ocular.*

ocular fundus See *fundus, ocular.*

ocular lubricants See *lubricants, ocular.*

ocular media See *media, ocular.*

ocular motility See *motility, ocular.*

ocularist (ok-yu-lar'ist) A skilled technician in the science of fabrication and fitting of artificial (plastic) eyes and orbital prostheses; from the Roman artificial eye maker Oculariarus.

oculi (ok'yu-lī) Plural of oculus.

oculi uterque (O.U.) (yoo'ter-ke) Both eyes.

oculist (ok'u-list) Latin term previously used to designate an ophthalmologist.

oculo- A combining prefix indicating relationship to the eye.

oculus (ok'yu-lus) The organ of vision; eye.

Ocusert (ok'yu-sert) Trade name for a slowly dissolving, soft, banana-shaped insert of medication placed under the eyelid to provide prolonged drug therapy to the eye.

-ogist Suffix to indicate an individual skilled in the specified subject area.

-ology Suffix indicating knowledge of.

180° line See *line, geometric center*; *bisector, horizontal lens.*

one-piece multifocal lens See *lens, one-piece multifocal.*

opacities, corneal (o-pas'i-tez) Areas of localized density in the front surface of the eye; named according to degrees of density: nebula, faint haze; macula, moderate haze; leucoma, dense white.

opacity (o-pas'i-te)

1. The relative capacity to obstruct the transmission of radiant energy.
2. The reciprocal of transmittance (transparency), T.
3. Opacity, O = 1/T. (cf. *transmittance.*)

opaque Impervious to light; non-transparent and non-translucent.

opening, lens The area of a spectacle frame front encompassed by the rim, either left or right, which conforms to the shape and A and B dimensions of the lens intended to be inserted therein.

ophthalm- Prefix meaning eye.

ophthalmia (of-thal′mia) A long-ago superseded term referring to extensive eye inflammation; in English use since the fourteenth century (e.g., gonorrheal ophthalmia; sympathetic ophthalmia).

ophthalmic (of-thal′mik) Pertaining to the eye; ocular.

ophthalmic community See *community, ophthalmic.*

ophthalmic glass See *glass, ophthalmic.*

ophthalmic lens See *lens, ophthalmic.*

ophthalmic prescription See *prescription, ophthalmic.*

ophthalmic technician/technologist See *technician/technologist, ophthalmic.*

Ophthalmic Pathology, Registry of The eye section (established 1922) of the Armed Forces Institute of Pathology (established 1862) for the study of ocular tissues, biopsies, and whole globes as surgically removed; located at Walter Reed Army Medical Center, Washington, D.C. 20305.

Ophthalmic Photographers Society (O.P.S.) A professional association of photographers interested in photography of the eye; established 1969; 1,200 members. Office: Buffalo, New York 14215.

ophthalmo- Prefix indicating relationship to the eye.

ophthalmodynamometer (of-thal″mō-dī″nah-mom′i-ter) A calibrated mechanical diagnostic ophthalmic instrument to measure blood pressure in the central retinal artery or ophthalmic artery by measured increases of the intraocular pressure necessary to induce pulsations in the central retinal artery; introduced and named in 1917 by Paul Bailliart (1877–1969), French ophthalmologist, as a spring-loaded, hand-held, piston cylinder device.

ophthalmologist A physician concerned with and specializing in the medical, optical and surgical care of the eye and its appendages; treats the structure, function, and diseases of the visual system. Older term is oculist.

ophthalmometer (of″thal-mom′i-ter) Keratometer. A diagnostic optical instrument to measure radii of curvature of the anterior corneal surface (specifically called keratometer); precision instruments for this measurement were introduced in 1728 by Pourfour du Petit

(1664–1741), French physician; simplified and popularized by French ophthalmologist Louis Emile Javal (1839–1907), later blinded by glaucoma.

ophthalmoscope (of-thal'mo-skōp) Diagnostic optical instrument to examine the interior of the eye, the ocular fundus, and media as follows:

1. Direct, hand-held, greater magnification, but smaller field examination in erect image; invented in 1851 by Hermann von Helmholtz (1821–1894), German physician and physiologist.
2. Indirect, allows binocular examination with a large field (including peripheral retina), but under less magnification and with inverted image; first developed in 1861 as binocular instrument by Felix Giraud-Teulon (1816–1887), French ophthalmologist.
3. Spectacle, indirect; a lightweight spectacle-mounted binocular ophthalmoscope and light source; developed in mid-1960s by G.W. Crock, ophthalmologist of Melbourne, Australia.

ophthalmotrope (of-thal'mo-trōp) A mechanical apparatus used to demonstrate the movements and positions of the eyeballs.

-opia Suffix denoting a condition or defect of sight or of the visual organs.

-opsia Suffix denoting a condition or defect in vision.

-opsis Suffix referring to sight or view.

Optacon A portable, print-reading optical scanner introduced in 1970, that translates print into mechanical vibrations in Braille configurations that are read on the pulp tip of the index finger; used by blind Braille readers; current model, Optacon II, introduced in 1990, is computer-compatible.

optic atrophy See *atrophy, optic.*

optic axis See *axis, optic.*

optic chiasma See *chiasma, optic.*

optic disc See *disc, optic.*

optic foramen See *foramen, optic.*

optic nerve See *nerve, optic.*

optical Pertaining to the science of optics or vision.

optical anisophoria See *anisophoria, optical.*

optical axis See *axis, optical.*

optical center height See *height, major reference point.*

optical center See *center, optical.*

optical cross See *cross, optical.*

optical density See *density, optical.*

optical medium See *medium, optical.*

optical mineralogy See *mineralogy, optical.*

optical protractor See *protractor, layout.*

optical radiations See *radiations, optical.*

optical surface See *surface, optical.*

optical tape measure Informal name for stereoscopic device used to measure distances to about 100 yards, based on optical principles of triangulation; trade name, Rangematic.

optical transfer function See *function, optical transfer.*

optical zone, OZ See *zone, optical (OZ).*

Optical Industry Association (O.I.A.) See *Optical Manufacturers Association.*

Optical Laboratories Association (O.L.A.) Established in 1962 from earlier organization dating to 1894. An association of about 350 member firms that fabricate and assemble prescription eyewear and related materials in approximately 1,400 business locations in the United States for delivery to dispensing opticians, ophthalmologists and optometrists (formerly Optical Wholesalers Association). Office: 11096-B Lee Highway, Unit 102, Fairfax City, Virginia 22030.

Optical Manufacturers Association (O.M.A.) Established in 1916. An association of firms which manufacture or import eyewear, eyewear components, and related products. Recently known as the Optical Industry Association. Office: 6055-A Arlington Blvd., Falls Church, Virginia 22044-2706.

Optical Products Code Council (O.P.C.C.) A trade group established in 1986 by the Optical Manufacturers Association, Optical Laboratories Association, National Association of Manufacturing Opticians, and other members of the optical industry to establish standards for bar coding of optical products.

Optical Society of America (O.S.A.) Professional association primarily of research scientists in the field of light and dioptrics, established in Washington, D.C. in 1916; 11,000 members. Publishes two monthly journals, *Applied Optics* and the *Journal of the Optical Society of America.* Office: 2010 Massachusetts Ave., N.W., Washington, D.C. 20036.

optician A skilled artisan who designs or manufactures lenses, appliances, or optical instruments and devices; one who compounds, adapts and dispenses ophthalmic prescriptions.

optician, apprentice A technician who is engaged in an on-the-job program to learn the knowledge and skills of a dispensing or manufacturing optician.

optician, certified In the field of ophthalmic optics, a craftsman who has been tested and on passing, been credentialed by the American Board of Opticianry. The designation of such a person is American Board Opticianry Certified (A.B.O.C.). Approximately 23,000 current certificants.

optician, dispensing A skilled, technical expert who takes anatomical measurements, analyzes lens formulas and the wearer's needs, sets forth specifications for finished eyewear, and verifies, fits, and adjusts finished eyewear to adapt lens formulas to the wearer's needs. Also referred to as an ophthalmic dispenser.

optician, licensed One who holds a valid license issued by a state government body, authorizing the practice of dispensing opticianry within its jurisdiction.

optician, manufacturing A skilled artisan who surfaces lenses and processes lenses and frames according to specifications into finished products.

optician, master A technical expert in ophthalmic optics who has been tested at an advanced level and on passing, been credentialed by the American Board of Opticianry. The designation for such person is American Board of Opticianry Master (A.B.O.M.).

opticianry (op-tish'ən-re) The skilled vocational field of work of one who designs, fabricates, or manufactures lenses, optical instruments, visual appliances, and devices; the field of work of one who compounds, adapts, and dispenses ophthalmic prescriptions.

Opticians Association of America (O.A.A.) Initially formed in 1926 as Guild of Prescription Opticians of America, and reorganized in 1972 into O.A.A.; professional society of retail optical firms, individual opticians, and state society members. Office: 10341 Democracy Lane, P.O. Box 10110, Fairfax, Virginia 22030.

optics The branch of physics dealing with the science of vision and light, and its reflection and refraction by lenses, mirrors, and the eye.

optics, Cartesian The science elaborated and summarized by René Descartes (1596–1650) in his book *Dioptrique* (1636), using only the principles of physics, geometry and mathematics to explain the functions of light, lenses, prisms, and mirrors.

optics, cosmetic The use of spherical, cylindrical, or prismatic lenses to alter or enhance the appearance of an eye or its eyelids, especially after distortion due to trauma or enucleation.

optics, crystal That part of the science of light and dioptrics dealing with angular solids of definite form, built from naturally or synthetically produced units that are systematically arranged. (cf. *mineralogy, optical.*)

optics, Euclidean The mathematical and geometric foundations of optical science; developed c. 300 B.C. by Euclid, the most prominent Greek mathematician in his volume *Optics.*

optics, fiber The component of optical science dealing with the transmission of light and images around bends and curves by closely packed transparent fibers (light pipes) of very small diameter (often 0.003 inch to 0.005 inch in diameter) and high refractive index; fibers are usually coated with material of lower refractive index and may be arranged in random or coherent position; may be jacketed or unjacketed optical wave guides (often written as one word, *fiber-optics).* Developed in 1966 by a pioneering fiber optical engineer Charles Kuen Kao (b. 1933) of China, the United States, and Hong Kong, with the assistance of G. Hockhorn.

optics, fibre See *optics, fiber.*

optics, Gaussian (gow'shun) A simplified approximation of exact physical optics in which lenses are assumed to be infinitely thin, and parallel rays are similar to principal or axial rays. Named for Carl Frederick Gauss (1777–1855), German mathematician and professor at Göttingen.

optics, geometric The study of reflection and refraction of light by mathematic derivation, ray tracing, and image formation; follows the laws of linear propagation. Fundamental ray tracing (point-by-point) introduced in the early 1600s by German astronomer Johann Kepler (1571–1630).

optics, linear That portion of optical science concerned with variables that occur only in the first degree, multiplied by a constant, and combined only by addition and subtraction.

optics, Maxwellian The science of three-dimensional electromagnetic waveform meeting the several equations to explain the propagation of light; first described by James C. Maxwell (1831–1879), Scottish physicist and mathematician.

optics, mirror In the science of catoptrics, the functions of light in relation to smooth or highly polished surfaces.

optics, non-linear That portion of optical science concerned with variables which in relation to one another, are not of constants, exponents, or first-degree mathematical order; generally these are of high-order field strengths derived from the advent of laser light in the range of 10^4 to 10^7 above conventional (prelaser) intensities; initiated in 1961 by Peter Alden Franken (b. 1928), American physicist, and his coworkers.

optics, ophthalmic That part of the science of optics dealing primarily with the eye and its relations to light and optical devices associated with vision in both its physiologic and pathologic conditions.

optics, physical The portion of the science of light and vision derived from the laws and phenomena of mechanics, radiation, and atomic structure; the dioptric structure of the eye.

optics, physiologic The functional processes of the eye concerned with reception and processing of light, converting it to neural and perceptual vision by photochemical and electrophysiologic actions. Pioneering investigator Thomas Young (1773–1829), London physician, advanced this field to create its scientific base.

optics, spectacle That branch of physical and geometric optics dealing particularly with the design, manufacture, and fitting of eyeglasses and eyewear.

optics, statistical The use of standard mathematical methods to evaluate functions (averages, means, frequency distributions, linear or non-linear components, specificity, exponential variables, and the like) to design, predict and evaluate dioptric and catoptric precision in an optical system.

optics, visual That part of the science of sight or seeing dealing with light, its dioptrics, and its processing in the acts of vision; a component of ophthalmic optics.

Optivisor Trade name for an inexpensive head-mounted, binocular magnifier usually 1.5X magnification (20" focal length) to 3.5X magnification (4" focal length); a low-vision or occupational visual aid using a single-lens magnifying system.

opto- Prefix indicating relation to vision or sight.

optometer Any of a large class of optical and mechanical instruments used to measure refractive errors of the eye, generally combining both subjective and objective elements in measurements; predecessors of current refractometers and automated refractors. Developed after the 1860s by a large group of optical clinicians, led by German ophthalmologist Hermann Schmidt-Rimpler (1828–1915).

optometrist (op-tom'i-trist) A person credentialed and licensed to practice the profession concerned with vision, the practice of which may include any part or all of the services and care involved in the determination and evaluation of the refractive status of the eye and of other optical attributes and functions directly subserving vision, as well as the selection, design, provision, and adaptation of optical and optically related corrective measures, aids, and counsel for the preservation, maintenance, improvement, and enhancement of ocular performance, and, where permitted by statute, to use diagnostic and therapeutic pharmaceuticals.

optotype (op'to-tīp) Test letter, character, or symbol standardized for quantitation of visual acuity or resolving power of the eye (e.g., Snellen letter since 1862, Landolt broken C since 1909); test types. First standardized by Herman Snellen (1834–1908), ophthalmologist of Utrecht who introduced the word "optotype" in 1862.

Optyl (op'til) Trade name for a thermosetting epoxy resin of high-dimensional stability. Optyl is brittle when cold but flexible when warm and has the ability to return to its original molded shape when heated; it is lightweight and capable of retaining its shape without adjustment for long periods of time. Because it requires higher temperatures than cellulose acetate to adjust or shape, once configured it tends to stay in shape. Optyl is resistant to perspiration and is hypo-allergenic. It is vacuum-molded as a clear product, but dying allows for a great variety of surface finishes, colors, and color densities.

ora serrata (ō'rah se-ra'tah) Anterior boundary of the retina where the retina is attached to the choroid. Its gross contour is notched or toothed, resembling a saw, hence its description as serrated; margo undulato-dentatus.

orbicularis oculi muscle See *muscle, orbicularis oculi.*

orbit One of the two pyramidal-shaped bony cavities in the frontal aspect of the skull containing the eye and its appendages.

ortho- Prefix meaning straight, upright, correct, normal.

orthogonal Having to do with right angles, perpendicularity, or rectangular structure.

orthokeratology (or"tho-ker"-ah-tol'o-je) The study of correcting or reducing ametropic conditions of corneal curvature by wearing "tight" contact lenses to alter the shape of the cornea; a controversial corrective procedure.

orthophoria (or"tho-fō're-ah) Normal neuro-muscular alignment of the two eyes with no tendency to deviate when fusion is interrupted.

orthophoric (or"tho-fōr'ik) Pertaining to, or having, orthophoria.

orthoptics (or-thop'tiks) Analysis and training of patients for the improvement of visual sensory mechanisms, functional amblyopia, symptomatic heterophorias, and related abnormalities by prescribed non-surgical methods such as glasses, prisms, occlusion, and exercises. Traced to 1743 when Comte George Louis Leclerc du Buffon (1707–1788), French naturalist, began logical-use therapy of deviating eyes.

orthoptist A technician skilled in the field of measuring positional deviations of the eyes and sensory alterations in the visual process; conducts remedial training exercises when prescribed; certified in the United States by the American Orthoptic Council.

orthoscope An optical device which neutralizes the refracting power of the cornea through the use of a small glass container filled with water and held in contact with the eye; hydrophthalmoscope introduced in 1851 by German ophthalmologist Wilhelm Czermak (1828–1873); such a water-bath technique has been used since the early 1960s almost exclusively as a coupling medium for ultrasound examination of the eye and orbit.

orthoscopic Allowing a true and undistorted image; an optical system that produces an image free of aberration.

orthotopic Occurring at the normal place or upon the proper part of the body; in tissue transplants said of a graft, as the cornea, transplanted to a position formerly occupied by tissue of the same kind.

os **1.** An opening, orifice, or mouth.
2. A general term to designate bone.

os opticus Ossicle of Gemminger. A ring or horseshoe-shaped cancellous bone found in the posterior cartilageous cup surrounding the distal optic nerve as it leaves the sclera, in about half of bird species. Described in 1852 by Zolpgut Gemminger of Switzerland.

osculate (os'kyu-lāt") To kiss or touch closely; said of two lens surfaces which match precisely.

Osteopathic College of Ophthalmology and Otolaryngology (O.C.O.O.) A voluntary professional association of physicians (derived from the doctrines of Andrew Taylor Still, who established a new medical school in 1892, Kirksville, Missouri, with an emphasis on bone and manipulative concepts) specializing in eye, ear, nose, and throat diseases. Established 1916; 385 members. Office: Dayton, Ohio 45405

OTC Abbreviation for over the counter; applies to drugs or pharmaceuticals that are not required by law to be sold only by perscription.

-otomy See *-tomy.*

outset, bridge A spectacle front configuration wherein the bridge-fitting surface is located in front of the plane of the lenses (farther from the face).

outset, temple See *angle, set-back.*

over-refraction A determination of additional refractive power needed over a pair of spectacles or contact lenses to correct a visual error completely.

overall length See *length, overall.*

oxygen An essential gaseous element, chemical symbol O, atomic number 8. Necessary for life, and the health of corneal epithelium under contact lenses. Discovered in 1774 by Joseph Priestley (1733–1804), English chemist; named in 1779 by Parisian chemist Antoine Laurent Lavoisier (1743–1794).

oz Abbreviation for liquid ounce (approximately 30 ml).

OZ Abbreviation for zone, optical; q.v.

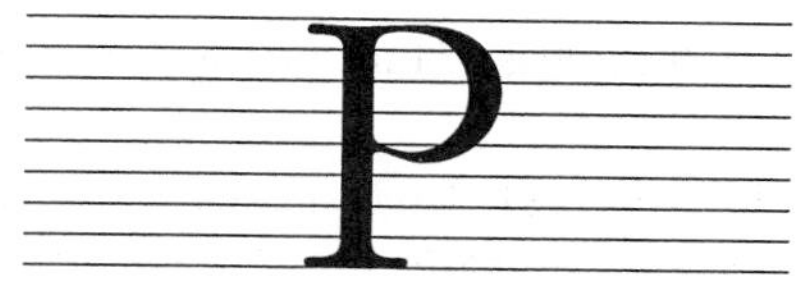

P.A. **1.** Posteroanterior direction, moving from back to front, as light reflected from the retina.
2. Abbreviation for physician's assistant.

PAC Acronym for curve, peripheral anterior; q.v.

pachometer; pachymeter (pah-kim'i-ter) An optical or ultrasonic instrument used to measure thickness; in ophthalmic use, an instrument to measure corneal thickness either optically (e.g., Ehlers and Sperling, 1977, manufactured by Haag-Streit) or by high-frequency A-scan ultrasound; trade names, Sonogage; XL Pach-Pen; Sonomed Pachymeter.

pachymetry The study of the measurement of thickness.

pad A cushion-like layer of soft material; (cf. *nosepad.*)

pad area See *area, pad.*

pad flair See *flair, pad.*

pad, rocking A nosepad mounted on a spectacle front that allows movement in one or more planes; a self-adjusting nose pad. Trade name, Flex Pad.

paddle tip See *tip, paddle.*

PAL Acronym for progressive addition lens. See *lens, progressive.*

palladium A rare, hard, inert metal of light weight and neutral color; chemical symbol Pd, atomic number 46; resembles platinum; used in dentures, orthodontic devices, and recently in spectacle frames. Isolated in 1804 by William Hyde Wollaston (1766–1828), English chemist, optical scientist, physicist, and physician.

palpebrae (pal'pe-brā) The eyelids.

palpebral (pal'pe-bral) Pertaining to, or of, an eyelid.

palpebral fissure See *fissure, palpebral.*

palsy (pawl'ze) Paralysis; loss of function of a muscle group.

PAM

1. Acronym for Potential Acuity Meter, an optical instrument to estimate post-cataract extraction visual acuity through a partial cataract; uses a reduced Snellen chart in the very near range; developed by David L. Guyton (b. 1944) and John S. Minkowski (b. 1951), Johns Hopkins ophthalmologists. (cf. *Visometer, Lotmar.*)
2. Acronym for Plasma Arc Machine; used in welding and metal cutting; may cause corneal burns in the unprotected eye.

pan- Prefix meaning all.

pannus Superficial vascularization of the cornea with infiltration of granulation tissue, particularly as seen from above in chronic trachoma; generally a contraindication to fitting contact lenses.

Panoptik (pan-op'tik) Trade name of a series of fused multifocal lenses made by Bausch & Lomb. Segment tops were slightly curved and corners rounded.

pantoscopic angle See *angle, frame pantoscopic (down angle).*

pantoscopic tilt See *tilt, pantoscopic.*

papilla A small protrusion or elevation; plural, papillae.

papillary conjunctivitis See *conjunctivitis, papillary.*

papilledema (pap"i-le-dē'mah) Elevation of the optic disc as visualized inside the eye, usually due to fluid accumulation in increased intracranial pressure, or malignant (grade IV) hypertension; choked disc; rarely due to extremely low pressure within the eye.

papin See *cleaner, contact lens, enzymatic.*

para- Prefix meaning beside; near; beyond; aside; amiss.

parabola The plane (two-dimensional) configuration outlined by a moving point that remains equally distant from a fixed point (focus) and from a fixed straight line (directrix); the curve formed by the section of a cone cut by a plane parallel to the side of a cone; (conic section).

parabolic In geometry, pertaining to a conic section or parabola, the aspheric curve formed by a section of a cone cut by a plane parallel to the side of the cone.

parafovea (par″a-fō′ve-ah) A capillary-free area in the retina about 2mm wide surrounding the fovea centralis or point of highest retinal resolving power; extends about 5° from fixation, but excludes the central 2° of the foveola.

parallax The apparent change in position of viewed objects when the viewing eye is moved from one position to another, or when the object is viewed alternately with one eye and then the other; a secondary factor or monocular clue to depth perception.

parameter A constant or variable whose value determines the specific form or performance of an object or procedure.

paraxial (par-ak′se-al) Close to the axis of an optical lens or system; close enough that in Gaussian optics, the trigonometric functions of ray slopes are essentially equal for ophthalmic purposes.

parfocal The optical condition of retaining the correct focus of an optical system when changing power of magnification.

parison (par′i-son)

1. Almost equal; evenly balanced.
2. A globular mass of molten glass taken from a furnace to be worked (molded, pressed, blown).

pars plana The posterior portion of the ciliary body which is non-secretory.

pars plicata ciliaris The anterior portion of the ciliary body from which the ciliary processes radiate; corona ciliaris; epithelium secretes aqueous fluid.

patho- Prefix meaning disease.

pathological diagnostics See *diagnostics, pathological.*

patient From the Latin, "patiens," to suffer; one who suffers or is ill (not a client or customer).

pattern, fluorescein A component of contact lens analysis aided by fluorescein in the tear film, and demonstrating the lens corneal relationship; the intensity of fluorescence is increased where the lens vaults over the cornea and is diminished where there is corneal bearing or touch; commonly assessed in diffuse slit-lamp illumination.

pattern, lens A cam, or template, used in lens-edging equipment to generate correct peripheral shape and geometric center location; also called lens former.

PCC Mnemonic for curve, posterior central; q.v.

pd ruler See *rule, millimeter.*

pd See *distance, interocular.*

Pd Chemical symbol for palladium; q.v.

pencil In geometric optics, a group of light rays emanating from a point or converging toward a point.

penumbra The partial illumination cast in the surround of an umbra (q.v.), or complete shadow (as in a solar eclipse).

perception The conscious mental or cortical registration of a sensory stimulus, generally in reference to the coordinates of one's own body and personal experience.

perception, depth Impression of relative or absolute differences in distance of objects from the observer; may be achieved with one eye or with two eyes. (cf. *stereopsis.*)

perception, light The ability of a patient to recognize the presence of a luminous source.

peri- Prefix meaning about; around; beyond.

perifovea (per″i-fō′ve-ah) A retinal band approximately 1.5mm wide, immediately surrounding the parafovea and representing the outer limit of the macular area of the retina; extends to approximately 10° from fixation, excluding the central 5° from the foveola.

perimeter An optical examining instrument usually of bowl or hemisphere configuration on which various light stimuli are displayed in order to test or quantify the sensitivity of the visual field. The standard reference perimeter since the late 1940s is the Goldmann bowl perimeter, developed by Swiss ophthalmologist Hans Goldmann (1899–1991), professor at the University of Bern.

perimeter, arc A mechanical device with a rotating portion of a circle, a chin or cheekrest, or other appliance for keeping the eye in the same position for testing of light sensitivity throughout the visual field; used for testing in the kinetic mode. Invented by Carl F. Richard Förster (1825–1902), professor of ophthalmology in Breslau.

perimeter, automated One of many variations in visual-field examining equipment that presents series of pre-programmed light stimuli to a patient at scattered locations in the visual field and then prints out a retinal sensitivity diagram within the radius of examination; usually based on static testing (variable stimulus intensity in fixed locations) rather than kinetic testing (variable position of a fixed intensity stimulus); trade names, Allergan Humphrey Visual Field Analyzer; Octopus; Squid; Dicon; Fieldmaster; Tomey; Synemed.

perimetry, kinetic (per-im'i-tre) Testing of the extent of the visual field using moving targets.

perimetry, static Testing of the extent (usually threshold) of the visual field using pre-programmed light stimuli of various intensities and areas in fixed locations.

peripheral

1. At or near the edge or outside margins.
2. Away from central or axial region; the outlying part, surface, structure, or portion of a system; applicable to the description of an ophthalmic lens, the retina, or a visual-field examination.

peripheral power error See *error, peripheral power.*

periscope An optical viewing instrument enabling an observer to see around an obstruction in the line of view; may incorporate multiple mirrors, multiple prisms, or fiber optics.

periscopic lens See *lens, periscopic.*

permeability Permitting passage of a substance; see *Dk.*

Petzval curvature of field See *curvature of field.*

Ph.D. Abbreviation for the academic degree, doctor of philosophy, a university terminal degree earned following the bachelor's or master's degree; held by most laboratory research scholars.

phaco- (fāk'o) Pertaining to the crystalline lens.

phacoemulsification (fāk"o-ē-mul"si-fi-kā'shun) A surgical procedure that shatters and breaks up the nucleus and cortex of the human crystalline lens; commonly employs ultrasonic vibrations and is used in extracapsular cataract removal Developed in 1966–1969 by Charles D. Kelman, ophthalmologist of New York, New York.

phakic (fā'kik) Refers to an eye possessing its crystalline lens. (cf. *pseudophakic.*)

-phoria (fō're-ah) A combining form meaning a tendency to turn or bear. See *heterophoria*; *orthophoria.*

phoropter (for-op'ter) Rotary-mounted trial assemblage of lenses and prisms used to determine the refractive state of the eye, its optical correction, and the binocular muscle balance; phoro-optometer.

phosphor Substance which has the property of absorbing energy and releasing it again in the form of luminescence; phosphorescence.

phosphorescence (fos"fo-res'ens) Property of emitting light, without any apparent rise in temperature, or the light so produced, due to absorption of radiation from another source, and lasting after exposure has ceased.

phot (fot) A psychophysical unit of illumination expressed as one lumen per square centimeter; equals 10^4 lux.

photo- A combining prefix indicating relation to light.

photobiology That part of the science of living organisms dealing with the effects of light on living tissues.

Photocentron Trade name for a special Polaroid camera that produces a picture showing the corneal reflexes in relation to the lens or lens opening of a spectacle mounting or frame being fitted; used for precise positioning of ophthalmic lens optics.

photochromatic lens See *lens, phototropic.*

photochromatic See *lens, phototropic.*

photocoagulation The use of monochromatic collimated light in the form of a laser beam to cauterize, seal, or destroy blood vessels within the eye; may also be used to repair detached tissue or for performing an iridotomy to improve the circulation of aqueous humor from the posterior to the anterior chamber.

photofrin A commercially available and enriched hematoporphrin derivative which localizes in malignant tissue and greatly increases photosensitivity; used to promote tumor death by laser energy.

PhotoGray Trade name for an ophthalmic lens made of photochromic glass varying in light transmission from approximately 45% to 85%; appears neutral gray in hue.

photomedicine The study and application of various light types to etiologic, diagnostic, and therapeutic roles in disease.

photometer (fo-tom′i-ter) An optical instrument designed for measuring radiant energy in the ultraviolet, infrared, or visible regions of the electromagnetic spectrum; light meter.

photometrics (fō″to-met′riks) The science of measuring light both in psychophysical units and in its ability to elicit visual sensation in the eye; is confined to the visible spectrum from 300nm or 400nm to 760nm or 780nm; distinguished from the purely physical, or radiometric, system that can be used across the entire spectrum of electromagnetic energy and is usually expressed in joules or watts per unit area.

photometry (fo-tom′i-tre) The measurement of the intensity or of the relative illuminating power of light.

photon (fō'ton) The basic quantum particle of electromagnetic energy; the particles of light that transmit electromagnetic force; concept evolved in the 1920s from theoretical quantum physics of Max Planck (1858–1947), German physicist, and Albert Einstein (1879–1955), naturalized U.S. citizen and physicist of Princeton, New Jersey; term coined in 1923 by American physicist Arthur Holly Compton (1892–1962).

photophobia Abnormal sensitivity or intolerance to light.

photopic vision See *vision, photopic.*

photosensitive lens See *lens, phototropic.*

photosensitizing drug See *drug, photosensitizing.*

phototropic (fō-to-tro'pic)

1. A response to light which may be mechanical or optical.
2. A tendency to change color when exposed to light, as the silver halides in light-sensitive lenses, which darken on exposure to ultraviolet light. (photochromic).
3. A tendency to movement of a part of a plant toward (or away from) light sources (heliotropic).

phototropic lens See *lens, phototropic.*

phthisis (ti'sis) In ophthalmology, a wasting away, shrinkage, or atrophy of the eyeball; may at times be managed for cosmetic improvement by fitting a reform prosthesis; phthisis bulbi.

physical optics See *optics, physical.*

physics The science dealing with the properties, changes, interactions, laws, and related phenomena of matter and energy, including optics.

physiologic optics See *optics, physiologic.*

physiological Of or pertaining to the science which deals with the functions of living organisms or their parts.

physiology The science of the functions of living organisms and their parts.

PIC Acronym for curve, posterior intermediate; q.v.; see *curve, intermediate.*

pico A combining form in measurement indicating one trillionth (10^{-12}) of a unit.

piece, center That portion of a rimless spectacle mounting that connects the two lenses together at the nasal side of each lens, usually using screws through drilled holes in the lens, set into a threaded hole in a strap extending from a spring type shoe or plate, on which the nasal side of the lens is held; sometimes called the bridge piece.

pilocarpine (pī″lo-kar′pin) A plant alkaloid drug of cholinergic activity widely used in the topical treatment of glaucoma; as a side effect, causes the pupil to become small (miotic); introduced for the medical care of glaucoma in 1876 by Adolf Weber (1829–1915), Darmstadt ophthalmologist.

pin A cylindrical piece of wood, metal, or other material used to fasten separate articles together.

pin bevel See *bevel, pin.*

pin-cushion distortion See *distortion, pin-cushion.*

pince-nez (pans′nā″) Eyeglasses, usually rimless, held before the eyes by a simple spring mechanism gripping the bridge of the nose; introduced in many forms beginning in the mid-1880s.

pinguecula (ping-gwek′yu-lah) A localized, yellowish-gray, elevated mass in the bulbar conjunctiva of the eye, nasal or temporal to the cornea in the exposed interpalpebral area. Generally innocuous and rarely becomes inflamed; plural, pingueculae.

pinhole A tiny (e.g., 0.05mm) opening or aperture, often used to estimate any potential improvement in visual acuity that might be achieved by refractive correction or other optical assistance.

pins, marking Small, metal, spring-mounted pointed cylinders on a focimeter, inked and used to mark the major reference point and horizontal lens bisector on an ophthalmic lens.

Placido's disc See *disc, Placido's.*

plane A surface, such that a straight line joining any two of its points lies wholly in that surface.

plane, face A plano surface representing the vertical orientation of the face tangent to the upper orbital ridges and the point of the chin; one of several facial planes.

plane, Listing's A vertical and equatorial plane penetrated by the anteroposterior Y axis of Fick, and containing both the X and Z axes of Fick; divides the globe into anterior and posterior halves. Originally described in 1854 by Johann Benedikt Listing (1808–1882), professor of optics at Göttingen.

plane, midsagittal (plane median) A vertical plane passing through the body from front to back and through the length of the (sagittal)

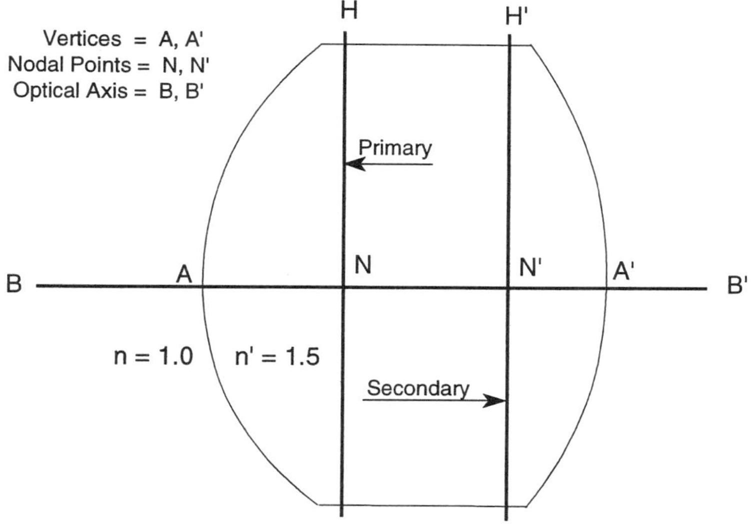

Figure 30 H, H' = Principal planes (thick lens).

suture line between the two parietal bones of the skull, dividing the body into right and left halves.

plane polariscope See *polariscope, plane.*

plane, primary principal The principal plane at which incident light rays from the primary focal point intersect and graphically are shown to be refracted parallel to the optical axis, then intersect the secondary principal plane. Also known as anterior principal plane (see Figure 30).

plane, principal In geometric optics, a plane perpendicular to the optical axis of a lens wherein incoming or emergent light rays are said to be refracted; one to one (1:1) magnification, also called unit plane; cardinal plane (Figure 30).

plane, sagittal In anatomical description, any vertical plane that passes through the body, or a component of the body, parallel to the median plane.

plane, sagittal focal In ophthalmic optics, the plane perpendicular to the tangential plane in oblique astigmatism; secondary plane.

plane, secondary principal The principal plane at which incident-parallel rays from infinity graphically are shown to be refracted, such that they focus at the secondary focal point; also known as the posterior principal plane. (See Figure 30.)

plane, spectacle A flat, geometric surface projected through the posterior lens vertices equidistant from corresponding points of a pair of mounted ophthalmic lenses; used as a reference for the orientation of ophthalmic lenses in front of the wearer's eyes.

plane, tangential In ophthalmic optics, a plane containing the optical axis of a lens system and an off-axis object, primary plane.

plano See *lens, plano.*

plano lens See *lens, plano.*

plano surface See *surface, plano.*

plaque

1. A decorative attachment for a spectacle frame.
2. On the skin, a flat area or patch of altered structure.
3. A patch or flat area of conjunctival thickening or premalignant change.

plaque, hyaline (hī'ah-lin) Localized, vertically oval areas of scleral yellowing, anterior to the insertion of the medial or lateral rectus muscles; generally without symptoms and appearing in older individuals (focal senile translucency of the sclera).

plasma

1. A high-intensity gas of electrons and positively charged ions, used for plasma welding and metal cutting; may cause corneal burns.
2. The fluid portion of the blood.

plastic A substance of linear or cross-linked organic polymers produced by chemical condensation or polymerization that can be molded or cut-formed (e.g., cellulose acetate, methyl methacrylate, polycarbonate).

plastic frame See *frame, plastic.*

plastic, thermolabile (ther"mo-lā'bil) A polymerized organic compound having long, linear carbon-carbon chains with two radicals on each carbon atom; will alter under heat (thermoplastic) (e.g., methacrylates).

plastic, thermostable (ther"mo-stā'bil) A polymerized organic compound having cross-linked or three-dimensional, carbon-carbon chains; when once hardened under heat, such compounds are not softened by heat (thermosetting) (e.g., allyl resins, polyesters).

-plasty Suffix meaning to form; usually referring to a type of plastic surgery on a specific part of the body (e.g., blepharoplasty—a reconstructive operation on an eyelid).

plate, rolled gold Thin sheets of at least 10K gold, bonded by heat and pressure to one or more surfaces of a supporting metal, and weighing less than 1/20th, by weight, of the total metal content.

plate, tritan A single test plate of 169 polychromatic color discs arranged contiguously in a square; developed in 1955 by Dean Farnsworth (1902–1959), color scientist of the U.S. Navy, to detect the rare congenital yellow/blue color deficiency.

plates, Arden A series of cards, usually seven, printed with sinusoidal gratings of varying contrast and displayed progressively from a slipcase at reading distance; used for clinically testing contrast sensitivity; developed in 1977 by G.B. Arden of New York and London. Not to be confused with the Arden index (1962); also developed by G.B. Arden as an electro-oculographic ratio obtained by dividing the dark trough potential by the light-peak potential and multiplying by 100.

plates, H-R-R Abbreviation for Hardy-Rand-Rittler; a series of 24 plates introduced in 1954 to test color vision against background of gray confusion dots; initially produced by American Optical Co.; developed by LeGrand H. Hardy (1895–1954), New York ophthalmologist, with Gertrude Rand and M. Catherine Rittler.

plates, Ishihara See *test, Ishihara.*

plates, Stilling's The first pseudoisochromatic plates to detect deficiencies of color perception; 10 plates originally introduced in 1883 by Jacob Stilling (1842–1915), clinical ophthalmologist of Strasbourg, Germany; twenty different editions were published by 1900.

pliers A hand-held tool consisting of two handles attached to jaws, pivoting about a fulcrum; used to grip, bend, cut, or otherwise manipulate materials.

pliers, crimping Hand-held gripping tool having two parallel jaws perpendicular to the length of the handle in the form of a T, with rough facing jaws used to grab and break glass away from an ophthalmic lens in a chipping manner. Also called "chipping" or "cribbing" pliers.

pliers, half-round Hand-held gripping tool with one round, tapered jaw and one flat-faced, tapered jaw; used in adjusting spectacle frame and mounting pad arms.

pliers, Numont arm Hand-held gripping tool with articulated jaws that have a small transverse groove for gripping the arm of a spectacle mounting; used for reshaping the arm or in angling the earpiece.

plus lens See *lens, plus.*

plus power See *power, plus.*

PMMA Mnemonic for the term **p**oly**m**ethyl **m**eth**a**crylate; q.v.

pneumotonometer See *tonometer.*

point

1. A minute mark, or dot, having a definite position, but no size, shape, or extension.
2. A location from which measures are made, as focal point.
3. An ambiguous term meaning 1/5mm (i.e., 0.2mm) in lens thickness measurements.
4. An ambiguous term for measuring type size that varies in different countries. See *Standard Revised Jaeger.*

point, distant intersection (DIP) That location on an ophthalmic lens where the fixation axis intersects the lens when the eyes are in the primary position (i.e., focused at 20 feet or beyond).

point, distant reference (DRP) That location on a progressive-power lens blank designated by the manufacturer at which the prescription specifications, except prism power, for the distant portion are to apply. If prism power applies, it must be verified at the prism reference point. See *lens, progressive.*

point, error-free The location on a lens at which the prism power actually corresponds to that prescribed, which should also be the location of the MRP. Any disparity between MRP and the error-free point indicates unwanted prism. This term facilitates communication concerning prism and centration measurement in lens manufacture. See *point, major reference.*

point, far Also P.R. (punctum remotum); that location upon the visual axis which is sharply imaged on the retina when accommodation is relaxed. In myopia it is less than infinity; in hyperopia it is a virtual point behind the retina.

point, fitting That location on a progressive-addition lens blank designated by the manufacturer as a reference location for positioning the lens in front of a patient's eye (see Figure 29). See also *lens, progressive.*

point, focal The locus of convergence of light rays.

point, major reference (MRP) That location on an ophthalmic lens at which the specified distant prescription requirements should apply (commonly, but less precisely referred to as the optical center, OC). When no prism is prescribed, the optical center, OC, is the major reference point, MRP. (See Figure 20.)

point, near Also P.P. (Punctum Proximum). The closest location at which accommodation can be momentarily maintained to achieve clear focus; the nearest point of clear vision.

point, near intersection (NIP) That location at the reading level on an ophthalmic lens where the fixation axis intersects the lens when the eyes are converged to focus on near objects, usually at the reading or working distance.

point, near reference (NRP) That location on a progressive power lens designated by the manufacturer at which, except for prism power, the specifications for the near portion are to apply. This location is at the center of the near verification circle. If prism power applies, it must be verified at the prism reference point. (See Figure 29; see also *lens, progressive.*)

point, nodal Singular for points, nodal; q.v.

point of incidence Location at which a ray of light strikes a refracting or reflecting surface.

point of regard A location in space upon which visual attention is directed while the eye is aligned foveally to such point of fixation; point of fixation.

point, primary focal

1. The actual location on the optical axis from which **real** (i.e., diverging) object rays, incident on a plus lens, are rendered parallel after refraction (Figure 31a).
2. The apparent location on the optical axis to which **virtual** (i.e., converging) object rays, incident on a minus lens, are rendered parallel after refraction (Figure 31b).

point, prism reference That location on a progressive lens where the lens manufacturer designates that prism values are to be determined. Prism measured at this point will be the resultant of the prescribed prism and the prism used for thinning (see Figure 29). (cf. *point, error free.*)

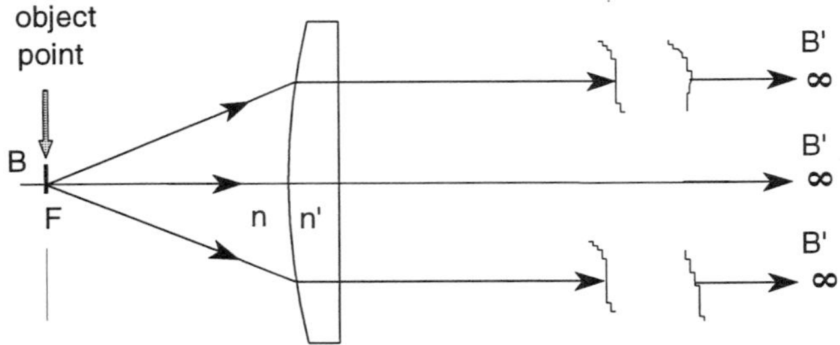

Figure 31a Primary focal point (F, plus lens).

point, secondary focal The location on the optical axis of a lens, at which incident parallel rays of light, as from a very distant object, after refraction converge in a plus lens (Figure 32) or appear to diverge in a minus lens, as a real or virtual image point, respectively.

points, cardinal The six points on the optical axis of a lens system (i.e., primary and secondary focal points, primary and secondary principal points, and primary and secondary nodal points); also known as principal points (Figure 33). See *optics, Gaussian.*

points, nodal A pair of conjugate points on the principal axis of an optical system at which any incident ray that passes through the first nodal point leaves the system as though from the second nodal point and parallel to the incident ray. Thus, the refracted ray is unchanged in direction, but is displaced along the optical axis (see Figure 33). The concept of nodal points introduced in 1844 by L.F. Moser (1805–1880).

polariscope, plane An optical inspection device consisting of two sheets of Polaroid film with axes of polarization at right angles to each other; positioned in front of a light source to produce attenuation of the light. The presence of strain-induced birefringence in a lens is visualized polariscopically by placing it between two such polarizing films and noting the colored (isochromatic) irregular lines that are a measure of the amount of strain present in the lens.

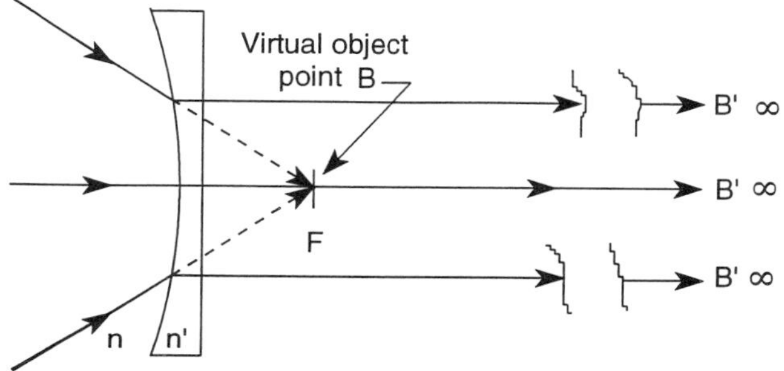

Figure 31b Primary focal point (F, concave lens).

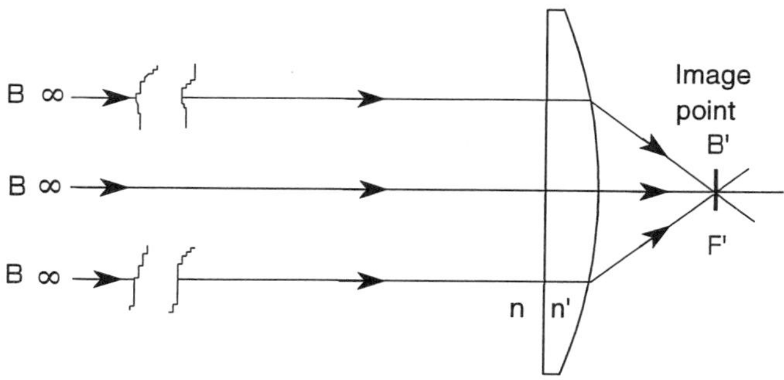

Figure 32 Secondary focal point (F')

polarity, image In light science, the display of opposite characteristics, such as bright characters on a dark background or dark characters on a light background.

polarization The act, process, or result of altering the transverse wave motion of radiant energy so that it is not uniform in amplitude in all directions in a plane perpendicular to the direction of propagation. See *lens, polarizing*.

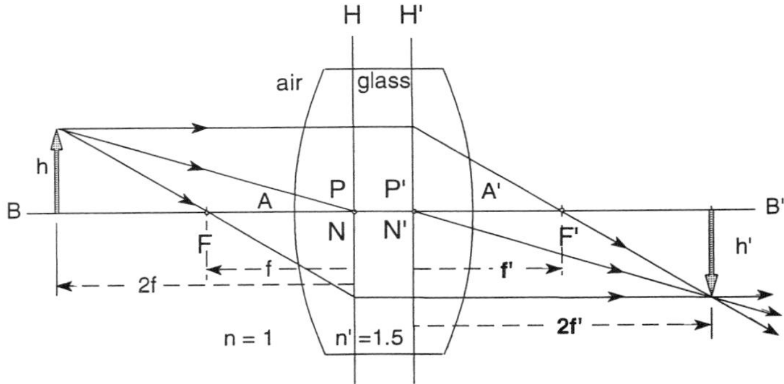

F = primary focal point; F' = secondary focal point; P = primary principal point; P' = secondary principal point; N = primary nodal point; N' = secondary nodal point; H = primary principal plan; H' = secondary principal plane.

Figure 33 Cardinal points of a lens and related principal planes.

polarizing lens See *lens, polarizing.*

Polaroid

1. A name coined in 1934 by Clarence Kennedy, Smith College professor, for a synthetic polarizing material made of plastic.
2. The name of a major company, incorporated in 1937, formed by Edwin H. Land (1910–1991), self-taught physicist of New York and Massachusetts.

Polaroid lens A trade name from one of 533 patents held by Edwin H. Land (1910–1991), American optical inventor. See *lens, polarizing.*

Polaroid vectograph See *vectograph, Polaroid.*

pole, aspheric (as-fer'ik) The point on the front surface of a non-spherical lens about which the asphericity is centered. The major reference point of the lens should be coincident with the axis of the aspheric pole or the visual benefits of the asphericity are negated and the field severely narrowed.

poliosis (pōl"e-o'sis) Loss of pigment in hair, particularly seen in eyelashes following certain inflammatory eye diseases.

poloxamines Hydrophilic surfactant polymers of various chain lengths used as contact lens cleaning, wetting, and soaking solutions.

poly- Prefix meaning much; many.

polyamide An organic compound of more than one amide (a class of compounds derived from ammonia by replacement of one hydrogen atom with a metal or acid radical); strong flexible material; used in sutures and ophthalmic frames; nylon-6,10.

polycarbonate An extremely long-chain thermolabile lens material with a 1.586 index of refraction. Because of the high index, lenses processed from this material are thinner and lighter than lenses of crown glass or CR-39. This material has good electrical insulating properties, dimensional stability, and very high impact resistance, but because of its softness, must be coated to resist scratching after surfacing or molding. Introduced as a safety material in mid-1970s; trade names, Gentex; Supershield. See *Table I, Index of Refraction* in the Appendix.

Polycarbonate Lens Council Trade association of polycarbonate manufacturers and laboratories fabricating polycarbonate lenses; established in 1989; approximately 60 group members. Office: Torrance, California 90503-2536.

polyimides Organic linear polymer compounds commonly synthesized from dianhydrides and diamines containing the bivalent group –NH, to which are attached only acid radicals; used as resins, adhesives, semi-conductors and high-temperature insulation.

polymacon A hydrophilic (soft) contact lens polymer $(C_6H_{10}O_3)_n$ first marketed by Bausch & Lomb, Inc., in 1971 following FDA clearance; water content, 38.6%; refractive index 1.43. Introduced in 1960 by Otto Wichterle and Drahoslav Lim of Czechoslovakia.

polymer A compound formed by joining smaller molecules, referred to as monomers. Organic plastics are macromolecules made up of a large number of monomers linked by covalent bonds.

polymethyl methacrylate (PMMA) (pol″e-meth′il meth-ak′ril-āt) A linear acrylic polymer of high optical clarity used to make hard contact lenses, artificial eyes, and intraocular implants; a thermolabile or thermoplastic which softens under heat at 122°F to 254°F; used to make certain ophthalmic frames; acrylic; methyl methacrylate. Introduced by Rohm & Haas Company of Philadelphia, Pennsylvania, as "Plexiglas" in 1935; by Imperial Chemical Industries, Ltd., of Bath, England, as "Perspex" in 1935, and by E.I. DuPont of Wilmington, Delaware, as "Lucite" in 1935.

polymide Any of a class of polymeric synthetic resins resistant to high temperature, wear, and corrosion; used in some spectacle frames.

polypropylene A polymerized gaseous hydrocarbon yielding a very clear optical plastic used in manufacture of haptics for intraocular lenses; also used for contact lens forceps; suitable for generation by molding.

polysiloxane Any of a class of polymerized organic compounds containing alternate silicon and oxygen atoms; made by hydrolysis of chlorosilanes or alkoxyl-silanes, stable over a broad temperature range; used as a lens coating to increase scratch resistance.

polyurethane Any of various linear polymers that contain $NHCO_2$ linkage of the type found in carbamic esters; obtained by reaction of isocyanate ester with polyester or glycol; used in making frames, elastomers (Spandex) and resins; resins are used as material for spectacle lens, index 1.56 to 1.6. Suitable for lens production by casting, similar to CR-39; density and refractive index are increased by addition of halogens to the molecular structure.

polyvinyl, alcohol A polymerization product of the univalent group CH_2CH– to which an OH radical is attached; in solution this is used to improve the wetability of a contact lens, or prolong contact of a pharmaceutical agent with the corneal surface; is also used as an ocular lubricating agent, or viscosity-increasing agent.

position, horizontal segment (HSP) The horizontal location of the vertical segment bisector (VSB) measured from the vertical MRP bisector (VMRPB); expressed as "inset" when located nasally from the VMRPB (see Figure 20). See also *inset, segment, SI.*

position, primary In visual physiology, the position of a viewer's head and eyes when standing with normal posture and focusing on a distant object directly in front of the viewer. This position determines where the viewer's visual axes intersect the spectacle lens planes when viewing a distant object.

position, vertical segment (VSP) The vertical location of the horizontal tangent to the top of a multifocal segment measured from the HLB, (horizontal lens bisector), being

1. A zero value, when coincident with the HLB, stated as being on.
2. A positive value (e.g., +4mm below the HLB), stated as 4B.
3. A negative value (e.g., –4mm above the HLB), stated as 4A.

Refer to Figure 20; formerly, but inaccurately, referred to as "below" and algebraically determined by the formula

$$\text{VSP} = \frac{B}{2} (-) \text{ segment height}$$

where

B = the boxed vertical dimension of the finished ophthalmic lens.

positive accommodation See *accommodation, positive.*

post- Prefix meaning behind; after.

posterior chamber See *chamber, posterior.*

potassium A silver-white, low-melting-point chemical element of the alkali metal group; chemical symbol K, atomic number 19; more reactive than sodium; oxidizes rapidly in air and reacts violently in water, releasing hydrogen to flame; must be preserved in kerosene or similar oil-based liquid; first extracted and named in 1807 by Humphry Davy (1778–1829), English experimental chemist.

potential acuity meter See *meter, potential acuity.*

power The ability or capability of effecting or doing something.

power, add See *addition (spectacle add).*

power, addition See *addition (spectacle add).*

power, angular magnifying (M) See *magnification, angular.*

power, corrective A general term comprising the spherical and/or cylindrical vertex power as well as the prismatic power of an ophthalmic lens.

power, cylinder The difference (plus or minus) between the powers measured in the two principal meridians of an ophthalmic lens.

power density See *density, power.*

power, dioptric The ability of a lens or lens system to change the vergence of incoming light rays. Unit dioptric power is the reciprocal of the secondary focal length of a lens of 1-meter focus (Figure 34).

power, dispersive An optical function indicated by a ratio; the ability of a transparent isotropic lens material to break up light into its component wavelengths (i.e., colors); specifically, the difference in the indices of refraction for the Fraunhofer F and C spectral lines divided by the difference in the Index of Refraction for the intermediate Fraunhofer D line (589.3) and unity, expressed as the Greek lowercase letter δ, delta. See *dispersion, relative.* Algebraically expressed as

$$\delta = \frac{(n_F - n_C)}{(n_D - 1)}$$

power, distant The refractive correction prescribed for improvement of visual acuity at infinity or when no accommodation is employed by the eye; expressed in diopters; the dioptric power of the distant portion of an ophthalmic lens.

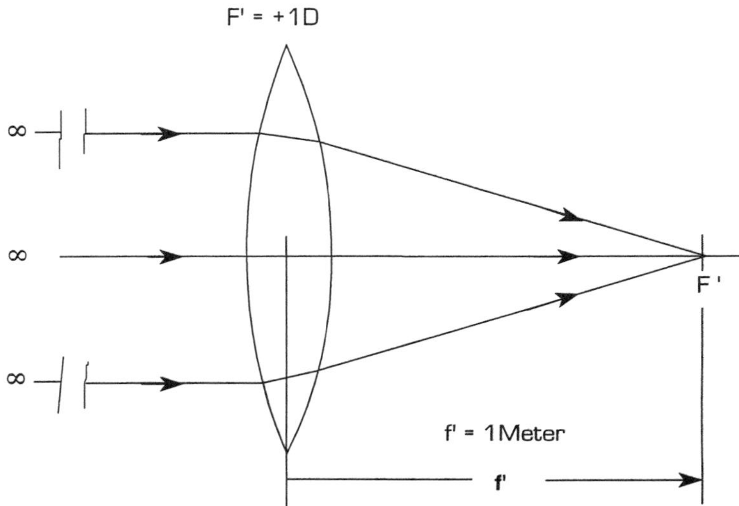

Figure 34 Diopter power. D = 1/f'; D = 1/1; D = +1 diopter.

power drum See *drum, power.*

power, effective The vergence power of an optical system designated at a point of reference other than the principal point; in an ophthalmic lens the back vertex power. The effective power of an ophthalmic plus lens is increased with increased vertex distance and decreased with decreased vertex distance. The effective power of an ophthalmic minus lens is decreased with an increase in vertex distance and increased with a decrease in vertex distance. In strong corrections, the refracting vertex and fitting vertex distances must be determined so that compensation in dioptric power can be made to provide an effective power equal to the refracted power. (cf. *minimum lash clearance (MLC).*)

power, equivalent

1. Reciprocal of the equivalent focal length in meters.

2. An expression of the power of a spherical magnifier.

power, focal Synonymous with vergence power. See *power, vergence.*

power, front vertex The refractive or vergence power of a lens as measured at its front surface (e.g., when measuring the power of a front surface fused multifocal segment).

power, linear magnifying (M) See *magnification, linear.*

power, magnifying The ratio of image size to object size. In a single-lens magnifier, roughly, the dioptric power of the lens divided by 4; more precisely, equivalent power or 1/equivalent focal length in meters. Sometimes abbreviated as P.

power, marked surface The nominal (i.e., indicated or marked) base curve of a semi-finished lens in diopters, as expressed by the manufacturer. The difference between the marked base and actual tool curve of the surface represents the manufacturer's compensation for that base curve. This compensation allows standard tooling to be utilized over a range of prescriptions with little or no further compensation required by the laboratory to produce accurate back vertex powers.

power, meridional (me-rid'e-o-nal) The refractive or surface power of a lens measured in a specified meridian.

power, minus The measure of the ability of a lens or optical system to diverge incident light.

power, nominal surface The named or designated base curve surface power of a lens as stated by the manufacturer. The nominal or indicated surface power is often used for purposes of lens inventory identification or as a means to determine the curves to be ground on the opposite side of the lens, whether spherical or toric.

power, plus The measure of the ability of a lens or optical system to converge incident light to a real focus.

power, prism A measure of the amount of deviation of a ray of light transmitted through a prism or the prismatic component in a lens. The amount of deviation is expressed in prism diopter ($^{\Delta}$) units, i.e., one, prism diopter, 1^{Δ}, deviates parallel rays of light 1cm at a distance of 1m. A prism may be specified in terms of its horizontal and vertical effects. For example, a 2.83^{Δ} prism base down and out at 45° (or 2.83^{Δ} prism, base at 225°), O.D. is equivalent to 2.0^{Δ} prism base-down and 2.0^{Δ} prism base-out O.D. When prism power is measured with a focimeter, the ray involved is normal to the back surface and coincides with the axis of the focimeter. It is specified in terms of the point on the front surface which it penetrates.

power, prismatic See *power, prism.*

power, reflective See *albedo.*

power, refractive The ability of an optical lens or an isotropic transparent body to produce a change in the vergence of a beam of light, usually expressed in diopters.

power, refractive, back vertex The reciprocal of the focal length of a spectacle or corneal contact lens when measured along the optical axis from the vertex on the posterior (ocular) side to the secondary focal point, expressed in diopters.

power, refractive, front vertex The reciprocal of the focal length of a spectacle or corneal contact lens when measured along the optical axis from the vertex on the anterior (objective) surface to the primary focal point, expressed in diopters.

power, refractive surface (F_T) Also called true power. The ability of an isotropic glass or plastic surface bounded by air to change the vergence of a beam of incident light, defined as

$$F_T = \frac{F_s\,(n_D - 1)}{(1.530 - 1)} = \frac{F_s\,(n_D - 1)}{(.530)}$$

where

n_D = the index of refraction of the material at the Sodium D line (i.e., yellow).

r = the radius of curvature of the refracting surface in millimeters.

F_s = the tool-marked surface power in diopters

1.530 = constant value based on original surfacing tools for glass of that index.

Since common ophthalmic materials do not have indices of refraction (n) equal to 1.530, there is no one-to-one correspondence between marked surface tool power and surface refractive power. For example, common ophthalmic crown glass has an index of refraction of 1.5230. Therefore, a one-diopter marked surface tool power (F_s) will produce an actual (i.e., true) refractive surface power (F_T) of 0.987 diopter. See *Table 5* in the Appendix.

power, required In ocular refraction, the dioptric power needed to bring parallel rays of light to a point focus on the retina. It is designated by the total dioptric powers found on the optical cross and determined by the prescriber's manifest prescription.

power, resolving The ability of the eye or a lens to image separately two small objects or stimuli that are close together; resolution, minimal separable power; minimal distance at which two adjacent objects can be distinguished as unconnected; sometimes expressed as line pairs per millimeter; visual acuity.

power, sphere The diopter power of a lens with a constant (uniform) radius of curvature; in a spherocylinder lens, the sphere power is located in the cylinder axis meridian.

power, surface (F_S) The ability of an optically polished refracting or reflecting face to change the vergence of a beam of light incident to its surface. The amount of vergence ability (i.e., power) can be determined algebraically

$$F_S = \frac{(n' - n)}{r}$$

where

- r = radius of curvature in millimeters
- n′ = index of refraction of the image medium (e.g., glass surface material)
- n = index of refraction of the object medium (e.g., air)

F_S, in diopters, is plus (+) for convex surfaces, minus (–) for concave surfaces. See *Table 3* in the Appendix.

power, tool surface A misnomer. A lens grinding or polishing tool made from any of a variety of opaque, non-refractive materials such as aluminum, brass, cast iron, plastic, etc., does not have the ability to change the vergence of light. However, once the surface of a lens or mirror attains the shape and curvature of the grinding and polishing tools, the lens or mirror gains the ability to change the vergence of light based on its own index of refraction and the radius of curvature imparted to it by the surfacing/polishing tool. By common usage, a grinding or polishing tool with a radius of curvature of 530mm has the capacity to produce a surface power (F_T) of one diopter if made on a lens that had an index of refraction of 1.530 and is marked and called a one-diopter tool. Tool power is determined as follows

$$F_T = \frac{530}{r}$$

where

- r = the actual radius of curvature in millimeters of the tool
- F_T = the marked surface power of the tool
- 530 = a constant based on obsolete crown glass, index n = 1.530

A convex surface tool is considered positive (i.e., plus, or +) to grind a minus surface power; a concave tool is considered negative (i.e., minus, or –) to grind a plus surface power. See *Table 3* in the Appendix.

power, vergence The ability of an optical system to change the convergence or divergence of a pencil of rays, usually designated quantitatively by the reciprocal of the focal length of the system expressed in meters.

power, vertex The inverse (i.e., reciprocal) of the distance in meters from the lens vertex to the corresponding focal point, stated in diopters. In an ophthalmic prescription, the spherical and cylindrical component of power are always expressed in terms of rear (or back) vertex power. Focimeters (lens meters) are designed to measure vertex power directly.

power wheel See *drum, power.*

POZ Mnemonic for zone, posterior optical; q.v..

PPC Mnemonic for curve, peripheral posterior; q.v.

pre- Prefix meaning before; prior to.

precipitates, keratic (K.P.s) Pigmentary, fatty, or cellular deposits on corneal endothelium, often due to inflammation of the iris or ciliary body.

precorneal film See *film, tear.*

preferential looking Test system to estimate visual acuity in infants, toddlers, handicapped, and non-verbal patients; uses grating acuity or striped stimulus plates (Teller acuity plates) from 20/15 to 20/2300; introduced in 1978 by Davida Y. Teller, Ph.D., U.S. research psychologist.

Prentice's law See *law, Prentice's.*

Prentice's rule See *law, Prentice's*

presbyopia (pres″be-ō′pe-ah) Impairment of vision due to advancing years. This includes reduction in accommodative ability, reduction in contrast sensitivity, need for additional light, increased light scattering, and reduced ability to cope with glare; usually becomes clinically significant after 40 years of age. First differentiated from hyperopia in 1855 by Vienna ophthalmologist Karl Stellwag von Carion (1823–1904).

prescribed prism See *prism, prescribed.*

prescription lens See *lens, prescription.*

prescription, ophthalmic The formula determined by an examiner to correct refractive anomalies in an individual patient, usually containing sphere power, cylinder and prism powers, and their direction as indicated. Other special instructions are part of the prescription. Prescription components may deviate from objective or instrumental findings based on tolerance of base curve, previously worn prescription, estimation of patient's tolerance for change, special work or avocational needs of the patient, request of the patient for near or distant lens only, type of lens mounting, and relation of spherical element to state of accommodation and muscle balance.

preservatives Chemicals that exert a toxic effect on a broad range of microorganisms and are used in contact lens disinfecting systems.

press, arbor A mechanical instrument or device for working or repairing spectacle frame parts; usually fitted with a centered shaft or round mandrel that holds a cylindrical bar connected to a rack and pinion operated by a lever handle to apply pressure to the frame or frame parts.

press-on prism See *prism, Fresnel.*

pressing Manufacturing process of glass ophthalmic lenses by which molten lens material is poured into a curved mold to form a lens blank of given base, diameter, and curvature; process known since the first century A.D.

pressure, intraocular The tension within an eyeball occurring as a result of the constant formation and drainage of the aqueous humor; measured with a tonometer. Pressure above 20mm or 25mm Hg usually indicates the pathologic condition of glaucoma. Pressure under 9mm or 10mm Hg usually causes fluctuation in acuity, because the optical curvature of the eye is unstable.

primary position See *position, primary.*

Prince's rule See *rule, Prince's.*

principal axis See *axis, principal.*

principal meridians See *meridians, principal.*

prism (optical) A wedge-shaped, transparent and isotropic body that deviates light. Its two major surfaces meet at an apex and have their greatest separation at the base. A prism deviates light toward its base causing the apparent image to be displaced toward its apex. (See Figure 5.)

prism apex See *apex, prism.*

prism ballast contact lens See *lens, contact, prism ballast.*

prism base See *base, prism.*

prism diopter See *diopter, prism.*

prism, double An optical test device consisting of two weak (about 4^{Δ}) prisms fixed together base-to-base and positioned over the visual axis of one eye, causing a double image and dissociating the vision of that eye from the other eye; used in measuring heterophoria, and particularly, cyclophoria; Maddox double prism. Devised in 1890 by Scottish ophthalmologist Ernest E. Maddox (1868–1933).

prism, Dove Internally reflecting prism, popularized by and imprecisely named for Heinrich W. Dove (1803–1879), Berlin professor of natural philosophy and author of *Optical Studies* (1859).

prism, face of Either of the two sides of a prism converging from the prism base to the prism apex. (See Figure 5.)

prism, Fresnel (fre-nel') A surface of narrow prism sections of specific prism power that gives the effect of a larger prism without the usual thickness and weight. Fresnel prisms may be made of a pliable, clear, plastic material that can be cut and applied to ophthalmic lenses as a diagnostic or compensatory aid. The ridged optical design was developed in 1822 by French physicist Augustine Jean Fresnel (1788–1827).

prism, induced The prism power created when the optical center of a lens is out of coincidence with the wearer's visual axes, or when the visual axis intersects any point on a lens with refractive power, away from the optical center.

prism, Nicol A beam-splitting prism made from two rhomboids of the birefringent crystal calcite (Iceland spar); the original crystal is cut in the longest diagonal and the halves cemented together; the prism is a high-precision polarizer; developed in the 1820s by Scottish physicist William Nicol (1768–1851).

prism, Porro Combination of two right-angle (totally reflecting) prisms used in field glasses and corneal microscopes that create four reflecting surfaces to permit shorter tube length and larger field with erect images; invented in 1851 by Ignazzio Porro (1795–1875), Italian optical scientist.

prism power See *power, prism.*

prism, prescribed A desired and ordered component of an ophthalmic lens producing specified displacement by refractive elements of the lens.

prism reference point See *point, prism reference.*

prism, reflecting Prism designed for total internal reflection of light; the incident and emergent chief ray of a light pencil is perpendicular to the prism base but makes 90° angles at each of the internal prism faces; total interal reflecting prisms as in a Porro prism; q.v.

prism, Rochon A three-prism (one equilateral and two right-angle) optical group for producing a variable angular separation between two beams of plane polarized light; prisms are made of calcite or quartz;

beam-splitting birefringent prism. Developed by A.M. Rochon (1741–1817) of France.

prism segment See *segment, prism.*

prism, slab-off See *grinding, bicentric.*

prism thinning (progressive lens) The reduction of inherent thickness in the upper portion of progressive lenses by grinding equal base-down prisms in each lens of a pair; the lower portions of progressive lenses, by virtue of the addition power, tend to be thinner than the upper portions. Thickness and weight may be reduced by prism thinning

prism, unwanted The amount of prism that exists in a prescription lens at the MRP when the error-free point is not coincident with the MRP; any amount of prism that exists at the MRP other than that prescribed.

prism, Wollaston A double-imaging prism constructed of two right-angle prisms of calcite or quartz cemented together to form a rectangular whole in which the optic axis of the first prism is parallel to the incident face, and at a right angle to the incident face in the second prism. A non-polarized bundle of light rays passing through it is split into two equally deviated emergent rays; the fundamental optic unit of a keratometer (e.g., B and L variable doubling keratometer). Devised by William Hyde Wollaston (1766–1828), English chemist, optical scientist, physicist, and physician.

prismatic imbalance See *imbalance, prismatic.*

prismatic power See *power, prism.*

pro- Prefix meaning priority in space or time; advancing or projecting forward or outward.

processes, ciliary Innermost portions of the finger-shaped vascular ciliary body containing blood vessels that are involved in the secretion of aqueous humor; the sites of attachment for the zonule of Zinn or suspensory ligament (zonules) of the crystalline lens.

professional A member of an occupational group requiring advanced education or training; a person making a living by letters, arts, or sports.

profile

1. The shape or contour of an object or surface.
2. Record constituting the history taken from an individual or class of people.
3. In ophthalmic optics, the shape or contour of an ophthalmic lens or contact lens in optical or sagittal section.

prognosis The prediction of the probable course of a disease.

progressive addition lens See *lens, progressive.*

progressive power lens See *lens, progressive.*

progressive power semi-finished blank See *blank, progressive power semi-finished.*

prolapse A falling down or protrusion of an organ or part from its normal position (e.g., a downward positioned lacrimal gland; a herniation of iris tissue through a wound in the eye).

proline A non-essential amino acid, one of the major (15% to 20%) constituents of tropocollagen, the molecular unit of collagen fibrils; used in the manufacture of haptics for some intraocular lenses. First isolated from casein in 1901 by the German chemist Emil H. Fischer (1852–1914).

propionate See *cellulose propionate.*

propylene A gaseous hydrocarbon of the olefin (unsaturated) series.

prosthesis (pros'thē-sis) An artificial substitute for a missing body part; plural, prostheses.

prosthesis, reform ocular The usual artificial or space-filling artificial eye fabricated to fit the conjunctival surface after a surgical enucleation.

prosthesis, shell ocular A thin artificial eye fabricated to cover a sightless and unsightly globe; commonly made of methyl methacrylate and hand-painted by an ocularist to match the sighted eye.

prosthetics (pros-thet'iks) The science of designing and fitting artificial replacement parts for lost anatomical components.

prot- A combining form Greek prefix meaning first.

protanomaly (prō"ta-nom'ah-le) A mild color deficiency of red receptors; present as a congenital defect in about 6% of American males and 0.5% of American females.

protanopia (prō"ta-nō'pe-ah) Total absence of the ability to perceive the color red; an absence of the first, or red-sensitive, pigment, erythrolabe.

protractor Any of a group of mechanical instruments used to construct or measure plane angles; simple, semicircular disc protractors, measuring from 0° to 180° are of ancient origin and were in use during the thirteenth century.

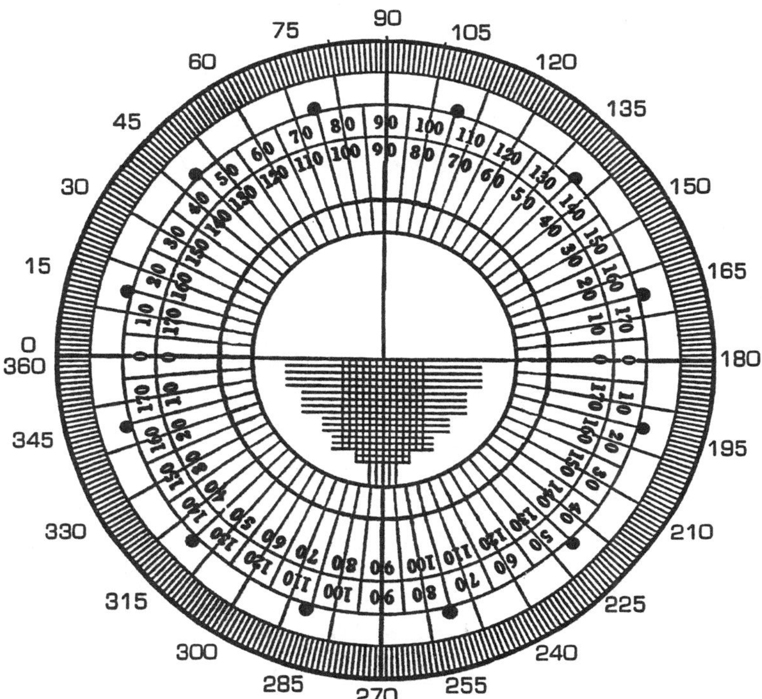

Figure 35 Layout protractor.

protractor, layout Lens protractor; optical protractor. A geometric gauge having a circle sectioned by degree markings from 0° to 360° for prism base location and from 0° to 180° in opposing directions, for cylinder axis location of astigmatic lenses; usually contains millimeter scales in the lower semicircle extending both vertically and horizontally from its center; used to position the major reference point and multifocal segment in laying out a lens for surfacing or edging (Figure 35).

With the lens held convex side up, the cylinder degree markings start from the right and progress counterclockwise; with the lens held convex side down, the cylinder degree markings start from the left and progress clockwise. Using the protractor sample to locate the prism base on a lens having prescribed prism, the lens must be held convex side down. The degree markings start on the left and progress clockwise from 0° to 360°. It also is common practice to relate the prism base location using the cylinder degree markings (e.g., a 3^{Δ} prism, base 225° in the right eye would equate to a 3^{Δ} prism base down and out at 45°. If prescribed for the left eye, a 3^{Δ} prism, base 225°, would equate to a 3^{Δ} prism base down and in at 45°.

protractor, optical See *protractor, layout.*

proximal (prok′si-mal) Nearest.

pseudo- Prefix meaning false.

Pseudomonas aeruginosa (soo″do-mō′nus er-roo″jin-o-sah) A form of gram-negative bacteria found in contaminated contact lens solutions or sodium fluorescein. Can result in major corneal infection, ulceration, or loss of the eye.

pseudomyopia (soo″do-mī-o′pe-ah)

1. A false appearance of myopia due to spasm of the ciliary muscle, failure of relaxation of accommodation, or, at times, induced by darkness.
2. An induced myopic shift associated with high blood-sugar levels as in a diabetic patient; usually transient.

pseudophake (soo′do-fāk) Informal designation of a patient who has a surgically implanted artificial lens in one or both eyes.

pseudophakia (soo″do-fā′ke-ah) The condition of an eye containing a surgically implanted artificial lens. Term introduced in 1959 by Netherlands ophthalmologist Cornelius D. Binkhorst.

pseudophakic

1. One who has pseudophakia.
2. Pertaining to or having pseudophakia.

pseudophakos (soo″do-fāk′os) A small plastic and substitute ophthalmic lens designed for implantation within the eye after cataract removal; usually manufactured of methyl methacrylate; intraocular lens (IOL) implant; commonly designated by eponym indicating name of the original designer. Governed by the A.N.S.I. Z80.7 standard. First designed and implanted in 1948–1949 by London ophthalmologist N. Harold Lloyd Ridley (b. 1906).

pseudoptosis (soo″do-tō′sis) A condition resembling prolapse or drooping, particularly applied to downward position of the upper eyelids; may be associated with small or deep-set eyes.

pseudostrabismus (soo″do-strah-biz′mus) Apparent or false deviation of one eye from the other eye; a condition resembling the deviation of one visual axis from the other; often associated with non-coincidence at the pupillary axis and fixation axis in one or both eyes; also associated with congenital skin folds over the medial canthi (epicanthal folds).

psychophysical Pertaining to the science of quantitative relationships between objective physical stimuli and resulting mental or cortical interpretations; said of photometric units in quantitation of light science, or of light stimuli and visual field awareness in static perimetry.

pterygium (ter-ij′e-um) A wing-like thickening of connective tissue and blood vessels beneath the bulbar conjunctiva which slowly grows from the inner canthus (rarely from the outer canthus) over the limbus and into the superficial cornea; particularly common among mature adults with chronic exposure to high levels of sunlight or adverse weather conditions.

ptosis (tō′sis)

1. Anatomical. Drooping or downward displacement of an organ or structure from its usual position.
2. Ophthalmic. Drooping of an eyelid below its normal position; more frequently occurring in the upper lid, but may occur in the lower lid; commonly associated with fatigue, orbital fat herniation, epicanthus, and similar lid defects.

ptosis crutch See *crutch, ptosis.*

puncta Plural of punctum.

punctum

1. A small spot or point.
2. Small opening located on the margin of the ciliary border of each eyelid near the medial canthus through which tears drain; lacrimal punctum; plural, puncta.

punctum, inferior Small opening found at the center of the lacrimal papilla on inside margin of the ciliary border of the lower eyelid near the inner canthus that provides a flow channel for drainage of tears from the eye (lower punctum). Similar opening on upper eyelid margin is called superior punctum (upper punctum).

punctum proximum See *point, near.*

punctum remotum See *point, far.*

Punktal lens See *lens, Punktal.*

pupil (pyoo′pil) The aperture or opening in the iris, normally circular and variable in size, through which light enters the lens of the eye.

pupil, cornpicker's Dilated pupil resulting from contact with dust from jimson weeds commonly found in cornfields.

pupill(o)- A combining form indicating relationship to the pupillary opening in the iris.

pupillary axis See *axis, pupillary.*

pupillary distance See *distance, interocular.*

pupillometer (pyoo″pi-lom′i-ter) An optical device for measuring the diameter, width, or area of the pupil of the eye; coreometer; coreoscope.

pupillometer, corneal reflection (CRP) Incorrect trade name for an optical instrument that measures interocular distances based on corneal light reflections seen on the fixation (visual) axes; device is not a pupillometer.

pupillometry (pyoo″pi-lom′i-tre) Measurement of the diameter or area of the pupil, usually expressed in millimeters or square millimeters; coreometry.

Pyrex Trade name for a heat-resistant borosilicate glass used at high temperatures, as in cooking or in laser optics.

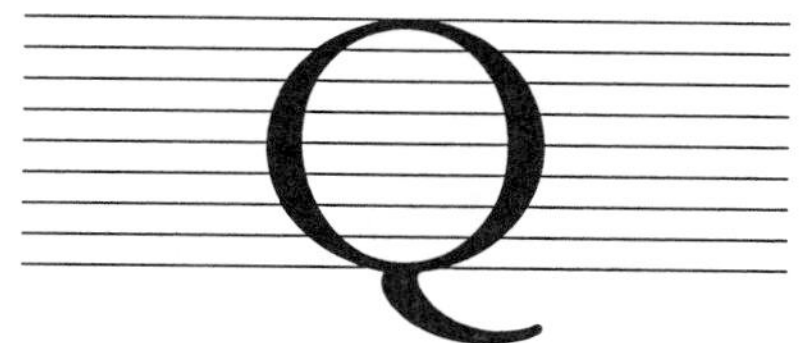

Q Abbreviation for the total radiant energy output of a pulsed laser measured in joules (J); term originally derives from the term *quality factor,* or Q factor, to indicate the ratio of energy storage to energy dissipation.

q.i.d. Abbreviation for Latin "quater in die," four times a day.

q.v. Abbreviation for Latin "quod vide," which see.

quadra-, quadri- Prefix meaning four.

quadrant One-fourth of a circle; that part which subtends an angle of 90°.

quadrifocal lens See *lens, quadrifocal.*

quantum (kwon'tum) In light science, the minimal energy unit of a photon (electron); expressed as Planck's constant (h), (6.626×10^{-27} erg seconds) times the frequency of the given wavelength.

quartz An hexagonal crystalline form of silicon dioxide (silica) naturally occurring as SiO_2; a hard (Mohs 7) transparent mineral which is doubly refracting; used in early Chinese and European lenses; sometimes called clear fused silica; has high transmission for ultraviolet and infrared lights; pebble lens.

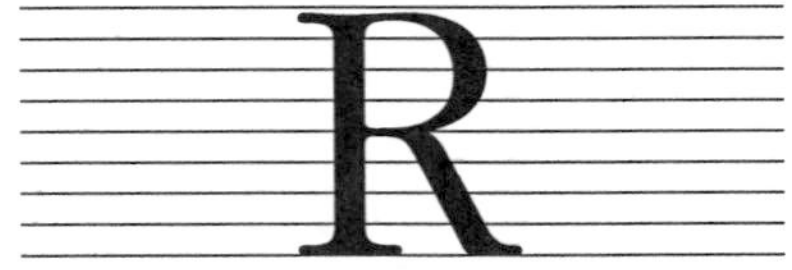

R Abbreviation for:
1. Ribbon segment.
2. Röentgen (Röntgen), the international unit for X-radiation.
3. The reciprocal of the radius of curvature of a surface r, in meters.

RGP Abbreviation for **r**igid **g**as **p**ermeable contact lens.

RP Abbreviation for retinitis pigmentosa; q.v.

R.P.B. Abbreviation for Research to Prevent Blindness; q.v.

Ra Chemical symbol for the radioactive element radium; q.v.

rack, skiascopy (retinoscopy) A hand-held, lightweight, elongated lens-holding device or frame, usually containing 16 to 24 individual spherical trial lenses for objective measurements of ocular refraction.

rad Acronym for *radiation absorbed dose*; a traditionally used unit of quantitation for X-ray energy transfer. Equals 100 ergs per gram of any absorbing tissue. Now being superseded by the unit *gray* (Gy) equal to 100 rads.

radial astigmatism See *astigmatism, radial.*

radian A unit of angular measurement, equal to the angle formed at the center of a circle by two radii cutting the circumference with an arc whose length is equal to the radius of the circle.

radiant exposure See *exposure, radiant.*

radiation Emission or transfer of energy in the form of electromagnetic waves or particles.

radiation, Lambertian Completely randomized light propagation in all directions with equal radiance; named in honor of Johann H. Lambert (1728–1777), German philosopher and mathematician.

radiation, monochromatic Electromagnetic energy of a single wavelength or color.

radiation, photochemical The part of the electromagnetic energy spectrum that produces chemical changes (e.g., ultraviolet light causing darkening of phototropic lenses).

Radiation Research Society (R.R.S.) A U.S.-based voluntary interdisciplinary association particularly interested in biological effects of electromagnetic energy; membership consists primarily of radiation biologists, radiation physicists, and physicians.

radiations, optical In neuroanatomy, nerve fibers transmitting visual impulses from the lateral geniculate body to the visual cortex (Brodmann's area 17) in the occipital portion of the brain; geniculocalcarine tract.

radium A radioactive chemical element used for treatment of cancer, but also causes cataract; chemical symbol Ra, atomic number 88. Discovered in Paris in 1898 by Polish research chemist Marie Sklodowska Curie (1867–1934) who received the Nobel Prize in physics (1903) and in chemistry (1911).

radius A straight line, one-half the diameter of a circle, emanating from the center and terminating at the circumference.

radius of curvature A straight line measured from the center of a circle to its circumference, usually used to express the curvature of a spectacle or contact lens in millimeters, or to compute the sagitta value and dioptric power of a corneal surface; abbreviated r or R, the latter for a specular surface. (See Figure 16.)

radius, posterior apical (PAR) See *curve, central posterior (CPC).*

Radiuscope Trade name for an optical inspection instrument used to measure back surface curvature of a contact lens.

Raman effect An optical function seen on irradiating a substance with monochromatic light; the spectrum of scattered light contains, in addition to the wavelength of the incident light, other wavelengths which are weak satellites of the primary wavelengths; used in spectroscopic studies of the crystalline lens and vitreous; discovered in 1928 by Sir C.V. Raman (1888–1970), Indian physicist who received the Nobel Prize in physics (1930) for diffusion discoveries.

Randot stereotest A set of red-green printed anaglyphs presenting a computer-generated random arrangement of dots in which figures emerge when viewed through red-green spectacles; test of stereopsis free of all monocular cues. Developed in 1960 by Hungarian-born Bela Julesz (b. 1928), research scientist in visual psychology at Bell Telephone Laboratories, New Jersey. (cf. *test, stereoacuity.*)

range of accommodation See *accommodation, range of.*

range of clear vision The linear measurement of the closest to the farthest point from the eye at which the viewer has distinct visual resolution; usually expressed in centimeters or inches.

Rapid eye movements (REM) Periodic, fast eye movements associated with the dream cycles that occur during deep sleep; occur in bursts lasting about 1 minute.

raster (rasterline) The well standardized line of the scanning pattern in a television picture proceeding from left to right and from top to bottom (from the Latin "rastrum," rake).

rate, blink The number of times that the eyelids completely close in a prescribed period of time; the average blink rate is 10 to 17 times per minute. May be increased or decreased by concentration. While reading, the blink rate may be reduced as much as 75%. Athletes in motion also experience a significant reduction in blink rate.

ratio An expression of the quantity of one substance or measure in relation to another; commonly expressed as a quotient of one divided by the other.

ratio, aperture The fixed relation in linear units of the diameter to the focal length of a lens.

ratio, contrast Difference between the luminance level (brightness) of two objects or images.

ray In optics, a linear representation of the direction of electromagnetic energy, particularly in the visible spectrum.

ray, cathode Negative particles of electricity streaming out in a vacuum tube at right angles to its surface; may be deflected by magnetic flux; may generate Röntgen (X) rays on a fluorescent screen; may produce lighted trace.

ray, chief In geometric optics, the ray in an incident beam of light that passes through the center of the entrance pupil of the optical system.

ray, emergent The ray of light in image space either after reflection (reflected ray) or after refraction (refracted ray).

ray, incident The ray in a narrow beam of light in object space striking a lens, prism, or reflecting surface at the interface of the object and image medium.

ray, reflected The ray in a narrow beam of light in image space after reflection at the surface of a mirror.

ray, refracted The ray in a narrow beam of light in image space after refraction.

ray, tracing Point-by-point analysis of linear propagation of light; introduced in 1611 as the foundation for geometric optics by the German astronomer Johann Kepler (1571–1630).

re- Prefix meaning again or back.

reaction, allergic An unexpected non-therapeutic response of an individual to a drug, chemical material, or other stimulus which may vary from a topical rash or irritation to systemic shock or death; especially considered as immediate type of hypersensitivity reaction (as in response to some mercurial compounds used as preservatives in solutions).

reading field See *field, reading.*

real image See *image, real.*

receptor, visual In ocular anatomy, a rod or cone cell of the outer layer of the retina.

reference

1. A beginning.
2. A person, place or thing to which comparisons are made.

reference line See *line, reference.*

reflected ray See *ray, reflected.*

reflection The turning back or rebounding of light which falls upon a surface.

reflection, angle of See *angle of reflection.*

reflection, specular A technique of illumination in ocular examination using a biomicroscope and slit-beam light, directed to a focus on the endothelial surface of the cornea; the angles of incidence and reflection are sufficiently narrow that only one viewing ocular of the microscope is used; affords evaluation of the pattern, size, and configuration of endothelial cells; introduced in 1918 by Alfred Vogt (1879–1943), Swiss ophthalmologist.

reflections, internal Subsequent and sequential returning of small and decreasing proportions of light from the glass-air surfaces of a lens; doubly reflected light.

reflections, retrodirective The action of a collimated incident beam of light being redirected along its original axis of propagation and remaining collimated regardless of the angle of incidence at the retroreflector; occurs in "cat's eye," "corner cubes," and Scotch-lite retrodirective screens; such retroreflection does not obey the laws of regular specular reflection.

reflections, veiling Diffuse glare from a light source falling on a reflective surface as on the inside of an automobile windshield or on a video display screen causing phosphores to appear "washed out," thereby reducing contrast and visibility.

reflective lens See *lens, reflective.*

reflectivity The degree to which an object can return incident light; reflectance. (cf. *albedo.*)

reflex, blink Episodic or periodic contraction of the orbicularis oculi muscles due to the stimulus of corneal or conjunctival irritation from foreign matter, sneezing, or corneal drying; also may be initiated by sudden sound.

reflex, corneal

1. Return of light from the corneal surface; a reflection of 4% to 6% of normal incident light occurs from the anterior corneal surface and a lesser amount may be detected from the posterior corneal surface. When derived from a small focal light source, this is used to estimate deviation of an eye from its normal position (Hirschberg test), or to determine the point where the visual axis intersects the cornea; more precisely, corneal reflection.
2. Irritation of the cornea resulting in reflex closure of the eyelids.

reflex, pupillary Reaction of the iris sphincter muscle to contract and narrow the pupil opening in the presence of bright light.

reform ocular prosthesis See *prosthesis, reform ocular.*

refracted ray See *ray, refracted.*

refraction

1. The change in direction of light as it passes obliquely from one medium to another of different optical density or refractive index. Concept first recorded c. 160 A.D. by the Greek astronomer and mathematician Claudius Ptolemy (c. 130–200 A.D.) in the fifth book of his volume *Optica.*
2. The act of determining the focal condition (emmetropia or various ametropias) of the eye and its correction by optical devices, usually spectacles or contact lenses.

refraction, cycloplegic The determination of a patient's need for refractive correction with the aid of topical drugs to paralyze all accommodative action within the eye.

refraction, double The change in an incident light ray, dividing it into two refracted rays so as to produce a double image, as through Iceland spar or a Nicol prism; birefringence. Discovered in 1669 by Erasmus Bartholin (1625–1698), Danish physician.

refraction, manifest The assessment or development of a refraction formula for an individual patient in prescription form for a specified vertex distance, without the use of cycloplegic eye drops.

refraction, objective Determination of the spectacle or contact lens formula without utilizing the response of the patient to determine the accuracy. Usually performed with a streak or spot retinoscope, or an automatic computerized refraction device.

refraction, subjective Determination of the spectacle or contact lens prescription utilizing the response of the patient to determine the accuracy of the prescription. Usually performed with a phoropter or trial frame in combination with a Snellen chart placed at a predetermined distance, usually 20 feet.

refraction, vectographic A binocular objective reflection system utilizing polarizing iodine-derived crystals in thin sheets of polyvinyl alcohol. Developed in 1967 by Massachusetts optometrist Bernard Grolman (b. 1923).

refractionist One skilled in determining the refractive state of the eyes, the state of binocularity, and the proper corrective lenses.

refractive error See *error, refractive.*

refractive power See *power, refractive.*

refractive surface power See *power, refractive surface.*

refractometer (objective optometer)

1. Diagnostic optical device to measure refractive state of the eye by objective means (e.g., Nikon Autorefractor). See *refractor, auto.*
2. Analytic optical device to measure glucose and the dissolved substances in the urine; Abbé refractometer.

refractometry (rē″frak-tom′i-tre)

1. The technical process of calculating the focusing state of the dioptrics of the eye; separate from judgment or interpretation.

2. A quantitative analysis of glucose and other dissolved substances in the urine.

refractometry, laser The use of a laser beam to generate an interference pattern (laser speckle pattern) in many planes in front of the retina and as virtual images behind the retina; plus and minus lenses are inserted to neutralize with and against movements of the pattern in the two principal meridians of the eye in order to establish the focusing state of the dioptrics of the eye.

refractor, auto A mechanical and optical diagnostic instrument usually of table-top design which makes objective measurements of the refraction of the human eye; sometimes includes subjective verification; trade names, Canon R-22; Auto-Refractor; Nikon NR 5100; Nikon Electronic Refractors OF8; Humphrey Automatic Refractor; Marco Automatic Refractor AR800 and AR1200; Topcon Autorefractometer; Topcon Pediatric Refractometer.

Register, Medical Device (International Edition) A one-volume, hardcover directory listing more than 6,000 non-U.S. medical device manufacturers and 20,000 medical devices by product category and manufacturer's profile; published by Medical Economics Co., Oradell, New Jersey 07649. Most recent edition is 1993.

Registry of Ophthalmic Pathology See *Ophthalmic Pathology, Registry of.*

regular astigmatism See *astigmatism, regular.*

Research to Prevent Blindness (R.P.B.) A voluntary corporate organization, founded in 1960 by Jules Stein, M.D. (1896–1981); committed to stimulate, sustain, and intensify a concerted research assault, with the goal of developing more effective methods of treatment, preventives, and cures for all diseases that damage and destroy sight. Thomas F. Furlong is the Director of Public Information. Office: 598 Madison Avenue, New York, New York 10022.

resin Any of various solid or semi-solid, usually clear, viscous, organic substances naturally exuded from various plants and trees, or as synthetic plastics.

resin, hard See *CR-39.*

resistance, corrosion The ability of a metal part to maintain the integrity of its surface finish without significant deterioration.

resistance, impact The ability of a material or object to sustain dynamically applied external forces without breaking. For street-wear lenses, this quantity has been regulated by the U.S. Food and Drug Administration since 1972, requiring that all lenses be capable of withstanding the impact of a 5/8-inch diameter steel sphere, freely falling from a height of 50 inches (F.D.A. Policy Section 804.410, A.N.S.I. Z80.1). For safety lenses, this quantity is regulated by the U.S. Occupational Safety and Health Administration which requires a similar impact test using a 1-inch diameter steel sphere (A.N.S.I. Z87.1).

resolution

1. In optics, sharpness, crispness, or clarity of an image; the ability to distinguish fine details from an object source.
2. In precision optics, graded in line pairs per millimeter.

resolving power See *power, resolving.*

resonance, optical The intensifying effect produced when the amplitude of oscillation of a single wavelength of the electromagnetic energy spectrum is greatly increased by external energy (electrical energy or light of the same, or nearly same, wavelength), and an emitted photon beam traverses the lasing material multiple times by reflection through the containing laser cavity (resonant cavity) which in length is a precise multiple of the laser light wavelength. Thus, a monochromatic, coherent, directional, and powerful light is generated. See *laser.*

resultant optical center See *center, resultant optical.*

retention, lens The ability of a spectacle front to keep a lens from dislodging from the rim groove under force.

reticle (ret′ih-kl) A series of lines, markers, or circles in the eyepiece of an optical instrument used to locate or measure details of an object being inspected; in a focimeter, usually a series of concentric rings and central cross to locate the optical center of an ophthalmic lens or to measure prism displacement.

retina The light-sensitive membrane lining the inner surface of the eye that receives the image formed by the optical system of the eye and is connected to the brain by the optic nerve; innermost layer of the eye. First described and named about 300 B.C. by Herophilus, Greek anatomist and surgeon.

retinitis pigmentosa (ret″i-nī′tis pig″men-tō′sa) Pigmentary degeneration of the retina. Hereditary degeneration of retina with migration of pigmentation, resulting in contraction of the visual field and night blindness. May be primary in the eye or secondary to single-

or multiple-organ-system disease; rod-cone or cone-rod dystrophy; hereditary patterns vary in different families; a three-generation history is desirable to establish genetic type.

retinol (ret'ih-nol) Vitamin A_1, a 20-carbon alcohol stored in the liver and possibly the retina; used by rods and cones as a photosensitive pigment, initiating the visual response in the eye.

Retinometer Trade name for a hand-held, battery-powered, potential-acuity meter to assess macular function in the presence of partial cataract formation.

retinopathy (ret"i-nop'ah-the) A diseased condition of the retina that is generally non-inflammatory in nature. May be caused by diabetes mellitus, drug abuse, hypertension, kidney failure, toxemia of pregnancy, and similar diseases.

retinoscope (ret'i-no-skōp) Hand-held, illuminated optical examining instrument to analyze a spot or streak of light reflected from the ocular fundus; intensity and movement of the reflected light, neutralized by trial lenses, indicates the refractive status of the eye (objective refraction).

retinoscope, spot Hand-held, illuminated optical device used in objective refraction to determine the manifest prescription. A spot of light is projected into the eye and lenses are used to neutralize the reflected light motion.

retinoscope, streak Hand-held, illuminated optical examining instrument to analyze light reflected from the ocular fundus; projection of a linear light image on the retina combined with trial lenses used to neutralize the reflected motion. This type of instrument is the most frequently used objective determinant of refraction in North America; Copeland retinoscope; earlier cylindrical (Angus Macnab) mirror retinoscope. Developed in 1927 by Wisconsin optometrist Jack C. Copeland (1900–1973).

retinoscopy (ret"i-nos'ko-pe) The optical technique of estimating refractive errors by projecting light on the ocular fundus and analyzing its reflected characteristics; previously called skiascopy (shadow test). First general application in 1873, by Ferdinand L.J. Cuignet (1823–1889), French ophthalmologist of Lille, France; refined and popularized by Edward Jackson (1856–1942), ophthalmologist of Philadelphia and Denver.

retro- Prefix meaning backward.

retro-illumination A technique of biomicroscopic ocular examination using slit-lamp illumination reflected from more posterior structures to delineate details in transparent or semi-transparent media; back lighting; particularly applicable to the lens and to evaluate the posterior cornea for precipitates or pigment deposits, or to view embedded transparent foreign bodies; may be direct or indirect. Introduced in 1919 by Swiss ophthalmologist Alfred Vogt (1874–1943).

retroscopic angle See *tilt, retroscopic.*

retroscopic tilt See *tilt, retroscopic.*

reversal, contrast Change from light to dark components as black letters on a white background to white letters on a black background.

reverse slab off See *slab off, reverse.*

reverse thermal coefficient See *coefficient, reverse thermal.*

Reversibility of Light Path, law of A general law in optics indicating that if light is interrupted by the placement of a plane mirror at a right angle to the path of the light, the light will retrace its path in a reversed direction.

Revised Jaeger Standard See *Standard, Revised Jaeger.*

Rh
1. Chemical symbol for the metallic element rhodium; q.v..
2. Symbol for rhesus factor, an agglutinogenic antigen present on the membrane of red blood cells.

rhodium A hard and rare metal of the platinum group; chemical symbol Rh, atomic number 45; used in construction of first-surface mirrors. First isolated in 1804 by English chemist and optical scientist William Hyde Wollaston (1776–1828).

rhodopsin (rō-dop′sin) A photosensitive protein pigment contained in the rods of the retina necessary for vision in dim light; visual purple. Term introduced in 1877 by the European photobiologist Willy Kühne (1837–1900).

ribbon A configuration of an add to a spectacle lens, narrow in vertical dimension and wider in horizontal dimension. (cf. *segment, compensated.*)

riding bow temple See *temple, riding bow.*

right eye See *eye, right; eye.*

rim Component of an ophthalmic spectacle front that surrounds the lens and into which a lens can be inserted, or to which the lens can be attached by screws, notching straps, or polyfilament line.

rim groove See *groove, rim.*

rimless bevel See *bevel, rimless.*

rimless lens See *lens, rimless.*

ring, Fleischer Superficial iron-containing deposits, usually brownish in color, found in incomplete circular pattern around the conical base in about 50% of kerataconic eyes. First described (1906–1916) by Bruno Fleischer (1874–1965), German ophthalmologist and professor at the University of Erlangen. (Not to be confused with the deep stromal, or pre-Descemet's copper-containing Kayser/Fleischer ring appearing in Wilson's hepato-lenticular degeneration, first reported by Fleischer in 1901.)

ring, Landolt A standardized optotype in C configuration for quantitating central visual acuity. A 1-minute gap in the C ring is presented in one of four alternating positions (up, down, right, or left); uses Snellen minimal visual angle for both strokes and gap width. Developed in 1888 by Edmond Landolt (1846–1926), Parisian ophthalmologist. (See Figure 17.)

rings, Newton's One of the basic examples of the interference phenomena of light. When a spherically surfaced lens is placed on an optical flat surface and viewed from above in monochromatic light, a series of concentric rings appear about a central dark spot and are shifted outward by pressure on the lens system; Newton's fringes. Reported in 1705 by Isaac Newton (1642–1727), English mathematician and optical scientist, who published *New Theory About Light and Color* (1672) and *Optics* (1704) and was president of the Royal Society from 1703 to 1727.

rivets Fasteners used to attach hinges or other frame components to a frame.

Robon spectacles Glass safety lenses introduced by Zeiss in 1924 to protect eyes from heat radiation.

rocking pad See *pad, rocking.*

rod, Maddox A cylindrical glass rod or multiple rods used in front of one eye to create gross image disparity and visual dissociation in order to measure the deviation (heterophoria or heterotropia) between the two eyes. The rod, when placed in front of one eye, converts the image of a small light source to a straight line perpendicular to the axis of the rod. Developed by ophthalmologist Ernest E. Maddox, M.D. (1863–1933), of Scotland, who also developed many other tests for strabismus.

rod monochromacy See *monochromacy, rod.*

rod vision See *vision, scotopic.*

rods (rod cells) Type of photoreceptor cells in the retina, consisting of an outer and an inner member in the layer of rods and cones, an outer rod cell body in the outer nuclear layer, and a rod fiber and end bulb in the outer plexiform layer. They contain rhodopsin in their outer components; their fibers synapse with a bipolar cell; involved in scotopic vision and detection of movement. There are about 120 million rods in the retina of each eye; retinal rods.

rolled gold plate See *plate, rolled gold.*

rose bengal A vital stain which produces red color in dead or degenerated epithelial cells of the cornea, conjunctiva, and mucous and epithelial filaments. Chemically is a dye described as dichlor, or tetrachlor erythrosin. Commonly used as sterile 1% aqueous solution preserved with 0.01% thimerosal. Though many attempts at staining the cornea have been reported since 1882, rose bengal was introduced shortly after World War II by Georges Kleefeld (1889-1979), ophthalmologist who practiced in Paris, Brussels, and New York. In 1933, Sjogren also recommended the use of 1% aqueous rose bengal to delineate the lesions of keratoconjunctivitis sicca; q.v.

rotation, optical The ability of certain minerals and chemical solutions to change the plane of incident polarized light in an arc characteristic of the substance, commonly specified as levorotatory (to the left), or dextrorotatory (to the right).

rouge (roozh) French for the word "red." A polishing compound of red oxide of iron (Fe_2O_2), though often applied to other polishing materials which are not red, such as "black rouge," "white rouge," etc.; also used as cosmetic preparation applied to eyelids, and as such, produces a distortion artifact to the anterior globe when seen in magnetic resonance imaging (MRI).

router A tool or machine for grooving, recessing, or gouging out recesses.

RPM Mnemonic for revolutions per minute.

Ru Chemical symbol for ruthenium; q.v.

rubber, silicone An organic elastic polymer in which all or part of the carbon has been replaced by silicon; used as an implant in scleral buckling to repair retinal detachment, and as a surgical implant within Tenon's capsule after enucleation of an eye.

ruby A naturally occurring precious stone of crystalline red corundum (aluminum oxide, Al_2O_3) containing a small amount of chromium (Cr); Mohs hardness approximately 9; used as an abrasive in grinding wheels and as the first successful laser material (1960).

rule, millimeter A linear measuring device conveniently marked in centimeters and millimeters, used to make linear optical measurements.

rule, Duane's A flat, wooden ruler notched at the proximal end to fit over the bridge of the nose, used to measure accommodation as devised by New York ophthalmologist Alexander Duane (1858–1926), an authority on motor anomalies of the eye.

rule, Kestenbaum's (kes'ten-baumz) Mathematical formula based on best Snellen distance acuity to estimate dioptric power of a magnifying low-vision aid; division of the Snellen numerator into the denominator gives the lower range of dioptric add to read conventional print in capital letters (e.g., 20/400 = 20D add needed); devised in 1956 by Alfred Kestenbaum (1890–1960), neuroophthalmologist of Vienna and later New York City; Kestenbaum formula.

rule, Knapp's A proper corrective lens located at the anterior focal point on the visual axis; in any axial ametropia will produce retinal images of the same size, no matter what the magnitude or sign (+ or –) of the ametropia; described by Hermann Jacob Knapp (1832–1911), ophthalmologist of Germany and New York.

rule, Prentice's See *law, Prentice's.*

rule, Prince's A hand-held linear scale usually marked in centimeters and inches to measure the distance from the eye to its near point of accommodation; accommodometer; near optometer; designed by Arthur Edward Prince, M.D. (1855–1930), practicing ophthalmologist of Jacksonville, Illinois. (cf. *rule, Duane's.*)

ruthenium A rare, very hard metallic element; chemical symbol Ru, atomic number 44; used as an alloy with other metals in spectacle frame manufacturing. Discovered in 1844 by Russian chemist Carl Ernst Claus (1796–1864).

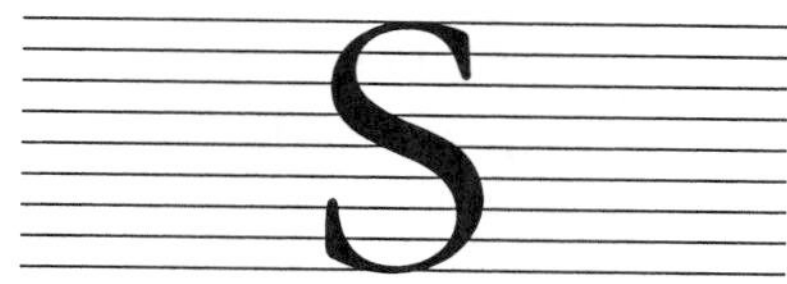

s Symbol for second, the Système Internationale (S.I.) base unit of time.

S Chemical symbol for the non-metallic element sulfur, atomic number 16. Used as a topical medication for skin diseases and scabies.

s.c. Abbreviation for without correction or without lenses.

S.I.D.U.O. Abbreviation for Society International for Diagnostic Ultrasound in Ophthalmology; q.v.

S.M.O. Abbreviation for Society of Military Ophthalmologists; q.v.

saccade (sah-kād′) A series of involuntary, abrupt, rapid, small movements or jerks of both eyes, especially seen in changing visual fixation from one point to another.

saddle bridge See *bridge, saddle.*

safety bevel See *bevel, safety.*

safety glasses See *glasses, safety.*

sagitta (saj′i-tah) Shaped like an arrow or arrowhead; a center line; the distance from the midpoint of an arc to the midpoint of its chord.

sagitta value See *value, sagitta.*

sagittal Pertaining to a straight line (arrow) or a straight plane; commonly, a vertical straight plane dividing the body into right and left halves.

sagittal depth See *depth, sagitta.*

sagittal plane See *plane, sagittal.*

salt, chemtempering Large, molecular configuration of acid-base combinations, such as potassium nitrate or lithium nitrate, used in heat-treating glass ophthalmic lenses to increase impact resistance.

SAM Mnemonic for steeper add minus. A fitting technique for contact lenses in which the plus power created by the tears trapped between a contact lens and the corneal surface is neutralized by the addition of an equal amount of minus (opposite) lens power.

sapphire stone A clear deep blue variety of corundum (aluminum oxide) near to diamond in hardness (Mohs 9), used for jewel bearings in Schiotz tonometers; available in both natural and synthetic form.

Sattler's veil See *veil, Sattler's.*

Sb Chemical symbol for the crystalline metallic element, antimony; q.v.

scalar Ladder-like; describable by a number that can be represented by a point in a system.

scale A scheme or device of units or steps at regular or graduated intervals, by which a specific property may be measured or evaluated.

scale, Baumé A measure of fluid density expressed in equal degrees for liquids heavier or lighter than water; used to express concentration of liquid polish or grinding compound slurries; range for lens-polishing slurries is usually graded from 0° to 50°; may be converted to specific gravity. Developed by the French chemist Antoine Baumé (1728–1804).

scale, Celsius A thermometric terminology expressing the degree centigrade (freezing point of distilled water at 0° and boiling point of water at normal atmospheric pressure at 100°); formerly expressed as degree centrigrade, but since 1948, adopted as preferred terminology. Developed in 1742 by Swedish astronomer Anders Celsius (1701–1744).

scale, centrigrade A thermometric measure expressed in degrees where the freezing point of distilled water is 0° and the boiling point of water at normal atmospheric pressure is 100°. See *scale, Celsius.*

scale, Fahrenheit A thermometric measure in degrees (°F) of the temperature of distilled water wherein its boiling point is 212°F and the freezing point at normal atmospheric pressure is 32°F. Developed in 1714 by German physicist Daniel Fahrenheit (1686–1736), who invented the first truly accurate thermometer.

scale, Kelvin An S.I. unit. A thermometric measure using the centigrade degree of measurement wherein absolute zero (0°K) equals approximately –273°C. Developed in 1848 by British physicist Lord William Thomson Kelvin (1824–1907).

scale, Mohs An orderly arrangement of minerals by their hardness characteristics from a low of talc at one (1) to a high of diamond at ten

(10); used at times to measure relative hardness of glass. Developed in 1822 by German mineralogist Friedrich Mohs (1733–1839).

scale, TABO conversion In keratometry, a nomogram to convert radius of curvature in millimeters to diopters of refractive power; used in all reflecting keratometers which read in diopters, based on presumed refractive index of 1.3375 in the human cornea. Mnemonic for the German committee, Technischer Ausschuss für Brillenoptik, established in 1917 to fix standards for cylinder axis notation and other optical measurements.

scatter, Tyndall Localized diffusion of light within a ray or beam due to presence of particulate matter such as proteins or cells in liquid, moisture in air; seen in the aqueous of the eye during inflammation; described by John Tyndall (1820–1893), physicist of Ireland and England.

scattered light See *light, scattered.*

Schirmer's test See *test, Schirmer's.*

scissors glasses See *glasses, scissors.*

SCL Mnemonic for lens, contact, soft; q.v.

sclera (sklā'rah) The white, opaque, fibrous, outer tunic of the eyeball, covering it entirely except for the segment covered anteriorly by the cornea.

sclera, blue (van der Hoeve's syndrome) Osteogenesis imperfecta. An hereditary syndrome with type-1 collagen disorder, brittle bones and multiple fractures often associated with deafness; may be confused with battered-child problems. The usually white sclera in such patients appears distinctly blue. Described by J. van der Hoeve (1878–1952), Dutch ophthalmologist, in 1917, though there are earlier, partial descriptions.

scleral zone See *zone, scleral.*

-scope Suffix meaning instrument for viewing.

scotoma (sko-to'mah) Blind area within the visual field. First described in practical detail and named by Julius Sichel (1802–1868), an Austrian ophthalmologist practicing in Paris.

scotopic vision See *vision, scotopic.*

scratch A slight mark, usually thin and shallow, caused by a sharp or pointed object moving against a surface.

screen, Harrington-Flocks, multiple pattern A series of 10 cards, each with a distinctive pattern printed in fluorescent ink and used under ultraviolet light for rapid testing of the central visual field. Developed in 1954 by California ophthalmologists David O. Harrington (1904–1990) and Milton Flocks (b. 1914).

screen, tangent Flat felt or unfigured dark surface usually positioned 1m from eye; used to test the central 60° diameter of the visual field for defects by the kinetic method; Bjerrum screen; campimeter; trade name, Autoplot. Popularized by Jannik Peterson Bjerrum (1851–1920), Danish ophthalmologist..

screw A threaded fastening device.

screw, hinge A threaded fastener used to join the front and temple barrel portions of a spectacle hinge.

screw, self-tapping A threaded mechanical fastening device, usually cylindrical or conical in shape, with a sharp, projecting thread (helical rib) that cuts its own reciprocal channel into the material into which it is inserted or twisted; used mainly on plastic spectacle frames.

sebaceous (se-bā'shus) Glands that secrete sebum or oil.

sebum (sē'bum) From the tarsal glands of the eyelids , a thick secretion that provides the outermost oily layer of the precorneal tear film; makes an airtight closure of the lids and prevents the lacrimal fluid from overflowing onto the outer surface of the eyelid, thus softening the skin.

second sight See *sight, second.*

secondary axis See *axis, secondary.*

seg measure An engraved measuring device of plastic or metal/plastic combination providing a millimeter scale that may be inserted or otherwise attached to the grooved rim of a spectacle eyewire to determine the proper segment height of a multifocal lens; segment measure.

segment In ophthalmic optics, a specified area of a multifocal lens having a different refractive power from the major portion. Also refers to the actual piece of material added to the lens in the case of a fused or cemented multifocal lens. See *addition (spectacle).*

segment, anterior In ocular anatomy, that portion of the eyeball contained between the surface of the cornea and the vitreous face encompassing approximately the front third of the globe.

segment, cemented An added power ophthalmic lens bound, usually by epoxy resin, to a carrier (i.e., distant corrective lens); paster,

Morck bifocal. (cf. *lens, bifocal cement.*) Also, Univision, a low--vision aid with a cemented add of high dioptric power.

segment clock See *clock, segment.*

segment, compensated Ribbon-shaped multifocal add ("R" type) ground with the segment center at different heights as prescribed to neutralize or minimize small amounts of vertical prismatic imbalance in a pair of anisometropic bifocal lenses.

segment drop See *drop, segment.*

segment height See *height, segment.*

segment inset See *inset, segment.*

segment line See *line, segment.*

segment optical center See *center, segment optical.*

segment, prism A reading portion of a bifocal lens into which prism has been ground before fusing. Formerly used to correct moderate amounts of vertical prismatic imbalance in a pair of anisometropic bifocals. Presently available with base in prism only. Used for the correction of convergence insufficiency.

segments, dissimilar Two differently shaped multifocal segments in a pair of anisometropic ophthalmic lenses, chosen so that their resultant reading optical centers neutralize or reduce the vertical prismatic imbalance at the reading level induced by the anisometropic correction.

segments, fused Component of an ophthalmic lens produced by heat-uniting a piece of glass of greater index of refraction into a countersunk area of a larger crown glass lens. Generally the segment is placed on the convex side of the lens, and the curves on this surface are then ground and polished uniformly. Developed between 1897 and 1908 by John F. Borsch, Jr.; télégic bifocal; trade name, Kryptok.

self-refraction Use of a modified phoropter (phoro-optometer) generally in over-refraction techniques with computer-assisted integration of patient's previous spectacle prescription; manually operated by both children and adults; developed by C. Norton Sims (b. 1937), Florida ophthalmologist.

semi- Prefix meaning half.

semi-finished blank See *blank, semi-finished.*

semi-finished lens See *lens, semi-finished.*

sensitivity, contrast The physiologic capacity of the eye to differentiate progressively subtle gradations in grayness between test lines and background; Vistech sine wave grating charts (1977); Regan mid-range spatial frequency charts (1975); Pelli-Robson large letter charts (1988); Arden mid-frequency plates (1977); Holladay contrast acuity test (1992) consisting of 10 charts at 5 different levels (100%, 50%, 25%, 12.5%, and 6.25%) of contrast.

sensory Pertaining to reception and transmission of an impression from a peripheral or end organ to the brain.

set-back angle See *angle, set-back.*

set, trial An ophthalmic examining kit including trial frames, trial lenses, prisms, Maddox rods, etc., for refraction. First known set of trial lenses, 1778, produced by the European optician Paul Hirn, Electoral Spectacle and Lens Maker.

shadowgraph An optical inspection device that uses magnification and projection to evaluate the surface, edges and curvature of a corneal contact lens; trade name, Neitz Projection Contacto-Screen.

sheath In fiber optics, a thin cover layer applied to the core fibers as a fluorine polymer of lower refractive index than the core material.

shell, casting A plastic molding cup 24mm to 30mm in diameter, perforated and fitted with a handle on its convex (outer) surface; used to make impression molds of an enucleation socket.

shell ocular prosthesis See *prosthesis, shell ocular.*

shield

1. A protective device, commonly made of aluminum or acrylic, taped over the eye following ocular surgery, e.g., Fox shield of malleable aluminum designed by L. Webster Fox, M.D. (1853–1931), Pennsylvania ophthalmologist.
2. A double rivet with an ornamental head joining both rivets, normally used to attach hinges or other components of a spectacle frame.

shield, collagen A temporary therapeutic bandage contact lens or drug-delivery device resembling a large cornea conformer 14mm to 16mm in diameter, made of porcine scleral collagen or bovine skin collagen; dissolves in 1 to 3 days; introduced in 1986 by Texas ophthalmologists J.H. Sheets and E.L. Wasserman. Trade names, Bio-Cor (Bausch & Lomb); Medilens.

shield, side A transparent protective device, usually attached to spectacle ear pieces to protect the eye from lateral injuries; usually made of CR-39 or polycarbonate and designed variously for wide or narrow ear pieces. Manufactured in three progressively larger styles, A, B and C.

shoe straps See *straps, shoe.*

short finish See *grayness.*

Si Chemical symbol for the non-metallic element silicon; q.v.

SI Acronym for segment inset; see *inset, segment.*

S.I. Système Internationale d'Unites, International System of Units. Established as Standard 1000 by the International Organization of Standards through General Conferences on Weights and Measures in 1954 with member bodies from 30 nations, including the United States; consists of seven base units, two supplementary units in 1960, and a growing number of more than 27 derived units.

sicca syndrome See *syndrome, sicca.*

side, nasal In spectacle optics, the side of a lens or frame closest to the nose.

sight, second An improvement in near-range acuity due to myopic shift occurring in early cataract or lens intumescence; may also be induced by elevated blood sugar in diabetic patients.

sign An objective manifestation or indication of a disease or abnormality, usually perceptible to an examiner.

sign, Munson's An abnormal forward bulging of the lower eyelid border observed when a patient looks downward; caused by high curvature of the cornea as deformed by keratoconus.

signature, optical Any characteristic feature of a substance created by the action of a given light.

Silastic (si-las'tik) Trade name for polymeric silicone substances having properties similar to rubber, but biologically inert. Used in some contact lenses and for surgical implants.

silica Silicon dioxide (SiO_2) or silicic anhydride, a naturally occurring hard stone in crystalline, amorphous, or colloidal form.

silica glass See *glass, silica.*

silicon A non-metallic element; chemical symbol Si, atomic number 14. Used as a major component of ophthalmic glass in the form of its oxide, SiO_2 (silica); also as a semiconducting crystal used in computer chips and diodes. Discovered in 1824 by Swedish chemist Jöns Jakob Berzelius (1779–1848).

silicone Any of a group of long-chain polymerized organic silicon compounds in which all or part of the carbon has been replaced by silicon; used in oxygen-permeable hard contact lenses, and as an implant material in the surgical correction of retinal detachments; organic derivatives of silica were produced in many forms for 40 years (1899–1939) by Frederic Stanley Kipping (1863–1949), English chemist.

silicone acrylate A combination polymer (or copolymer), used in contact lens fabrication providing high oxygen permeability with the rigid characteristics of PMMA; has poor wetting characteristics; introduced in mid-1970s.

silicone rubber See *rubber, silicone.*

silver A white, malleable metallic chemical element; chemical symbol Ag, atomic number 47; used as a halide in binary compounds with a halogen in phototropic lenses; used as a coating in mirrored sunglasses; also used in production of glass lenses to give a yellow tint.

simple hyperopic astigmatism See *astigmatism, simple hyperopic.*

simple myopic astigmatism See *astigmatism, simple myopic.*

single binocular vision See *vision, single binocular.*

single cut lens See *lens, single cut.*

single vision lens See *lens, single vision.*

single vision semi-finished blank See *blank, single vision semi-finished.*

sintercast To make into a cohesive mass by heating without melting; used for powdered or granular substances as polycarbonates.

size, blank The overall dimensions in millimeters of a rough, semi-finished, or finished lens as produced by the lens manufacturer, given either as round, horizontal, vertical, or a combination of same, as in the Boxing System.

size, bridge

1. In spectacle optics common usage, the designated horizontal distance between lenses on a spectacle front; e.g., 52❑22 are "boxed" measurements in millimeters, the latter measurement (22mm) being the indicated "bridge size."
2. That portion of the nominal frame front size measurement marked on the packaging envelope for inventory purposes, not always the actual DBL. (See Figures 19 and 20.)

size, lens The linear measurements A and B in millimeters between the vertical tangents and between the horizontal tangents to the apex of the finished lens bevel; erroneously called "eye" size. (See Figures 19 and 20.)

Sjogren's disease See *keratoconjunctivitis sicca.*

skiascopy From the Greek "skia," meaning shadow. Superseded term for retinoscopy. Introduced by Ernst Pfluger (1848–1903), chief of ophthalmology at University of Bern, Switzerland. See *retinoscopy.*

skiving A slicing or shaving operation in spectacle frame construction yielding greater precision than sawing or cutting; skive.

skull temple See *temple, skull.*

slab-off See *grinding, bicentric.*

slab-off, reverse A molding process on a plastic lens which produces base-down prism in the reading portion of the lens. This prism direction is the opposite of base-up prism produced in bicentric grinding of a glass lens. Developed by California optician Irving Rips. See *grinding, bicentric.*

slit lamp See *biomicroscope.*

slit, stenopaic See *disc, stenopaic.*

SLK Mnemonic for keratitis, superior limbic; q.v.

slurry A watery mixture of insoluble material; in optical lens surfacing is usually designated on Baumé Scale from 0° to 50°.

Snell's law of refraction See *law of refraction, Snell's.*

Snellen chart See *chart, Snellen.*

Society International for Diagnostic Ultrasound in Ophthalmology (S.I.D.U.O.) A voluntary professional association of ophthalmologists, acoustic engineers and related scientists in the field of high frequency echography, above the audible range. Established in 1964; approximately 500 members; convenes International Congress every two years and publishes *Proceedings*; governed by an executive board of 27.

Society of Military Ophthalmologists (S.M.O.) In the United States, a professional organization of approximately 1,500 individual ophthalmologists in the Army, Navy, and Air Force.

sodium fluorescein See *fluorescein, sodium.*

solution, balanced salt (BSS) A sterile isotonic solution of sodium chloride in water, but also containing other physiologic components, such as potassium chloride, dibase sodium phosphate, sodium carbonate, sodium hydroxide, and similar ions essential for cell metabolism.

solution, physiologic saline A sterile isotonic, preserved, or nonpreserved solution of distilled water containing 0.9% sodium chloride; used to rinse or store soft contact lenses, and as a surface irrigant for the eye.

solution, soaking/wetting A sterile, buffered, isotonic solution of distilled water containing potassium sorbate as preservative; used before the insertion of rigid contact lenses to increase lens wettability and wearing comfort.

Solution, Boston Advance Conditioning A sterile, buffered, slightly hypertonic solution by Polymer Technology, Wilmington, Massachusetts, containing a cationic, cellulose-derivative polymer with 0.0015% polyaminopropyl biguanimide and 0.05% editate disodium as preservatives; used as a wetting agent for rigid gas-permeable contact lenses. Lenses require a minimum of 4 hours of soaking then rewetting with fresh conditioner before insertion.

sonochemistry The interface of chemical structure with that aspect of vibration physics leading to cavitation and luminescence; ultrasonic cavitation; important in clinical echography of the eye.

sorbate, potassium A chemical compound, 2,4-hexadienoic acid potassium salt, occurring as a white crystal or powder, which is a mold and yeast inhibitor. In solution, may be used as a preservative for pharmaceutical preparations or contact lens solutions. May cause discoloration of soft contact lenses with water content greater than 50%. Generally superseded by benzalkonium chloride, a synthetic quaternary ammonium compound; q.v.

soulé (soo-lā′) To cut off a portion of a lens.

spall A small chip or fragment; characteristically having at least one feathered edge; seen in broken glass.

Spar, Iceland A transparent, colorless calcite found especially in Iceland and used to make double-refracting optical media; a rhombohedron crystallization of calcium carbonate.

spectacle blur See *blur, spectacle.*

spectacle plane See *plane, spectacle.*

spectacles An optical device to retain lenses in front of the eyes, consisting of a front, a bridge and two temples or earpieces. Worn to correct, assist, or protect vision, and, at times, for cosmetic reasons.

spectacles, divers (underwater spectacles) Ophthalmic lenses specially designed to neutralize the induced hypermetropia of the cornea when underwater; usually double construction including a refractive element.

spectacles, lift-front A conventional spectacle with an additional permanent, detachable, or hinged-front that can be raised or lowered to provide for special visual needs such as sunglass protection or additional lens power for near vision.

spectacles, rimless A pair of ophthalmic lenses joined together by a bridge (i.e., centerpiece), and having temple bows separately attached, with no rims to connect any of the parts to one another, thus reducing weight; Waldstein spectacles. Introduced by the Vienna optician Waldstein in about 1840.

spectacles, tube Special goggles or special fitted spectacles with opaque, hollow cylinders extending forward 1 to 2 inches to limit the energy of eccentric light into the eyes. Described by Samuel Pepys (1633–1703), politician and naval administrator with poor vision. Reintroduced in 1970s by John Win, ophthalmologist from Melbourne, Australia as "docking glasses" for astronauts.

spectrum, electromagnetic An ordered arrangement of radiant energies including all known radiations from very short (nanometer) to very long (kilometer) (i.e., cosmic rays, gamma rays, X-rays, ultraviolet rays, visible rays, infrared rays, microwaves and radiowaves).

spectrum, visible That portion of the electromagnetic spectrum which contains wavelengths capable of stimulating the retina, 380nm to 760nm.

specular Pertaining to a smooth or highly polished reflecting surface.

sphere See *surface, spheric.*

sphere, far point The curved surface described by the optical far point of an eye as it rotates.

sphere power See *power, sphere.*

spheric surface See *surface, spheric.*

spherical Relating to, or of the nature of, a curve with uniform radius of curvature.

spherical aberration See *aberration, spherical.*

spherical equivalent See *equivalent, spherical.*

spherical lens See *lens, spherical.*

spherical plus lens See *lens, spherical plus.*

spherocylinder See *lens, spherocylinder.*

spherocylindrical lens See *lens, spherocylinder.*

spindle, Krukenberg's (kroo'ken"bergz) A fusiform configuration of pigment deposits on the inner surface of the cornea, commonly between the corneal center and the 6 o'clock limbus; originally described in 1899 by Friedrich Ernst Krukenberg (1871–1946), German pathologist.

SPK Mnemonic for keratitis, superficial punctate; q.v.

splay To spread out or apart; sloping or spreading of a broad and flat surface.

splay angle See *angle, splay.*

spring-hinge temple See *temple, spring-hinge.*

SPX Trade name for a plastic material used in spectacle frame construction; requires no heat to adjust.

SRC Mnemonic for **c**oating, **s**cratch **r**esistant; q.v.

stain, stipple Fine, dot-like speckling in the corneal epithelium following application of sodium fluorescein solution.

staining, punctate A pattern of corneal epithelial damage that appears as small depressions when highlighted by sodium fluorescein solution.

staining, 3- and 9-o'clock Punctate staining of Bowman's membrane following the loss of epithelial cells along the horizontal margins of the cornea during contact lens wear. Most often caused by thick lens edge, corneal dehydration, and incomplete blinking. Demonstrated by topical application of sodium fluorescein solution.

standard eye See *eye, standard.*

Standard, Revised Jaeger (yā'ger) A critical notation of visual acuity in the near (reading) range based on a precise application of the 1-minute arc-resolving power as used in Snellen distant charts; introduced in 1958 by A.H. Keeney, M.D., and H. Lyle Duerson.

Standards, National Bureau of See *National Bureau of Standards.* In 1989, renamed National Institute for Standards and Technology.

static perimetry See perimetry, static.

steel, stainless A carbon steel alloyed with chromium and sometimes nickel, rendering the material practically immune to rust and corrosion. Commonly used in surgical instruments and sometimes in spectacle frames.

steeper than K Contact lens parlance for a contact lens fitting technique in which the central posterior curve of the lens to be fitted has a shorter radius of curvature (higher central vault) than the flattest meridian of the cornea.

steno- Prefix meaning narrow; close.

stenopaic slit See *disc, stenopaic.*

stent A mold, device, or container to hold a skin graft or control other tissues, as after a burn or corrective surgery. Named from the London dentist, Charles R. Stent (d. 1901), who introduced this device and impression compounds in 1857.

steradian (ste-rā'de-an) In solid geometry, a unit solid angle derived in three dimensions from a point source; in the Système Internationale (S.I.), one of the supplemental (non-base) units adopted in 1960; equivalent to the angle subtended at the center of a sphere by an area on its surface equal to the square of its radius. A full sphere subtends 4 π steradians.

stereo- Prefix meaning solid in reference to area and depth; solidity; three-dimensionality.

stereo-acuity Graded measurement of binocular ability to see in stereopsis with small differences in image configuration; graded in degrees or seconds of arc disparity between the two presented images; requires good visual acuity in each eye.

stereogram Visual test cards with slightly differing printed images for each eye; usually used in a steroscope that keeps each eye optically separated from the other in order to study stereo-acuity of a patient.

stereopsis (ste"re-op'sis) True, three-dimensional depth perception achieved by slightly dissimilar images falling on corresponding retinal points in the two eyes.; not obtainable with one eye. Stereoscopic vision; third-degree fusion.

stereopter, Verhoeff A hand-held mechanical device for qualitative estimation of near stereopsis. Developed in 1942 by Frederick Herman Verhoeff (1874–1968), Boston ophthalmologist; manufactured by American Optical Co.

stereoscope Binocular optical device that separates field of view of each eye; tests or trains binocular coordination, fusional amplitudes (vergence ability), and stereopsis; invented and named in 1838 as mirror stereoscope by Charles Wheatstone (1802–1875), English scientist and experimenter; improved as prism stereoscope (1844–1852) by David Brewster (1781–1868), scientific experimenter of Edinburgh.

stilb (stil′b) A psychophysical unit of luminance expressed as one candela per square centimeter; equals 10,000 nits.

Stilling's plates See *plates, Stilling's.*

stock lens See *lens, stock or factory finished uncut.*

Stokes' lens See *lens, Stokes'.*

stop, lens

1. The specified diameter of the available aperture in a lens.
2. In a focimeter, a mechanical holder to position the lens at a fixed position, thereby providing a uniform measuring aperture.

strabismic (stra-biz′mic) Having or pertaining to strabismus.

strabismus (stra-biz′mus) Misalignment of the eyes, manifest in extraocular muscle imbalance; binocular fixation is absent; squint; heterotropia.

strabismus, alternating Positional deviation of an eye (inward, outward, upward, or downward) in which there is frequent switching between the fixing and deviating eye and generally good acuity in each eye.

strabismus, concomitant Ocular deviation which is the same in all directions of rotation at a given distance (strabismus comitant). Term coined by German oculophysiologist Johannes Müller (1801–1858).

straight-top bifocal lens See *lens, straight-top bifocal.*

strain To stretch or force by applying pressure. In a lens, such forces may be from tempering processes, poor annealing, or induced by casting and molding during manufacturing; may also be created from the improper (i.e., tight) mounting of lenses in metal frames, or rimless or semi-rimless mountings which apply external stress.

strain, birefringence (bī″re-frin′jens) Multiple refraction seen in clear isotropic materials such as optical glass or plastic when subject to tensile or compressive stress; may appear as isoclinic (isotropic) lines in polarized light.

strap thickness See *thickness, strap.*

strap(s) Fittings used in eyeglasses, or rimless or semi-rimless spectacle frames to lock endpieces or center pieces to lenses.

straps, shoe Metal fasteners used to attach bridge and endpiece components to the lenses of rimless spectacle mountings; at ends of saddle bridge are sometimes described as *shanks.*

streak retinoscope See *retinoscope, streak.*

stress A force applied to an object; the tendency within a body to be deformed by other forces.

stria (strī'ah)

1. Optical. A lens defect characterized by elongated areas of localized variation of index of refraction caused by chemical nonhomogeneity in the body of the material.
2. Anatomical. A narrow streak or line; plural, striae.

striae (strī'ā) Plural of stria; q.v.

striae atrophicae (a-tro-fē'kā) Linear, thin, white bands commonly on skin that has been stretched.

striking To make or impress by a blow or stamping; used in spectacle frame manufacture, especially metal frames.

stroma, corneal Thickest layer of the cornea; located between Bowman's membrane, anteriorly, and Descemet's membrane, posteriorly. Represents 90% of the total corneal thickness and gives the cornea its strength. Consists of layers of parallel collagen fibrils and scattered, small, flattened cells (keratocytes).

Sturm, conoid of See *conoid of Sturm.*

stye See *hordeolum.*

sub- Prefix meaning under; below.

subluxation of the lens Incomplete loss of usual suspension of the crystalline lens; one of the causes of monocular diplopia; commonly expressed as anterior or through the pupil, and posterior or behind the pupil; induces major visual distortion. (cf. *Luxation.*)

subnormal vision See *vision, subnormal.*

subtends That which extends under or is opposite to; commonly expressed in regard to an angular extent or fixed vertex; indicated as the included cord or arc.

subtilisin See *cleaner, enzymatic.*

Sunglass Association of America (S.A.A.) A voluntary association of approximately 90 optical manufacturers, import distributors, and visual scientists concerned with development, standardization, research, good manufacturing practices and labeling practices in the sunglass industry. Established 1970. Office: Norwalk, Connecticut 06851.

sunglasses Ophthalmic lenses designed to reduce light transmission. Standardized by A.N.S.I. Z80.3 as cosmetic, general purpose, and special purpose.

super- Prefix meaning excessive; more than normal.

superior Upper or upper direction.

suppression Visual physiology. Process of ignoring what one sees, particularly the vision in a deviating or strabismic eye; more intense than the psychological level of *disregarding*..

supra- Prefix meaning above; over.

supraduction An upward rotation of the eye.

surface The outer face, outside, or exterior of something.

surface, aspheric (a-sfer'ik) A non-uniform surface curvature commonly used to improve optical lens performance, particularly for high refractive powers. Conic surfaces are widely used for this purpose; each is radial symmetrically with respect to an axis of symmetry. A meridianal section of such a surface is a conic section.

surface, Cartesian An ellipsoidal surface, mathematically calculated to be free of all spherical aberration; also, Cartesian lens. Calculated and proposed by René Descartes (1596–1650), French philosopher and mathematician.

surface, combining In ophthalmic optics, the other or opposite face from the base curve of an ophthalmic lens; sometimes called the second surface. For a plus base-curve lens, sometimes called the minus surface, back surface or ocular surface.

surface, concave A surface which is both hollow and curved resembling the inner surface of a sphere; the opposite of a convex surface; the back surface of a spectacle lens is commonly concave.

surface, convex A surface which is both protruding and curved; the opposite of concave surface; the front surface of a spectacle lens is usually convex.

surface, first One of the two refracting surfaces between two media of differing refractive index; interface; designated according to the direction of incident light.

surface, optical A surface at which uniform refraction occurs, especially one designed for this purpose in a lens system.

surface, Petzval A mathematically designed optical surface to reduce curvature of field; described in 1843 by Jozsef Miska Petzval, Hungarian mathematician and optician. Mathematical treatment of the curvature of the image was calculated and published in 1830 by George Biddell Airy (1801–1892), English mathematician and astronomer.

surface, plano A flat surface having zero surface power or infinite radius of curvature.

surface power See *power, surface.*

surface, second One of the two refracting surfaces between two media of differing refractive index; designated as the subsequent or following surface, according to the direction of incident light.

surface, spheric A curved surface having the same radius of curvature in all meridians.

surface, toric The form of a portion of a torus having different curvatures in the two principal meridians. The shape may be visualized as a small part of the surface of a doughnut or of a football containing both principal meridians of a torus. A toric surface is generated by rotating an arc of a circle around an axis which does not pass through the center of the circle. See *torus.*

surfactant An agent which is primarily active on the surface and does not penetrate into tissues (e.g., soap or synthetic detergents); often contain phospholipids; used in contact lens cleaning solutions to dislodge accumulated lipoprotein and similar deposits from the anterior and posterior lens surface. May be classified chemically as cationic (protein precipitant), anionic (cytolytic) and nonionic (possessing neither of the previous actions).

suspensory ligaments See *zonule of Zinn.*

swarf In grinding and cutting operations, debris of fine dust and particles, particularly of metal, but commonly extended to include plastics and glass.

sym-, syn-, sys- Prefix meaning with; in union; associated.

symblepharon (sim-blef'ah-ron) A congenital, disease-induced, or post-traumatic lid defect in which the lids are fused with the anterior aspect of the globe, usually uniting the palpebral with the bulbar conjunctiva; may be complete or incomplete. (cf. *ankyloblepharon.*)

symptom Subjective evidence, feeling, or perception of disease or disorder by a patient.

synapse (sin'aps) The place where a nerve impulse is transmitted from one neuron to another.

syndrome A set of symptoms and signs generally occurring together, but not a clearly defined, specific disease.

syndrome, carpal tunnel A complex of symptoms and discomfort in the wrist and hand resulting from compression of the median nerve and the flexor tendons against the carpal bones; associated with repetitive hand motions while the wrist is flexed.

syndrome, overwear (OWS) Pain, corneal edema, photosensitivity, and the erosion of the corneal epithelium as a result of wearing contact lenses over an extended period of time.

syndrome, sicca (sik'ah) Abnormal tear deficiency causing dry eyes; frequently associated with dry mouth and dry joints, especially in middle-aged females; Sjogren's syndrome; keratoconjunctivitis sicca. A contraindication to fitting contact lenses, unless specifically prescribed as a therapeutic or bandage device; sometimes called Gougerot-Sjogren. Originally described in 1933 by Swedish ophthalmologist Henrik Samuel Conrad Sjogren (1899–1986).

syndrome, sucked on Informal designation of a condition in which a contact lens is firmly adhered to the corneal or conjunctival surface, often the result of a steep fitting or large diameter lens. Removal may result in loss of corneal epithelium.

synechia (si-nēk'e-ah) Adhesions of the iris to the cornea (anterior) or the crystalline lens (posterior); plural is synechiae.

synechia, anterior An adhesion of the front surface of the iris to the corneal endothelium.

synechia, posterior An adhesion of the back surface of the iris to the anterior surface of the crystalline lens capsule.

system, boxing A technique that circumscribes a box about a lens, or frame lens opening to standardize the method of determining frame and lens measurements and to locate prescription requirements in relation thereto; technique adopted January 1, 1962, by the O.L.A. The vertical sides of the box are tangents to the lateral extremities, and the horizontal sides are tangents to the vertical extremities, with the center (i.e., the intersection of diagonals from opposite corners of the box), designated as the geometric center of the box so formed. The method specifies that all measurements must be taken from the geometric center or bevel apexes, and be expressed in millimeters. See *diagram, boxing system.*

system, Grolman fitting A mechanical device and schema to assist dispensing opticians in precise vertical and horizontal measurements to fit progressive-power multifocal lenses; devised by Massachusetts optometrist Bernard Grolman (b. 1926).

system, metric A decimal system of weights and measures legislatively sanctioned by the U.S. Congress in 1866 for general and scientific purposes and preferentially adopted by the U.S. National Bureau of Standards in 1964; governed by the S.I. system. The unit most commonly used by the optician is the millimeter (mm), and its value may be obtained from the following table of equivalents:

1 meter (m)	=	1000 millimeters (mm)
1 meter (m)	=	100 centimeters (cm)
1 meter (m)	=	39.37 inches (in., ")
25.4mm	=	1 inch
1mm	=	1,000 nanometers (nm)

system, Vistech An optical test of contrast sensitivity determined by subtle shades of grayness and interval between the test markings and their background; developed from 1977 by Arthur P. Ginsburg, U.S. military investigator in psychophysics.

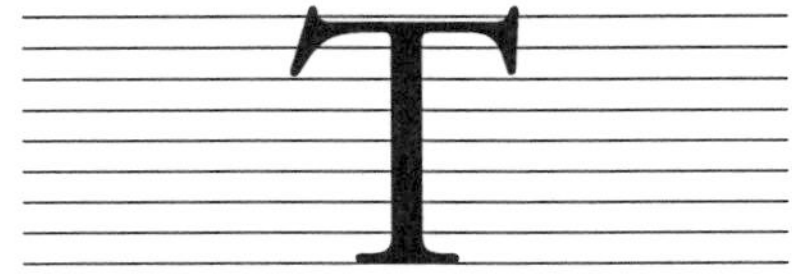

T **1.** Physiology. Symbol commonly used for intraocular tension.
2. Engineering. Symbol for Tesla, the derived S.I. unit of magnetic flux density; used to indicate strength of ophthalmic magnets; one Tesla equals 10,000 gauss.
3. Optics. Symbol for transmission factor of an optical medium.

Ta Chemical symbol for tantalum; q.v.

Table, Javal List of approximate dioptric powers converted from anterior keratometric readings as radius of curvature in millimeters, plus estimated value of posterior corneal astigmatism and corrected to a spectacle plane 14mm in front of cornea. Developed in 1881 by French ophthalmologist L. Emil Javal (1839–1907).

TABO See *scale, TABO conversion.*

TABO conversion scale See *scale, TABO conversion.*

tachistoscope An optical, mechanical, or electronic device used to display images for controlled brief moments of time, usually less than 1/10 of a second.

tangency In geometry, the state of a line and curve being tangent.

tangent In geometry, a line (or plane) touching, but not intersecting, a curve at only one point.

tangent screen See *screen, tangent.*

tangential plane See *plane, tangential.*

tantalum A rare metallic element, chemical symbol Ta, atomic number 73; non-corrosive and malleable; used to replace orbital and cranial defects and for wire sutures to unite bones. Discovered and named in 1802 by Anders Gustaf Ekeberg (1767–1813), Swedish chemist.

target

1. A mark or device, sometimes concentric circles, with which to align objects. In a focimeter, commonly, a set of lines crossed perpendicularly; the three narrow lines close together comprising the sphere part of the target, and the broad, farther apart lines being the cylinder part of the target; mires.
2. An object or area toward which something is directed, as the metal plate in an X-ray tube on which the electron beam impinges, or a titanium or similar plate in a lasing generator on which the light beam impinges.
3. Critical devices of optical scaling used to confirm resolving accuracy of lenses (e.g., U.S. Air Force 1951 Resolution Targets, currently available in both chromium and silver gray elements of 1 to 228 line pairs/mm).

target, vanishing resolution Visual-acuity test targets with closely similar detection and resolution thresholds; generally includes two luminance levels, one above and the other below background level, adjusted so that the space average equals the background; when presented with size below resolution threshold, target blends invisibly into the background. Technique originally developed for astigmatic charts in 1924 by Johns Hopkins ophthalmologist Jonas Friedenwald (1897–1955). Also known as high-pass resolution target.

tarsal

1. Pertaining to the tarsus or connective tissue framework of the eyelids.
2. Pertaining to the joints between the foot and the leg.

tarsal glands See *glands, Meibomian.*

tarsitis Inflammation of the tarsal or Meibomian glands of the eyelids.

tarsus Thin, flat plate of dense connective tissue situated one in each eyelid, which gives the lid shape and firmness. Contains the Meibomian or tarsal glands. Named by Claudius Galen of Pergamun (c. 130–c. 200 A.D.).

tear Salty, clear, watery fluid that helps to maintain a moist and healthy environment for the conjunctiva and cornea; secreted primarily by the lacrimal gland; often in the plural, tears.

tear break up time See *test, break up time (BUT).*

tear film See *film, tear.*

tears, artificial Ocular solution approximating the viscosity, tonicity, and pH of normal tears; useful as a tear replacement in dry-eye syndrome, Sjogren's syndrome, or following surgical removal of the lacrimal gland.

technician/technologist, ophthalmic Trained ophthalmic medical personnel who perform ocular measurements and data-gathering, assist in office management of patients, and may assist in surgery. Examined and certified by the Joint Commission on Allied Health Personnel in Ophthalmology (J.C.A.H.P.O.), since 1969, in three grade levels; approximately 15,000 certificants.

technologist, Certified Industrial Hygiene (C.I.H.) Credentialed individual engaged in measurement of toxic and industrial hazards; established in 1963; superseded in 1986 by Certified Occupational Health and Safety Technologist (O.H.S.T.); governed by an 18-member Joint Committee.

technologist, Certified Occupational Health and Safety (O.H.S.T.) A credentialed individual in the field of measurement and assessment of toxic and industrial hazards. Established in 1986 as successor to Certified Industrial Hygiene Technologist (C.I.H.) established in 1963; governed by an 18-member Joint Committee.

tele- Prefix meaning distant.

telecentric The optical condition in which identical focal distances are maintained with differing lens systems (commonly producing differing magnifications), as in the rotating power drum or zoom lens system in a corneal microscope; parfocal.

telemicroscope A Galilean telescope with additional plus power in the objective lens to give a comfortable near working distance (e.g., a surgical loupe). Both size of field and depth of focus are reduced in proportion to magnification; compare BITA—mnemonic for bi-level telemicroscope apparatus, a miniature adjustable Galilean microscope of similar magnification and light weight mounted in a spectacle carrier lens as a low-vision aid, 2X to 6X M.

telescope A compound lens magnifying system; may be adapted as a distal low-vision aid and with an auxiliary plus lens cap used for proximal (near range) visual activities.

telescope, astronomic A compound lens magnifying system in tubular arrangement; both ocular and objective lens are plus power and image is inverted and reversed; sometimes called Keplerian, in honor of Johann Kepler (1571–1630) of Germany who modified the Galilean ocular in 1611.

telescope, Galilean A compound lens magnifying system in tubular arrangement; objective lens is plus power; ocular lens is minus power; image is erect and not reversed. Developed and refined in 1609 by Galileo Galilei (1564–1642) of Italy, but possibly based on earlier Dutch observations.

telescopic lens See *lens, telescopic.*

Teller acuity plates or test See *preferential looking.*

temperature The property or degree of heat or absense of heat (i.e., cold) in a system in relation to a standard as the freezing point of distilled water (0° Celsius) or absolute zero (0° Kelvin).

temperature scale See *scale, Celsius*; *scale, centigrade*; *scale, Fahrenheit*; *scale, Kelvin.*

tempered lens See *lens, impact-resistant.*

template A gauge. In ophthalmic lens processing, a metal plate, usually brass, with a given radius of curvature used for measuring the curves of lenses or lap surfaces.

temple

1. The lateral region on either side of the upper part of the head directly behind the frontal bone.
2. Component of a spectacle or ophthalmic frame connected to the front at the endpiece and extending over the side of the skull; introduced in 1752 by London optician James Ayscough; also by the Parisian optician Thomin about 1746, and by the London optician Edward Scarlett between 1727 and 1730. Imprecisely called earpiece. See *frame (ophthalmic or spectacle).*

temple bow See *bow, temple.*

temple butt See *butt, temple.*

temple, cable Component of an ophthalmic frame made of metal, plastic, or a combination thereof consisting of wound wire, with or without a core. The distal portion is in contact with the ear. Typically bent in the shape of a semicircle and adjusted to fit securely and comfortably around the external ear; more precisely, cable earpiece.

temple, center line See *center line of temple.*

temple, comfort cable Earpieces made of flexible metal wire wound singly or in two layers around a flexible core and covered with a plastic such as acrylic; used to enhance the security of spectacles by firm attachment around the ears.

temple, convertible A spectacle earpiece of skull design or the like, which stores a comfort cable end in its shank; this may be extended around the ear when the wearer is engaged in vigorous activity.

temple fold angle See *angle, temple fold.*

temple head curve See *curve, temple head.*

temple, Hibo A spectacle earpiece attached to the spectacle front close to its uppermost point (fulvue).

temple, library A flattened earpiece without an ear bend or down bend.

temple outset See *angle, set-back.*

temple, riding bow An earpiece with its distal portion in contact with the ear, bent in a semicircle to fit securely around the external ear; introduced in England c. 1850.

temple, skull An earpiece with an ear bend or down bend; skull earpiece.

temple, spring-hinge An earpiece which has a tension device as an integral part of the hinge to maintain lateral pressure against the side of the head.

temple tip See *tip, temple.*

temporal

1. Pertaining to or in close proximity to the temple.
2. The side of a lens or frame which is more lateral or closer to the side of the head.

temporal edge See *edge, temporal.*

tension In ocular physiology, physical expression of the expansive force or pressure within an eyeball, usually measured by a tonometer and expressed in millimeters of mercury. Very low tension (8mm or less) impairs the support of the cornea and leads to shifting refraction and acuity; high pressure indicates glaucoma.

terminal, visual display (VDT) An image screen used to communicate with a computer. It consists of a display, usually a cathode ray tube (CRT), coupled to a keyboard.

Tesla (T) An S.I. unit of magnetic flux or density equal to 10,000 gauss; since 1934, supersedes the unit Oersted. Named for Coratian-born and naturalized American citizen (1884) electrical engineer Nikola Tesla (1856–1943).

test, break-up time (BUT) A timed observation of the dissipation of the sebaceous pre-corneal tear film while the lids are held open; determined visually with the assistance of a topical sodium fluorescein solution; usually expressed in seconds.

test chart, Bailey-Lovie See *chart, Bailey-Lovie test.*

test chart, ETDRS See *chart, ETDRS.*

test chart, geometric Gradation and logarithmic notation. A highly standardized series of optotypes for quantifying central visual acuity; derived in 1966 from earlier geometric letter size in equal steps. Popularized by Chinese ophthalmologist Tian-Yung Mizo.

test, drop-ball A low-velocity, impact-resistance test, commonly using a solid steel sphere free-falling 50 inches. For A.N.S.I. Z80.1, a 5/8-inch steel ball falling 50 inches; for A.N.S.I. Z80.7, a 1-inch steel ball falling 50 inches. See *resistance, impact.*

test, Duochrome The use of opaque Snellen test letters set in two illuminated glass panels, one red and the other blue or blue-green to assess residual refractive correction of about 1/4 diopter. Introduced in 1929 by the French ophthalmologist René Imbert; originally manufactured by Clifford Brown of London, England; sometimes called "bichrome" (a near-range duochrome test was introduced about 1929 by ophthalmologist Ernest E. Maddox (1860–1933) of Scotland.

test, Farnsworth D-15 test A simple pigment-matching test (1943) in which the patient arranges fifteen differently colored discs according to their similarity of hue. All discs are of equal saturation and brightness; color discs are selected from the Albert Henry Munsell (1859–1918) *Atlas of the Munsell Color System* (1913). Does not identify minor degrees of color deficiency. Developed by U.S. Navy color scientist Commander Dean Farnsworth (1902–1959), New London, Connecticut.

test, Farnsworth-Munsell 100 hue An elaborate pigment-matching test (1943, revised 1957) for subtle defects in color matching in which the patient arranges 86 differently colored discs (between 445nm and 633nm) into four separate hue panels. All discs are of equal saturation and brightness (selected from the Albert Henry Munsell (1859–1918) *Atlas of the Munsell Color System* (1913). Does not identify minor degrees of color deficiency. Developed by U.S. Navy color scientist Commander Dean Farnsworth (1902–1959), New London, Connecticut.

test, Farnsworth-Munsell 28 hue Intermediate range modification of pigment-matching test using 28 different colored discs arranged in oval fashion in a retaining box; after colored discs are aligned by the test subject, box is closed, turned over, and scored from sequential numbers on the back of each disc.

test, high-velocity impact A lens safety standard (A.N.S.I. Z87) using 1/4-inch steel balls propelled by an air gun at high rates of speed.

test, Ishihara (ish-i-hah'rah) A series of plates with pseudoisochromatic dotted numbers of one color against an equal intensity dotted background of other colors; used to test for types and degrees of color blindness; detects minor degrees of color deficiencies; most recent publication (15th edition), 1990, available in three series of 15, 24 and 38 plates. Should be used with standard illumination as New London Easel Lamp or C.I.E. "C" filter over 100-watt tungsten bulb. First edition developed in 1917 by ophthalmologist Shinobu Ishihara (1879–1963) of Tokyo University.

test, Jones An examination to determine flow through the tear ducts; a drop of sterile fluorescein dye solution is placed in the lower conjunctival sac; fluorescein appearing in the nasal cavity indicates open ducts; if no fluorescein passes through, there is obstruction in the outflow tear channels (dye-passage test). Introduced in 1961 and popularized by Oregon ophthalmologist Lester T. Jones (1894–1983).

test letters (equal difficulty) See *letters, test (equal difficulty).*

test letters (test types) See *letters, test (test types); optotype.*

test, Nertheim Opaque disc used as an occluder with 9 pin holes centered over the pupil; used to determine (by apparent improvement in acuity) if further refractive correction will help the patient. Based on the original pinhole test (1619) by the Jesuit anatomist and astronomer Christophorus Scheiner (1575–1650) of Germany.

test, Schirmer's A diagnostic procedure to quantitate tear production; tip of filter paper strip (5mm x 30mm) is folded over the lower lid border and inserted into the lower conjunctival sac, away from the cornea; the length of strip moistened in a 5-minute period is a measure of the rate of lacrimal secretion. May be done with topical anesthesia (basic secretion test, Schirmer II) or without anesthesia (reflex secretion test, Schirmer I). Developed in 1903 by Otto Schirmer (1864–1908), ophthalmologist of Germany and New York.

test, statistical batch A sampling technique in which a group of identical products (e.g. ophthalmic lenses), is removed from a larger number of like products to represent reliability by testing characteristics expected in the total series; Military Standard 105 D (1975) for sampling procedures.

test, stereo-acuity An optical or optical-mechanical device to quantify binocular stereopsis or true, three-dimensional depth perception; Wirt-Titmus test consists of two pages of double-printed polarizing vectograms viewed through a pair of polarizing glasses, with axes at 90° to one another; quantitates stereopsis from 3000s to 40s (seconds) of arc disparity; steps are at 800s, 400s, 200s, 140s, 100s, 80s, 60s, 50s, and 40s of disparity. Developed in 1947 by S.E. Wirt, optical engineer at Titmus Optical Company of Virginia.

test, taco A manual examination of a soft contact lens held convex side down, squeezed gently between thumb and forefinger to determine whether the lens has been inverted; if edges curl inward like the edges of a taco, orientation is correct; if edges flare outward like wings of a bird, lens is inverted.

test, Worth 4 dot A clinical test for first-degree fusion in which a patient wears a green filter over one eye and a red filter over the other while observing at 20 feet one red, one white, and two green lights; developed in 1903 by Claud Worth (1869–1936), London ophthalmologist; a Hardy (1937) modification for near-range use is available in flashlight form.

tetrafilcon A A complex hydroxyethyl methacrylate polymer used in the manufacture of soft hydrophilic contact lenses; refractive index 1.40; 25% water content.

Th Chemical symbol for the element thorium; q.v.

thalamus (thal'ah-mus) Anatomical designation of two large, ovoid masses, chiefly composed of gray matter in the base of the brain; a major center of sensory integration and emotion.

therapeutics Therapy; the treatment or curing of diseases.

Therminon lens See *lens, Therminon.*

thermo- Prefix meaning heat; hot.

thermometer An instrument for measuring heat (temperature).

thermolabile (ther"mo-lā'bil) Subject to the change, destruction, or loss of characteristic properties by the action of heat; heat labile.

thermosetting A type of material or complex, high-polymer plastic that solidifies under heat and cannot be remolded by heating; thermostabile.

thermostable plastic See *plastic, thermostable.*

thickness caliper See *caliper, lens.*

thickness, center The front-to-back measurement of a lens at its optical or geometric center; usually expressed in 0.1mm units.

thickness, geometric center The front-to-back measurement of a contact or spectacle lens at the intersection of the horizontal and vertical lens bisectors.

thickness, strap The front-to-back measurement of a rimless lens at the hole or point over which the strap of the mounting fits.

thimerosal An organomercurial antiseptic and preservative used in some contact lens disinfection systems and eyedrops; an antifungal and bacteriostatic for non-spore-forming bacteria. Historically a significant number of exposed contact lens wearers have demonstrated allergy or sensitivity to this chemical.

Thinlite lens See *lens, Thinlite.*

thinning prism See *prism, thinning.*

thorium A rare, heavy, grey metal of low radioactivity; chemical symbol Th, atomic number 90; has been used in glass sunlenses particularly of rose tint. Discovered in 1829 by Jöns Jakob Berzelius (1779–1848), Swedish chemist.

thread diameter See *diameter, thread.*

3 and 9 o'clock staining See *staining, 3 and 9 o'clock.*

Ti The symbol for the chemical element, titanium; q.v.

tilt, pantoscopic (pan″to-skop′ik) A temple to frame-front adjustment resulting in the angle formed by the intersection of the spectacle lens plane and the face plane wherein the superior lens edge is farther forward of the face than is the inferior edge; sometimes called pantoscopic angle (Figure 36). See also Figure 2. (cf. *angle, frame pantoscopic (down angle).*)

tilt, retroscopic A temple to frame-front adjustment resulting in the angle formed by the intersection of the spectacle lens plane and the face plane wherein the inferior lens edge is farther forward of the face than is the superior edge; sometimes called retroscopic angle (Figure 37). See also Figure 2. (cf. *angle, frame pantoscopic (down angle).*)

tinted lens See *lens, absorptive.*

tip, paddle A flattened portion of a spectacle earpiece fitting over and behind the ear.

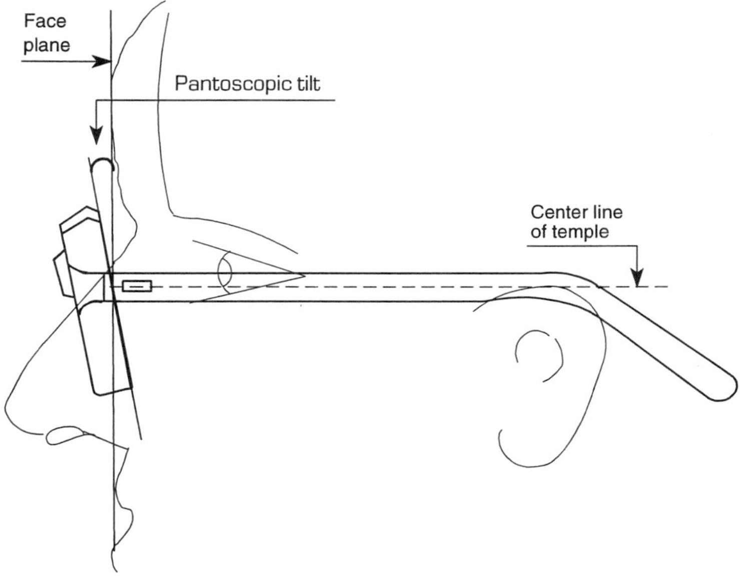

Figure 36 Pantoscopic tilt.

tip, temple The extreme distal portion of an earpiece fitting over and behind the ear.

tissue An aggregation of similarly specialized cells united in the performance of a particular function (e.g., the cornea, the retina).

tissue, granulation An exuberant new growth of vascularized connective tissue in small nodular masses in a secondary or abnormal healing process; seen under irritative artificial eyes; proud flesh.

titanium A lightweight, dark gray, metallic element; chemical symbol Ti, atomic number 22; used to toughen steel alloys; popular as a frame material for its strength, durability and fashion finishes. A titanium frame may be up to 40% lighter than comparable gold-filled or gold-plated frames. Easy to adjust, titanium frames hold their adjustment well and resist deteriorization caused by body chemicals. Also used as a replacement for lead in some high-refractive index optical glass; also used in surgical instruments. Discovered in

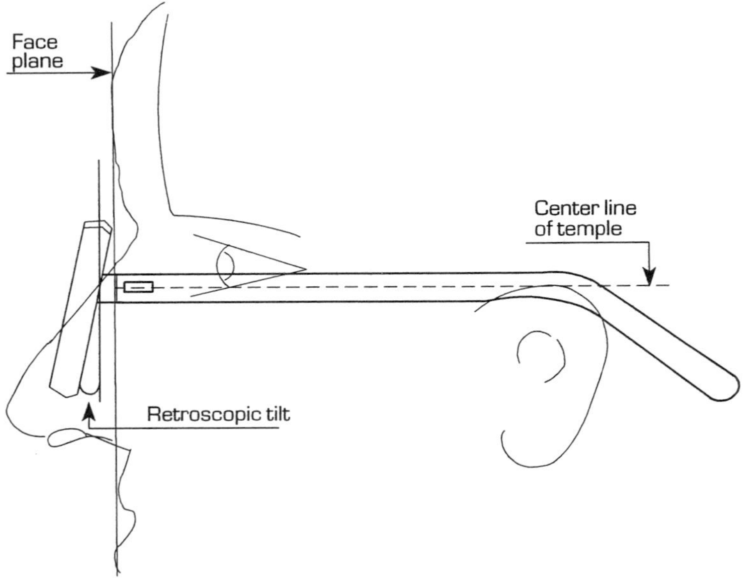

Figure 37 Retroscopic tilt.

1791 by William Gregor (1761–1817), English mineralogist, and named in 1795 by German chemist Martin Heinrich Klaproth (1743–1817).

titanium dioxide A white powder (TiO_2) used as a topical protection against sunburn.

titanium, Elasta Trade name for spectacle frame made from pure titanium with a patented "Elasta spring" hinge incorporated into the earpiece.

titanium oxide A high-grade, white powder compound used to polish ophthalmic lenses.

tolerance A permissible allowance for variation from standard. The allowable optical variation in a prescribed parameter (e.g., sphere power +1.00D +/–0.03D, where +1.00 is the specified sphere power and +/–0.03D is the allowable variation).

-tomy Suffix meaning cutting; division; incision.

Tono-Pen Trade name for a small, hand-held, rapid-reading, mechanical applanation tonometer which gives generally accurate readings of intraocular pressure in common clinical situations; manufactured by Mentor O. & O., Inc. (formerly Bio-Rad Laboratories, Inc.).

tonography (to-nog′rah-fe) Technique of continuously measuring intraocular pressure over a 4-minute period, to quantitate outflow facility of the eye. Popularized in the 1950s by Boston ophthalmologist W. Morton Grant (b. 1915) using the continuously recording electronic tonometer. Now infrequently used.

tonometer (to-nom′i-ter) A class of mechanical and optical instruments that measure intraocular pressure (mm Hg). Applanation (simplified and refined in 1954 by ophthalmologist Hans Goldmann of Switzerland), flattens small area of cornea; most accurate; available in hand-held Perkins model developed in 1970 by Prof. E.S. Perkins, ophthalmologist of London. Indentation Schiotz—developed in 1905 by Hjalmar A. Schiotz (1850–1927), a professor of ophthalmology at Oslo and later Paris; indents cornea. Air-puff, non-contact instrument (developed in 1972 by Massachusetts optometrist Bernard Grolmann, b. 1923) that senses deflection of the cornea in response to a very short puff of pressurized air (pneumotonometer); trade names, Keeler Pulsair 2000; Tomey ProTom.

tonometry, applanation Measurement of intraocular pressure determined by the amount of pressure, measured in millimeters of mercury (mm Hg), needed to flatten a specific area of the corneal surface; see *tonometer.*

tool, staking A miniature, or table-top, mechanical device (e.g., arbor press) used to make repairs or additions to spectacle frame hinges, plaques, or pad arms; punch holes in plastic frame parts; peen rivets or press out broken temple/hinge screws; mechanical arbor incorporating a shaft, mandrel, spindle, or axle.

tool surface power See *power, tool surface.*

topical anesthetic See *anesthetic, topical.*

topogometer An illuminated, mechanical/optical, or laser-assisted contour measuring device to chart the curvatures of the anterior corneal surface. May read in traditional "K" values, or when automated, generate multicolored isoclinic or contour maps (toposcope); trade names, Topographic Modeling System; Marco SK2000; EyeSys Corneal Analysis System.

topography Graphic delineation of a surface showing relief, relative position, or elevations, as in examination of the front of the cornea.

topography, corneal Precise measures of anterior corneal surface contours, displayed graphically and used as guides for refractive corneal surgery.

toprims The components of a combination ophthalmic frame front that are attached to the upper portion of a spectacle chassis.

tore **1.** A geometric configuration obtained by rotating an oval or ellipsoid about an axis lying in its own plane.
2. An ornamental knob on the surface of furniture or a saddle, commonly of toric shape.

toric Of or pertaining to a tore or torus.

toric lens See *lens, toric.*

toric peripheries Edge treatment to a back surface toric or bitoric rigid contact lens designed to reduce lid pressure and drag. Is sometimes used in conjunction with a spherical CPC in an effort to provide better lens centration.

torsion In ocular physiology, wheel-like motion of the eye on its anteroposterior axis. Intorsion, rotation of superior limbus toward the nose; extorsion, rotation of superior limbus away from the nose. (Cyclotorsion)

torus Latin architectural term for a surface or solid shaped like an inner tube or doughnut and formed by revolving a circle about a line in its plane without intersecting the line.

total hyperopia See *hyperopia, total.*

total inset See *inset, total.*

total myopia See *myopia, total.*

trabecular meshwork See *meshwork, trabecular.*

trachoma (trah-kō'mah) Chronic, contagious, chlamydial infection of the conjunctiva and the cornea. One of the main causes of blindness. Most commonly encountered in hot regions with poor hygienic conditions. Easily transmitted by direct contact of common things such as a wet towel or mascara brush. The causative bacteria, chlamydia, also causes a wide range of sexually transmitted diseases in the male and female. Usually responds well to appropriate antibiotic therapy.

tracing, ray See *ray, tracing.*

tract, uveal The vascular or nutrient middle coat of the eye (between the retina and the sclera) including pigmented cells, the iris, choroid, and ciliary body; a major blood supply to the outer retina; first described and named by the Greek anatomist Herophilus of Alexandria (c. 344–280 B.C.).

trademark A symbol, device, or logotype used by a manufacturer or seller of merchandise to identify the origin of his product. To be valid, must be formally registered (in the United States with the Patent and Trademark Office of the Department of Commerce); must be uncontested for 3 to 7 years, depending on the nation of registry; and must not become a generic term. Under protection by both the U.S. Constitution, and, internationally, by the Paris Convention of 1883.

trans- Prefix meaning across; beyond; through.

translating bifocal contact lens See *lens, contact, translating bifocal.*

translucent Pertaining to a medium which transmits light diffusely, so that objects viewed through it are not clearly distinguished.

transmissibility The ability of inert gases to pass through a finished contact lens; a measurement of the diffusion coefficient divided by the lens thickness (Dk./L); decreases with increasing lens thickness.

transmission In spectacle optics, the transit or passing of radiant energy (e.g. light), through a transparent medium.

transmittance Transparency. The ratio of emerging radiant energy, intensity (I_T), transmitted through a medium, to the incident radiant energy, intensity (I); transmission factor (T); algebraically, $T = I_T/I$. (cf. *opacity (O).*)

transmittance properties, luminous Ratio of the visible radiant energy emerging through a lens or from a lens system to the incident radiant energy; symbol τ (tau). A quantitative function of light propagation through an optical medium weighted by the corresponding ordinates of the photopic luminous efficiency distribution of the 1931 C.I.E. standard colorimetric observer and by the spectral intensity of C.I.E. standard illuminant C.

transparent Pertaining to an optical medium having uniform light transmission without scatter so that objects can be seen clearly through it.

transposition An algebraic change in writing a spectacle lens prescription giving equal optical performance but specifying the cylinder form in opposite sign and axis rotation of 90°; the converting of a prescription written in minus (–) cylinder form to plus (+) cylinder form, or vice versa.

trauma Any injury, wound, or shock.

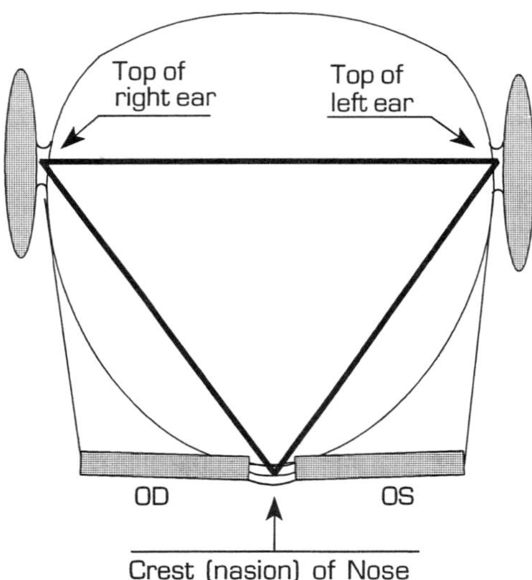

Figure 38. The fitting triangle.

tri- Prefix meaning three.

trial lens See *lens, trial.*

trial set See *set, trial.*

triangle, fitting In spectacle optics, a geometric construction from the three points where spectacles contact or put pressure against the head. The apex of the triangle is the pressure point on the crest (nasion) of the nose, and the base of the triangle is the two pressure points just above the external ears, on each side of the head. When nosepads are used, there will actually be two pressure points at the apex of the triangle, rather than one, as with a saddle bridge (Figure 38).

trichiasis (tri-kī'a-sis) Turning in of one or more eyelashes.

trichromat (tri'kro-mat) Normal color perception; responds to all three primary colors.

tricurve A contact lens design containing three concentric curves on its posterior surface.

trifocal lens See *lens, trifocal.*

tritanomaly (tri″tah-nom′ah-le) A mild color deficiency of yellow and blue receptors; rare as a congenital or hereditary defect; most usually seen as result of drug or toxic reaction.

tritanopia (tri″tah-nō′pe-ah) A rare absence of yellow and blue sensitivity with preservation of red and green sensitivity; may be associated with drug reaction or nervous system disease.

trochlea (trok′le-ah)

1. A pulley or pulley-shaped part.
2. A ring of cartilage attached to the frontal bone on the nasal side of the upper orbital rim that serves as a pulley for the tendon of the superior oblique muscle. First described by Gabriel Fallopius (1523–1562), Italian anatomist.

troland A psychophysical unit of illumination on the retina of the human eye; one troland is the intensity stimulation experienced by a normal observer when the entrance pupil of the eye has an area of 1mm^2 and is observing a surface illuminated at 1 lumen (international candle) per m^2; named for Leonard Thompson Troland (1889–1923), American psychologist and optical inventor.

-tropia Suffix meaning to turn.

true power See *power, refractive surface.*

truncation

1. The act of cutting off a component or edge.
2. In contact lens design, the cutting off of an edge of a lens, thus creating a plane or flat surface in its place; used to stabilize the rotation of a toric lens.

Tscherning's curve See *curve, Tscherning's.*

Tscherning's orthoscopic lenses See *lens, Tscherning's orthoscopic (corrected curve).*

TSI Mnemonic for total segment inset; q.v.

tube

1. In spectacle optics, a closure device attached to a metal eyewire; also known as an eyewire tube or split-joint barrel.
2. The opaque cylinder supporting the objective and ocular lenses of a telescope or a microscope.

tube, cathode ray The component of a visual display terminal that generates the display; the picture tube in a television set; abbreviated CRT.

tungsten A gray-white, heavy, high-melting-point metal, chemical symbol W (for the mineral Wolframite from which it is extracted); atomic number 74; used in incandescent lamp filament and as an alloy in hardened steel; isolated in 1783 by Spanish chemists Fausto d'Elhuyar (1755–1833) and his older brother Juan.

tunnel vision See *vision, tunnel.*

turbidity A quantitative description of the light-scattering power of an optical medium and the consequent loss of intensity of a primary light beam per unit of distance traversed; the intensity of the primary beam decreases exponentially with the distance traveled; cloudiness.

type, Jaeger test (yā'ger) A loosely arranged series of near-vision test types with 1 being average/normal and higher numbers indicating poorer near acuity. Schriftscalen, developed in 1854 by Eduard von Jaeger (1818–1884), Vienna ophthalmologist.

type, test Variously designed quantitated visual stimuli; usually in the form of letters to assess visual acuity or contrast sensitivity; optotypes; q.v..

typology The study of types or letter characteristics with the assistance of the science of classification.

typoscope A black shield which covers a reading page except for a horizontal slit aperture to expose one or two lines of print; reduces light scatter or glare from the page.

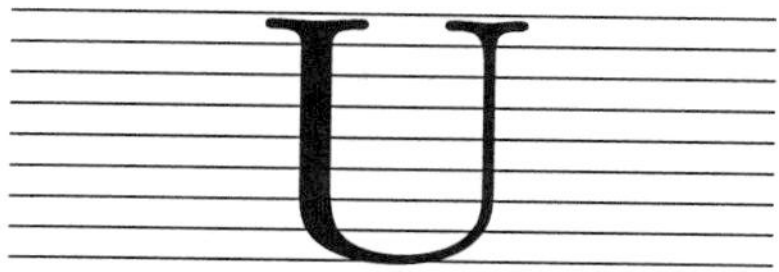

U.C.C. Abbreviation for Uniform Code Council, Inc.; q.v.

UPC Acronym for Universal Product Code; see *code, bar.*

U.S.A.N. Abbreviation for United States Adopted Names Council; q.v.

U.S.P. Abbreviation for United States Pharmacopeia; q.v.

ulcer Surface lesion with erosion or loss of substance; commonly described in cornea and in stomach.

ulcer, dendritic A corneal surface breakdown of branching configuration which usually stains with fluorescein; is commonly due to type I herpes simplex (a DNA virus) invasion, and is associated with reduced corneal sensitivity; a contraindication to fitting or wearing contact lenses.

ulcer, disciform (dis″i-form) A rounded or oval-shaped excavation of the corneal surface and stromal tissue, often subsequent to infection by the herpes simplex virus; generally associated with anesthesia of the cornea.

Ultex Trade name for a one-piece form of multifocal ophthalmic lens made by grinding two or three different spherical curves on one surface, generally the ocular side of a lens, so as to produce two or three foci with little or no chromatic aberration through the reading portion of the lens; a type of one-piece bifocal or trifocal having variable segment diameters. Originally designed in 1910 by Indianapolis optician Charles W. Conner and introduced by Continental Optical Co., now Textron. Trade names, Ultex A; Ultex B; Ultex AL; Ultex K; Ultex T.

ultra- Prefix meaning excessive; extreme; beyond.

ultrasonography (ul″tra-son-og′rah-fe) Echography. The use of pulsed sonic waves above the hearing range at frequency of 20 thousand to 10 million Hertz (cycles per second) to measure the length of the eye or diagnostically explore deep into opaque structures; visualization of structures of differing acoustic density by their ability to absorb or reflect ultrasound; variously displayed as "A" (linear), "B" (two-dimensional), "M" (motion) or holographic (three-dimensional) images. Developed at end of World War I from naval underwater instrumentation, SONAR (Sonic Aid to Navigation and Ranging).

ultrasound Mechanical energy of alternating condensations and rarefactions (longitudinal pressure waves) at frequencies above the upper limit of perception of the human ear, generally above 20,000 cycles per second; may be pulsed (for echography) or continuous wave (for destruction).

ultraviolet See *light, ultraviolet.*

ultraviolet absorbing lens See *lens, ultraviolet absorbing.*

ultraviolet light See *light, ultraviolet.*

umbra In optics, a complete shadow within which no light is received from a given source; see *penumbra.*

uncut lens See *lens, uncut.*

uncut plastic lens blank See *lens, uncut.*

uni- Prefix meaning one.

uniform density lens See *lens, uniform density.*

Uniform Code Council, Inc. A non-profit administrative and educational organization that develops and issues universal product codes, identification numbers, and electronic data interchange standards. Office: Dayton, Ohio 45459.

unilateral Pertaining to or affecting only one side of the body.

uniocular Pertaining to or affecting only one eye.

unit, Finsen A physical measure of intensity of uv radiation, 10^5 watts per m^2 at wavelength 2.967×10^{-7}m. Named for Niels Ryberg Finsen (1860–1904), Danish physician who received the 1903 Nobel Prize in medicine and physiology.

United States Adopted Names Council (U.S.A.N.) A voluntary professional association formed in 1961 by the American Medical Association and the U.S. Pharmacopeial Convention Inc. to organize non-proprietary names for drugs, contact lens materials, and the like; joined in 1964 by the American Pharmaceutical Association and in 1967 by the U.S. Food and Drug Administration. Official names must be approved by U.S.A.N. for labeling and advertising.

United States Pharmacopeia (U.S.P.) A private, nonprofit periodical initiated in 1820 that publishes a compilation of clinical pharmacology providing standards of identity, quality and useful strengths of drugs representing the best practice of medicine; jointly produced by the American Medical Association, American Pharmaceutical Association, and the U.S. Food and Drug Administration; 14th edition published in 1994. Ophthalmology division chaired by New Orleans ophthalmologist Herbert E. Kaufman, M.D.

unitless radiometric values Relations that are generally expressed as ratios (or percentages); e.g., absorptance, reflectance, trasmittance, and emissivity.

uv Abbreviation for ultraviolet. See *light, ultraviolet.*

uv-absorbing lens See *lens, ultraviolet absorbing.*

uv-400 Ultraviolet wavelength of 400 nanometers. Refers to lenses or lens treatments that absorb nearly all radiation with wavelengths of 400 nanometers or shorter.

uvea See *tract, uveal.*

uveitis (yoo″vē-ī′tis) Inflammation of the uveal tract: iris, ciliary body, or choroid; may include iritis, cyclitis, and choroiditis.

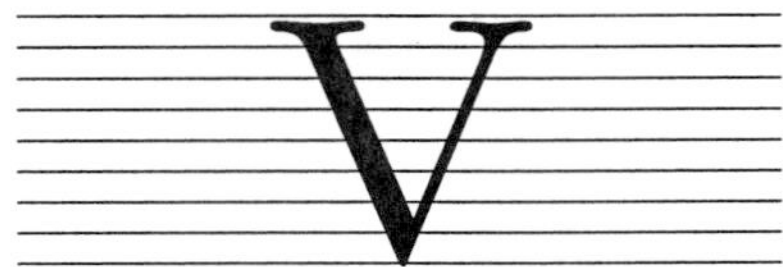

V **1.** Chemical symbol for the rare earth, metallic element, vanadium; q.v.

2. Symbol for the derived S.I. unit for electromotive force, volt, named for the Italian physiologist and physicist Alessandro Volta (1745–1827).

3. Sometimes used as the symbol for the dispersion value of an optical material; see *number, Abbé.*

V.A. Abbreviation for visual acuity or Veterans Affairs (name changed in 1991 from Veterans Administration).

V.D. Abbreviation for vertex distance; venereal disease (VD).

VDT Acronym for **v**isual **d**isplay **t**erminal; sometimes referred to as video display terminal. See *terminal, visual display.*

VDU Acronym for video display unit. See *terminal, visual display.*

V.I.C.A. Abbreviation for Vision Industry Council of America; q.v. Formerly, Vision Council of America (V.C.O.A.).

V.O.D. Abbreviation for vision right eye (oculus dexter).

V.O.S. Abbreviation for vision left eye (oculus sinister).

V.O.U. Abbreviation for vision with both eyes open (oculus uterque).

value, Abbé See *number, Abbé.*

value, f See *number, f.*

value, Nu See *number, Abbé.*

value, sagitta See *depth, sagitta.*

value, sagittal The linear distance from the posterior surface of a contact lens to the anterior surface of the cornea. Determined by the curvatures of both surfaces. Lacrimal lens profile is partly controlled by this value.

vanadium A rare-earth, grey, metallic element, chemical symbol V, atomic number 23; on chronic exposure is an irritant to the conjunctiva and lining of the respiratory passages; used at times to give a pale green tint to glass lenses. Discovered in 1831 by Nils Gabriel Sefstrom (1787–1845), Swedish physician and chemist.

variable Changeable; capable of being changed.

variation Deviation from the norm; the amount or rate of deviation.

vault General term for an arched configuration, commonly referenced to height.

vectograph

1. A chart or diagram expressing direction.
2. An instrument for writing or recording directional relationships.
3. A polarized double-printed display with axes at right angles affording a stereoscopic picture to binocular observers viewing through single polarizing filters at corresponding (opposite) angles in front of each eye. Developed in 1940 by E.H. Land and J. Mahler.

vectograph, Polaroid A visual function test chart with overlying, polarized components at right angles to each other; when viewed through corresponding polarized glasses, each eye can see figures invisible to the other. Basis of stereo-acuity test (1947) designed by S.E. Wirt and published by Titmus Optical Co.

veil, Sattler's Hazy obscurance of visual acuity due to corneal edema, mainly stromal, usually from overwear of contact lenses; due to anoxia of tight contact lens fit; observed in 1888 by Eugen Fick (1853–1937), ophthalmologist of Zurich, and in 1889 by Albert Carl Mueller (1864–1923), optician of Germany, but studied in detail by Charles Hubert Sattler (1844–1928), ophthalmologist of Konegsberg, Germany; see also *bedewing, corneal.*

veiling reflections See *reflections, veiling.*

velocity

1. The rate of change of position in relation to time.
2. In electromagnetic energy physics, a standard (referenced to the speed of light) that is a temperature-free constant in a vacuum (186,000 miles/second), but is variably reduced by the density of other media through which it may pass.

vergence (ver'jens)

1. The amount of divergence (negative) or convergence (positive) of a pencil of light rays entering or leaving a lens; the power, expressed in diopters, is inversely proportional to the distance in meters between a reference source and a focal plane.
2. Disjunctive movement of the two eyes in opposite directions, as in convergence and divergence.

vergence power See *power, vergence.*

vernier A precise two-part sliding mechanical scale, usually for linear measurements, in fractional divisions; utilizes aligning (not resolving) power of the eye to read. Developed by the French physicist Pierre Paul Vernier (1580–1637); forerunner of the micrometer. See *caliper, vernier.*

vernier caliper See *caliper, vernier.*

Versalite Trade name for a phototropic polycarbonate lens that darkens slowly over a period of about 15 minutes on exposure to ultraviolet light.

version A conjugate movement of the eyes in the same direction. Dextroversion, right (→); levoversion, left (←); supraversion, up (↑); infraversion, down (↓).

vertex

1. The highest point, summit or apex.
2. In optics, that point at which the optical axis of a lens intersects the surface.

vertex distance See *distance, vertex.*

vertex distance compensation See *compensation, vertex distance.*

vertex distometer See *distometer, vertex.*

vertex power See *power, vertex.*

vertical imbalance See *imbalance, prismatic.*

vertical lens bisector (VLB) See *bisector, vertical lens.*

vertical segment bisector (VSB) See *bisector, vertical segment.*

vertical segment position (VSP) See *position, vertical segment.*

Vertometer (ver-tom'i-ter) Trade name of a focimeter (lensmeter) manufactured by Bausch & Lomb.

vessels, ghost Small, empty, transparent blood channels found in areas that were previously vascularized; particularly seen after chronic corneal inflammation.

vibration

1. A steady and rhythmical movement occurring within a medium that is not in equilibrium.
2. An instance of undulation measured from one corresponding point to another; causes reduction in resolving power of the eye.

videokeratoscope An optical device for measuring corneal topography and recording it on video tape.

ViewMaster stereo reels A patented system of stereoscopic displays using a rotating disc for 7 stereopairs of color transparencies 10mm by 12mm in size; manufactured by GAP, New York, New York.

viewing angle See *angle, viewing.*

viewing distance See *distance, viewing.*

VIP Trade name used by SOLA Lens Co. for their progressive addition lens.

virtual image See *image, virtual.*

visible iris diameter (VID) See *diameter, visible iris (VID).*

visible spectrum See *spectrum, visible.*

vision

1. The act or facility of seeing.
2. The sense by which objects, their form, color, position, etc., in the external environment are perceived; the exciting stimulus being light from the objects striking the retina of the eye; the process of seeing; sight; a combined function of the eyes and the brain.

vision, alternating Vision in which there is cyclical suppression of one eye while the images from the other eye are utilized. A significant factor in the analysis and correction of anisometropia, aniseikonia, or alternating strabismus.

vision, binocular See *vision, single binocular.*

vision, form (form sense) The unitary psychological precept or mental interpretation of a pattern or object without regard to its image size or angle of view; the cortical ability to perceive the shape and meaning of an object or pattern based on experience.

vision, low A significant impairment of seeing, either centrally (brain) or peripherally (eye) which limits a patient's ability to read, to travel with visual guidance, or accomplish usual visually guided tasks of living, but retaining a level of sight distinctly better than blindness; by definition this is usually a fixed or permanent impairment which cannot be reversed or relieved by optimal medical or surgical care.

vision, mesopic (mes-op'ik) Seeing under conditions of dim light; between photopic and scotopic levels.

vision, near point Visual acuity or resolving power for objects at distances corresponding to the normal reading distance; clinical standards vary from about 33cm to 40cm, usually specified in inches or centimeters from the spectacle plane.

vision, photopic (fō-top'ik) Seeing under conditions of usual light or daylight.

vision, rod See *vision, scotopic*.

vision, scotopic (skō-top'ik) Seeing under conditions of unlighted nighttime (night vision). Vision in which the cones of the retina play little or no part (differentiated from the laboratory condition of absolute scotopic vision in which all visible light is totally excluded).

vision, single binocular Vision in which both eyes contribute to produce a single fused image; a necessary substrate for stereopsis; first-degree fusion.

vision, subnormal Vision inferior to or less than average in respect to visual acuity, fields, or color discrimination; cannot be corrected with conventional ophthalmic lenses. Subnormal vision can often be assisted by special optical systems, lenses, or other visual aids; low vision.

vision, tunnel An abnormal condition of sight in which the visual fields are severely constricted; remaining vision is described as central or macular vision.

vision, yellow An abnormal condition of the retina usually due to drug reaction in which a yellow color permeates most of the visual field, xanthopsia.

Vision Fund of America A voluntary charitable organization formed by professionals in the visual media industry of the U.S.; established in 1983 primarily from the fields of television, film and video production, book publishers, and equipment manufacturers. Office: White Plains, New York 10604.

Vision Industry Council of America (V.I.C.A.) An international nonprofit trade association for the optical industry founded in 1985; name changed in 1990 from the Vision Council of America (V.C.O.A.), which merged with the Better Vision Institute in 1989. Its purpose is to educate and inform the public about the importance of vision care. Office: 1800 N. Kent St., Suite 1210, Rosslyn, Virginia 22209.

Visolett Trade name for an improved paperweight and light-gathering magnifier which may be fitted with a round, +10.50D bifocal segment on its convex surface; in small diameters, high-index glass increases magnification. Developed in 1933 by Berlin ophthalmologist Jack Jaeckel (1880–1960).

Visometer A slit-lamp mounted optical instrument positioned in the very near range; used to estimate postcataract extraction visual acuity through a partial cataract; uses sine-wave gratings in various axes; developed by W. Lotmar of Haag-Streit, Switzerland. (cf. *meter, potential acuity (PAM).*)

Visorgogs Trade name for all plastic, one-piece, fit-over safety shield with unitized bridge and end piece; has attached combination brow bar and visor with either direct (18 hole) or screened ventilation.

Vista Trade name for a computer-driven, image-magnification system used by patients with major visual impairment.

Vistech system See *system, Vistech.*

visual Pertaining to vision; sight; seeing.

visual acuity See *acuity, visual.*

visual adaptation See *adaptation, visual.*

visual angle See *angle, visual.*

visual axis See *axis, visual.*

visual cortex See *cortex, visual.*

visual display terminal (VDT) See *terminal, visual display.*

visual field See *field, visual.*

visual hallucinations See *hallucinations, visual.*

visual purple See *rhodopsin.*

visual receptors See *receptors, visual.*

VISX Trade name for an excimer laser manufacturing corporation, Sunnyvale, California, formerly Taunton Technologies Co. of Monroe, Connecticut.

Vitalite Trade name for a "full spectrum" fluorescent tube illuminant manufactured by Durotest Corp., North Bergen, New Jersey.

vitrectomy (vi-trek"to-me) The surgical removal of all or part of the vitreous humor and contained blood or other foreign material.

vitreous chamber See *chamber, vitreous.*

vitreous hemorrhage See *hemorrhage, vitreous.*

vitreous humor See *humor, vitreous.*

VLB Mnemonic for bisector, vertical lens; q.v.

Volk, lens See *lens, conoid.*

Voltaren Trade name for an effective non-steroidal, anti-inflammatory drug which inhibits prostaglandin synthesis; introduced for oral administration, but effective topically to control ocular pain; generic name, diclofenac.

voluntary convergence See *convergence, voluntary.*

VSP Mnemonic for position, vertical segment; q.v.

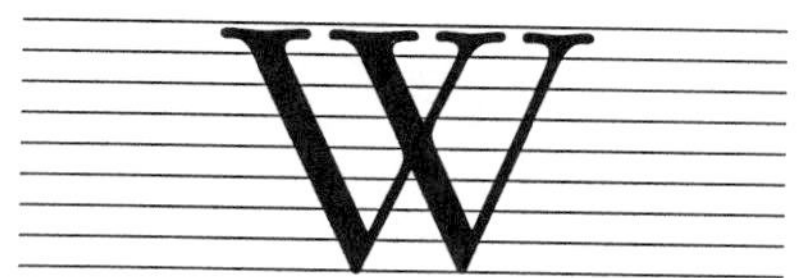

W Chemical symbol for the metallic element tungsten (Wolframite); q.v.

wafer A very thin lens which may be cemented to another lens to provide a different focus, a color absorption, or to reduce an aberration.

warpage A mechanical lens defect in which a surfaced lens (usually plastic) is bent or twisted in processing.

water content The percentage of water contained within the matrix of a hydrogel lens. Water of hydration; as water of hydration increases, there is a logarithmic increase in oxygen permeability.

watt A derived S.I. unit of power or radiant flux delivered at the rate of one joule per second; equals 1000 microwatts; used in quantifying laser or other light energy. Named in honor of James Watt (1736–1819), Scottish engineer and inventor of the first practical steam engine.

wave

1. A local, ripple-like irregularity in a lens surface; see *distortion.*
2. A uniformly advancing disturbance in which the parts moved undergo a double oscillation.

wavelength The linear distance occupied by one complete cycle of vibration of an energy form from any given point to the next point characterized by the same phase; frequency in cycles per second (Hertz) is an inversely related variable (Figure 39).

wax A plastic substance deposited by insects or obtained from plants; usually an ester of a fatty acid with higher, monohydric alcohols; as casting wax, an impression medium.

welding, arc A high-temperature gas or plasma stream used industrially to melt, fuse, or cut metal components; emits varying amounts of

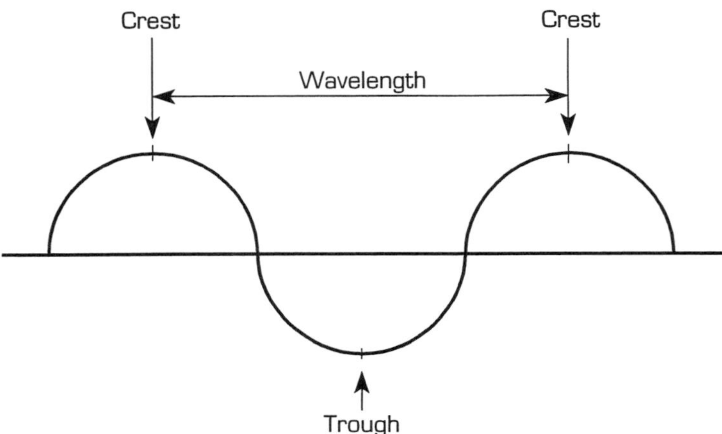

Figure 39. Wavelength.

light energy across the spectrum from ultraviolet through infrared; uv radiation increases approximately as the square of the electric current in amperes. May cause painful damage to unprotected epithelial cells of the cornea.

welding goggles See *goggles, welding.*

wheel, power See *drum, power.*

window The portion of a protective face shield or helmet through which the wearer sees; fitted with various optical protective materials corresponding to intended use.

Wirt-Titmus test See *test, stereo-acuity.*

with motion See *motion, with; retinoscopy; retinoscope, streak.*

Wood's light See *light, Wood's.*

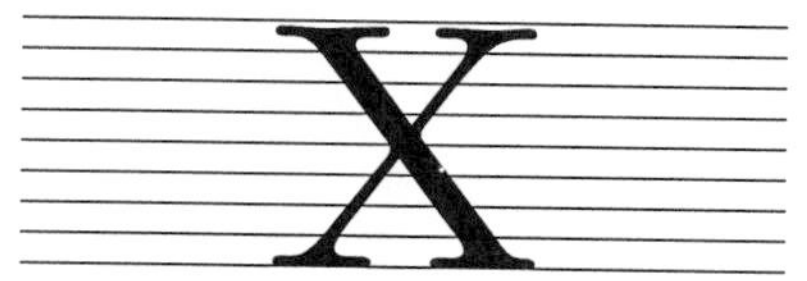

x axis See *axis, x of Fick.*

X-Chrom lens See *lens, contact, X-Chrom.*

xanthelasma (zan"thel-az'mah) Yellow deposits in the skin of the lids, usually near nasal (inner) canthus ; associated with elevated blood lipids.

xanthopsia (zan-thop'se-ah) See *vision, yellow.*

Xe Symbol for the chemical element xenon; q.v.

xenon A chemically unreactive gaseous element found in the atmosphere; chemical symbol Xe, atomic number 54; used in high-intensity lamps and in lasers in combination with ruby or YAG; discovered in 1898 by Sir William Ramsey (1852–1916), Scottish-born chemist.

xero- Prefix meaning dry.

xerophthalmia (zē"rof-thal'me-ah) Pathologic dryness of conjunctiva and corneal epithelium due to Vitamin A deficiency; may lead to blindness; associated with increased risk of pulmonary death.

XL Trade name for a progressive-addition spectacle lens; particularly suggested for use by early presbyopic patients.

XLC Trade name for a progressive-addition spectacle lens; suggested for use by presbyopic contact lens wearers.

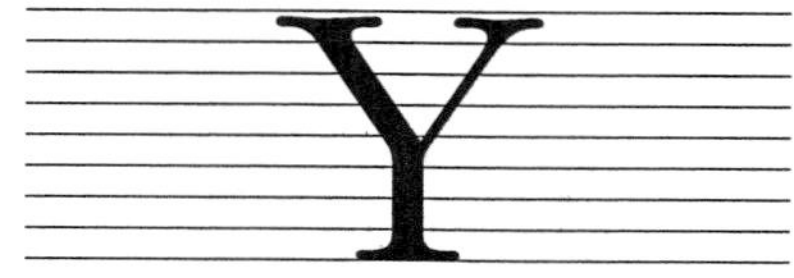

Y The symbol for the chemical element yttrium; q.v.

y axis See *axis, y of Fick.*

YAG laser See *laser, YAG.*

yellow lens See *lens, Kalichrome; lens, Noviol.*

yellow vision See *vision, yellow.*

yttrium A very rare metal of the rare earth group, allied to cerium; chemical symbol Y, atomic number 39; used in some protective lenses to absorb potentially hazardous wavelengths of light. Now commonly used in the crystal of a neodymium laser emitting at 1060nm; named for the Ytterby quarry where it was first isolated in the 1840s by Swedish chemist Carl Gustav Mosander (1797–1858).

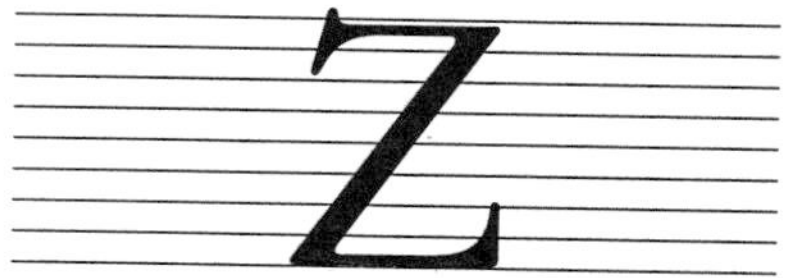

z axis See *axis, z of Fick.*

zinc A blue-white metallic element, chemical zymbol Zn, atomic number 30. Many salts of zinc are used as anti-infectives and astringents; a trace element nutrient, commonly promoted for macular health.

Zn Chemical symbol for zinc; q.v.

zone

1. An encircling band, stripe, girdle, belt, region, or the like.
2. In geometric optics, the portion of the surface of a sphere included between two parallel planes.

zone, anterior optical (AOZ) In contact lens optics, the usable refractive area of the front surface of the lens. Determined in common practice by subtracting twice the width of the anterior peripheral curves from the overall lens diameter; specified to nearest 1/10mm.

zone, apical The most forward portion of the anterior corneal surface; delimited by the area (usually 3mm to 4mm in diameter) over which the steepest corneal curvature in each of its principal meridians is constant.

zone, optical (OZ) In contact lens optics, the central area of a contact lens containing the power needed to correct ametropia; the area inside the peripheral curves of a contact lens. Term also used to describe the central area of the cornea and the refractive portion of a lenticular spectacle lens (e.g., "Myo-Disc").

zone, posterior optical (POZ) The central area on the back of a corneal contact lens that contains the refractive power. The POZ is measured with a measuring magnifier and is determined by subtracting two times the width of the peripheral curves from the overall lens diameter.

zone, scleral That part of a contact lens or prosthetic shell designed to lie in front of the white of the eye. Sometimes abbreviated s.z; see *haptic*.

zone, transitional On the surface of the cornea or a contact lens, the portion (ring) involved in the change or passage from one fixed radius of curvature to another.

zonule (zōn'yul) A small zone, belt, or band; small fibrous strands.

zonule of Zinn A system of radially arranged suspensory fibers that connect the crystalline lens capsule to the ciliary body. The tension of these fibers varies with the state of contraction of the ciliary muscle and thus affects the convexity of the lens. Originally described in 1753 by Johann Gottfried Zinn (1727–1759), a German anatomist. The flower Zinnia was named by Carolus Linnaeus (1707–1778) in honor of Johann Zinn.

zoom lens See *lens, zoom.*

zygo- Prefix meaning yoke, yoke-shaped.

zygoma (zī-gō'mah) The cheek bone; forms part of the bony orbital floor.

zylonite (xylonite) (zī'lo-nīt) A highly flammable synthetic substance resembling celluloid; manufactured from pyroxylin or guncotton; formerly used in the manufacture of spectacle frames and camera film; voluntarily discontinued in 1950 because of fire hazard.

Selected References

Borror DJ. *Dictionary of Word Roots and Combining Forms.* Mt. View, Calif.: Mayfield Publishing Co.; 1960.

British Standards Institution. *Glossary of Terms Relating to Ophthalmic Lenses and Spectacle Frames.* London: British Standards Institute; 1984.

Bynum WF, Browne EJ, Porter R. *Dictionary of the History of Science.* Princeton: Princeton University Press; 1985.

Cassin B, Solomon SAB (Rubin ML, Ed.). *Dictionary of Eye Terminology.* 2nd ed. Gainesville, Fla.: Triad Publishing Co.; 1990.

Esterling K. *Advanced Materials in Sports Equipment.* New York: Chapman and Hall; 1993.

Hailman JP. *Optical Signals, Animal Communication and Light.* Bloomington: Indiana University Press; 1977.

Heath RJ, Birley AW. *Dictionary of Plastics Technology.* Glasgow: Blackie & Son; 1992.

Hoad, TF. *The Concise Oxford Dictionary of English Etymology.* New York: Oxford University Press; 1986.

International Council of Ophthalmology. *Perimetric Standards and Perimetric Glossary of the International Council of Ophthalmology.* The Hague: W. Junk; 1979.

Jablonski S. *Dictionary of Medical Acronyms and Abbreviations,* 2nd ed. St. Louis: C. V. Mosby; 1993.

Jakuba S. *Metric (S.I.) in Everyday Science and Engineering.* Warrendale, Penn.: Society of Automotive Engineers; 1992.

Jerrard HG, McNeill DB. *A Dictionary of Scientific Units,* 6th ed. New York: Chapman and Hall; 1992.

Klein HA. *The Science of Measurement: An Historical Survey.* New York: Dover Publications; 1988.

MacIntrye JD (Ed.). *Dictionary of Inorganic Compounds.* New York: Chapman and Hall; 1992.

Phillips WR, Griffen DT. *Optical Mineralogy: The Non-Opaque Minerals.* San Francisco: W. H. Freeman Co.; 1981.

Ravault M. *Syndromes en Ophthalmologie, Guide—Dictionnaire.* Paris: Deren; 1970.

Scarborough J. *Medical Terminologies: Classical Origins.* Norman, Okla.: University of Oklahoma Press; 1992.

Skeat WW. Etymological *Dictionary of the English Language.* New York: Oxford University Press; 1959.

Smith WJ. *Modern Optical Engineering: The Design of Optical Systems,* 2nd ed. New York: McGraw-Hill; 1990.

Stedman TL. *Stedman's Abbreviations, Acronyms and Symbols.* Baltimore: Williams & Wilkins; 1992.

Taylor EJ (Ed.). *Dorland's Illustrated Medical Dictionary,* 27th ed. Philadelphia: W. B. Saunders; 1988.

Tulloch S. *Oxford Dictionary of New Words.* New York: Oxford University Press; 1991.

Turner G.L'E. History of optical instruments: Survey of sources and modern studies. In: Crombie AC, Hoskin MA, *History of Science.* Cambridge, England: Heffer and Sons; 1969; 8:53-93.

U.S. Department of Energy. *Dictionary and Thesaurus of Environment, Health and Safety.* Boca Raton: Lewis Publishers; 1992.

Winkler W (Ed.). *A Spectacle of Spectacles.* Leipzig, Germany: Druckerei Fortschritt Erfurt; 1988.

Zupko RE. *A Dictionary of English Weights and Measures.* Madison: University of Wisconsin Press; 1968.

Appendix

Table 1
Index of Refraction of Common Ophthalmic Materials

Material Trade Name	*Index, n*	*Sp Grav*	*Abbé No.*
Resin			
Polymethyl methacrylate	1.490	1.20	57
CR-39	1.498	1.32	58
Glass			
Spectacle/ophthalmic crown	1.523	2.52	59
High index resin			
Sola Spectralite™	1.537	1.21	47
Index 1.56	1.556	1.42	39
Index 1.58	1.578	1.47	37
Polycarbonate	1.586	1.20	31
Index 1.60	1.60	1.34	37
Index 1.66	1.66	1.35	32
High index glass			
Index 1.6	1.601	2.73	42
Barium crown (for segments)	1.616	2.96	52
Index 1.7	1.701	2.99	32
Index 1.8	1.801	3.37	25

Table 2

Focal Power (F′) in Diopters Converted to Focal Length (f′) in Millimeters and Inches

Where: $f' = \dfrac{1000\,mm}{F'}$ or $f' = \dfrac{39.37''}{F'}$

Diopters	mm	inches	Diopters	mm	inches
0.125	8000.0	315.0	5.125	195.1	7.7
0.250	4000.0	157.5	5.250	190.5	7.5
0.375	2666.7	105.0	5.375	186.0	7.3
0.500	2000.0	78.7	5.500	181.8	7.2
0.625	1600.0	63.0	5.625	177.8	7.0
0.750	1333.3	52.5	5.750	173.9	6.8
0.875	1142.9	45.0	5.875	170.2	6.7
1.000	1000.0	39.4	6.000	166.7	6.6
1.125	888.9	35.0	6.125	163.3	6.4
1.250	800.0	31.5	6.250	160.0	6.3
1.375	727.3	28.6	6.375	156.9	6.2
1.500	666.7	26.2	6.500	153.8	6.1
1.625	615.4	24.2	6.625	150.9	5.9
1.750	571.4	22.5	6.750	148.1	5.8
1.875	533.3	21.0	6.875	145.5	5.7
2.000	500.0	19.7	7.000	142.9	5.6
2.125	470.6	18.5	7.125	140.4	5.5
2.250	444.4	17.5	7.250	137.9	5.4
2.375	421.1	16.6	7.375	135.6	5.3
2.500	400.0	15.7	7.500	133.3	5.2
2.625	381.0	15.0	7.625	131.1	5.2
2.750	363.6	14.3	7.750	129.0	5.1
2.875	347.8	13.7	7.875	127.0	5.0
3.000	333.3	13.1	8.000	125.0	4.9
3.125	320.0	12.6	8.125	123.1	4.8
3.250	307.7	12.1	8.250	121.2	4.8
3.375	296.3	11.7	8.375	119.4	4.7
3.500	285.7	11.2	8.500	117.6	4.6
3.625	275.9	10.9	8.625	115.9	4.6
3.750	266.7	10.5	8.750	114.3	4.5
3.875	258.1	10.2	8.875	112.7	4.4
4.000	250.0	9.8	9.000	111.1	4.4
4.125	242.4	9.5	9.125	109.6	4.3
4.250	235.3	9.3	9.250	108.1	4.3
4.375	228.6	9.0	9.375	106.7	4.2
4.500	222.2	8.7	9.500	105.3	4.1
4.625	216.2	8.5	9.625	103.9	4.1
4.750	210.5	8.3	9.750	102.6	4.0
4.875	205.1	8.1	9.875	101.3	4.0
5.000	200.0	7.9	10.000	100.0	3.9

Table 2 *(continued)*

Where: $f' = \frac{1000\,mm}{F'}$ or $f' = \frac{39.37''}{F'}$

Diopters	mm	inches	Diopters	mm	inches
10.125	98.8	3.9	15.125	66.1	2.6
10.250	97.6	3.8	15.250	65.6	2.6
10.375	96.4	3.8	15.375	65.0	2.6
10.500	95.2	3.7	15.500	64.5	2.5
10.625	94.1	3.7	15.625	64.0	2.5
10.750	93.0	3.7	15.750	63.5	2.5
10.875	92.0	3.6	15.875	63.0	2.5
11.000	90.9	3.6	16.000	62.5	2.5
11.125	89.9	3.5	16.125	62.0	2.4
11.250	88.9	3.5	16.250	61.5	2.4
11.375	87.9	3.5	16.375	61.1	2.4
11.500	87.0	3.4	16.500	60.6	2.4
11.625	86.0	3.4	16.625	60.2	2.4
11.750	85.1	3.4	16.750	59.7	2.4
11.875	84.2	3.3	16.875	59.3	2.3
12.000	83.3	3.3	17.000	58.8	2.3
12.125	82.5	3.2	17.125	58.4	2.3
12.250	81.6	3.2	17.250	58.0	2.3
12.375	80.8	3.2	17.375	57.6	2.3
12.500	80.0	3.1	17.500	57.1	2.2
12.625	79.2	3.1	17.625	56.7	2.2
12.750	78.4	3.1	17.750	56.3	2.2
12.875	77.7	3.1	17.875	55.9	2.2
13.000	76.9	3.0	18.000	55.6	2.2
13.125	76.2	3.0	18.125	55.2	2.2
13.250	75.5	3.0	18.250	54.8	2.2
13.375	74.8	2.9	18.375	54.4	2.1
13.500	74.1	2.9	18.500	54.1	2.1
13.625	73.4	2.9	18.625	53.7	2.1
13.750	72.7	2.9	18.750	53.3	2.1
13.875	72.1	2.8	18.875	53.0	2.1
14.000	71.4	2.8	19.000	52.6	2.1
14.125	70.8	2.8	19.125	52.3	2.1
14.250	70.2	2.8	19.250	51.9	2.0
14.375	69.6	2.7	19.375	51.6	2.0
14.500	69.0	2.7	19.500	51.3	2.0
14.625	68.4	2.7	19.625	51.0	2.0
14.750	67.8	2.7	19.750	50.6	2.0
14.875	67.2	2.6	19.875	50.3	2.0
15.000	66.7	2.6	20.000	50.0	2.0

Table 3
Radius of Curvature (r) in Millimeters (mm) of Standard Surface Grinding Tools

Where: $r = \frac{(1000\,\text{mm})(n' - 1)}{F'}$

$n' = 1.530$ glass, c. 1900; and F' = marked tool surface power.

Marked Power	Radius mm	Marked Power	Radius mm
0 or plano	>6100		
0.125	4240.0	3.125	169.6
0.250	2120.0	3.250	163.1
0.375	1413.3	3.375	157.0
0.500	1060.0	3.500	151.4
0.625	848.0	3.625	146.2
0.750	706.7	3.750	141.3
0.875	605.7	3.875	136.8
1.000	530.0	4.000	132.5
1.125	471.1	4.125	128.5
1.250	424.0	4.250	124.7
1.375	385.5	4.375	121.1
1.500	353.3	4.500	117.8
1.625	326.2	4.625	114.6
1.750	302.9	4.750	111.6
1.875	282.7	4.875	108.7
2.000	265.0	5.000	106.0
2.125	249.4	5.125	103.4
2.250	235.6	5.250	101.0
2.375	223.2	5.375	98.6
2.500	212.0	5.500	96.4
2.625	201.9	5.625	94.2
2.750	192.7	5.750	92.2
2.875	184.3	5.875	90.2
3.000	176.7	6.000	88.3

Table 3 *(continued)*

Where: $r = \frac{(1000\,\text{mm})(n' - 1)}{F'}$

$n' = 1.530$ glass, c. 1900; and F' = marked tool surface power.

Marked Power	Radius mm		Marked Power	Radius mm
6.125	86.5		9.125	58.1
6.250	84.8		9.250	57.3
6.375	83.1		9.375	56.5
6.500	81.5		9.500	55.8
6.625	80.0		9.625	55.1
6.750	78.5		9.750	54.4
6.875	77.1		9.875	53.7
7.000	75.7		10.000	53.0
7.125	74.4		10.125	52.3
7.250	73.1		10.250	51.7
7.375	71.9		10.375	51.1
7.500	70.7		10.500	50.5
7.625	69.5		10.625	49.9
7.750	68.4		10.750	49.3
7.875	67.3		10.875	48.7
8.000	66.3		11.000	48.2
8.125	65.2		11.125	47.6
8.250	64.2		11.250	47.1
8.375	63.3		11.375	46.6
8.500	62.4		11.500	46.1
8.625	61.4		11.625	45.6
8.750	60.6		11.750	45.1
8.875	59.7		11:875	44.6
9.000	58.9		12.000	44.2

Table 3 Radius of Curvature *(continued)*

Where: $r = \frac{(1000\,mm)(n' - 1)}{F'}$

$n' = 1.530$ glass, c. 1900; and F' = marked tool surface power.

Marked Power	Radius mm		Marked Power	Radius mm
12.125	43.7		15.125	35.0
12.250	43.3		15.250	34.8
12.375	42.8		15.375	34.5
12.500	42.4		15.500	34.2
12.625	42.0		15.625	33.9
12.750	41.6		15.750	33.7
12.875	41.2		15.875	33.4
13.000	40.8		16.000	33.1
13.125	40.4		16.125	32.9
13.250	40.0		16.250	32.6
13.375	39.6		16.375	32.4
13.500	39.3		16.500	32.1
13.625	38.9		16.625	31.9
13.750	38.5		16.750	31.6
13.875	38.2		16.875	31.4
14.000	37.9		17.000	31.2
14.125	37.5		17.125	30.9
14.250	37.2		17.250	30.7
14.375	36.9		17.375	30.5
14.500	36.6		17.500	30.3
14.625	36.2		17.625	30.1
14.750	35.9		17.750	29.9
14.875	35.6		17.875	29.7
15.000	35.3		18.000	29.4

Table 3 *(continued)*

Where: $r = \frac{(1000\,mm)(n' - 1)}{F'}$

$n' = 1.530$ glass, c. 1900; and F' = marked tool surface power.

Marked Power	Radius mm		Marked Power	Radius mm
18.125	29.2		21.125	25.1
18.250	29.0		21.250	24.9
18.375	28.8		21.375	24.8
18.500	28.6		21.500	24.7
18.625	28.5		21.625	24.5
18.750	28.3		21.750	24.4
18.875	28.1		21.875	24.2
19.000	27.9		22.000	24.1
19.125	27.7		22.125	24.0
19.250	27.5		22.250	23.8
19.375	27.4		22.375	23.7
19.500	27.2		22.500	23.6
19.625	27.0		22.625	23.4
19.750	26.8		22.750	23.3
19.875	26.7		22.875	23.2
20.000	26.5		23.000	23.0
20.125	26.3		23.125	22.9
20.250	26.2		23.250	22.8
20.375	26.0		23.375	22.7
20.500	25.9		23.500	22.6
20.625	25.7		23.625	22.4
20.750	25.5		23.750	22.3
20.875	25.4		23.875	22.2
21.000	25.2		24.000	22.1

Table 4

Power of a One-Diopter Cylinder* at 1° Intervals from the Axis

Where: partial cylinder power, $D = \sin^2 \theta$

Degrees away from The cylinder axis in 1 degree steps Column A	Cylinder power, D in the meridian away from the axis Column B	Degrees away from The cylinder axis in 1 degree steps Column A	Cylinder power, D in the meridian away from the axis Column B
0 or 180	0.000		
1 or 179	0.000	46 or 134	0.517
2 or 178	0.001	47 or 133	0.535
3 or 177	0.003	48 or 132	0.552
4 or 176	0.005	49 or 131	0.570
5 or 175	0.01	50 or 130	0.59
6 or 174	0.011	51 or 129	0.604
7 or 173	0.015	52 or 128	0.621
8 or 172	0.019	53 or 127	0.638
9 or 171	0.024	54 or 126	0.655
10 or 170	0.03	55 or 125	0.67
11 or 169	0.036	56 or 124	0.687
12 or 168	0.043	57 or 123	0.703
13 or 167	0.051	58 or 122	0.719
14 or 166	0.059	59 or 121	0.735
15 or 165	0.07	60 or 120	0.75
16 or 164	0.076	61 or 119	0.765
17 or 163	0.085	62 or 118	0.780
18 or 162	0.095	63 or 117	0.794
19 or 161	0.106	64 or 116	0.808

20 or 160	0.12	65 or 115	0.82
21 or 159	0.128	66 or 114	0.835
22 or 158	0.140	67 or 113	0.847
23 or 157	0.153	68 or 112	0.860
24 or 156	0.165	69 or 111	0.872
25 or 155	0.18	70 or 110	0.88
26 or 154	0.192	71 or 109	0.894
27 or 153	0.206	72 or 108	0.905
28 or 152	0.220	73 or 107	0.915
29 or 151	0.235	74 or 106	0.924
30 or 150	0.25	75 or 105	0.93
31 or 149	0.265	76 or 104	0.941
32 or 148	0.281	77 or 103	0.949
33 or 147	0.297	78 or 102	0.957
34 or 146	0.313	79 or 101	0.964
35 or 145	0.33	80 or 100	0.97
36 or 144	0.345	81 or 99	0.976
37 or 143	0.362	82 or 98	0.981
38 or 142	0.379	83 or 97	0.985
39 or 141	0.396	84 or 96	0.989
40 or 140	0.41	85 or 95	0.99
41 or 139	0.430	86 or 94	0.995
42 or 138	0.448	87 or 93	0.997
43 or 137	0.465	88 or 92	0.999
44 or 136	0.483	89 or 91	1.000
45 or 135	0.50	90 or 90	1.00

* For other cylinder powers, multiply the actual cylinder times the partial cylinder power (D) shown in column B.

Table 5
True Surface Power of Various Refractive Index Lenses Surfaced Using Standad Marked Grinding and Polishing Tools Made for n′ = 1.530

Where: $TP = \frac{(MP)(n' - 1)}{0.530}$

True Power n′=1.498	True Power n′=1.523	MARKED POWER n′=1.530	True Power n′=1.586	True Power n′=1.701	True Power n′=1.801
0.12	0.12	0.125	0.14	0.17	0.19
0.23	0.25	0.250	0.28	0.33	0.38
0.35	0.37	0.375	0.41	0.50	0.57
0.47	0.49	0.500	0.55	0.66	0.76
0.59	0.62	0.625	0.69	0.83	0.94
0.70	0.74	0.750	0.83	0.99	1.13
0.82	0.86	0.875	0.97	1.16	1.32
0.94	0.99	1.000	1.11	1.32	1.51
1.06	1.11	1.125	1.24	1.49	1.70
1.17	1.23	1.250	1.38	1.65	1.89
1.29	1.36	1.375	1.52	1.82	2.08
1.41	1.48	1.500	1.66	1.98	2.27
1.53	1.60	1.625	1.80	2.15	2.46
1.64	1.73	1.750	1.93	2.31	2.64
1.76	1.85	1.875	2.07	2.48	2.83
1.88	1.97	2.000	2.21	2.65	3.02
2.00	2.10	2.125	2.35	2.81	3.21
2.11	2.22	2.250	2.49	2.98	3.40
2.23	2.34	2.375	2.63	3.14	3.59
2.35	2.47	2.500	2.76	3.31	3.78
2.47	2.59	2.625	2.90	3.47	3.97
2.58	2.71	2.750	3.04	3.64	4.16
2.70	2.84	2.875	3.18	3.80	4.35
2.82	2.96	3.000	3.32	3.97	4.53
2.94	3.08	3.125	3.46	4.13	4.72
3.05	3.21	3.250	3.59	4.30	4.91
3.17	3.33	3.375	3.73	4.46	5.10
3.29	3.45	3.500	3.87	4.63	5.29
3.41	3.58	3.625	4.01	4.79	5.48
3.52	3.70	3.750	4.15	4.96	5.67
3.64	3.82	3.875	4.28	5.13	5.86
3.76	3.95	4.000	4.42	5.29	6.05
3.88	4.07	4.125	4.56	5.46	6.23
3.99	4.19	4.250	4.70	5.62	6.42
4.11	4.32	4.375	4.84	5.79	6.61
4.23	4.44	4.500	4.98	5.95	6.80
4.35	4.56	4.625	5.11	6.12	6.99
4.46	4.69	4.750	5.25	6.28	7.18
4.58	4.81	4.875	5.39	6.45	7.37
4.70	4.93	5.000	5.53	6.61	7.56

Table 5 *(continued)*

Where: $TP = \frac{(MP)(n' - 1)}{0.530}$

True Power n'=1.498	True Power n'=1.523	MARKED POWER n'=1.530	True Power n'=1.586	True Power n'=1.701	True Power n'=1.801
4.82	5.06	5.125	5.67	6.78	7.75
4.93	5.18	5.250	5.80	6.94	7.93
5.05	5.30	5.375	5.94	7.11	8.12
5.17	5.43	5.500	6.08	7.27	8.31
5.29	5.55	5.625	6.22	7.44	8.50
5.40	5.67	5.750	6.36	7.61	8.69
5.52	5.80	5.875	6.50	7.77	8.88
5.64	5.92	6.000	6.63	7.94	9.07
5.76	6.04	6.125	6.77	8.10	9.26
5.87	6.17	6.250	6.91	8.27	9.45
5.99	6.29	6.375	7.05	8.43	9.63
6.11	6.41	6.500	7.19	8.60	9.82
6.23	6.54	6.625	7.33	8.76	10.01
6.34	6.66	6.750	7.46	8.93	10.20
6.46	6.78	6.875	7.60	9.09	10.39
6.58	6.91	7.000	7.74	9.26	10.58
6.69	7.03	7.125	7.88	9.42	10.77
6.81	7.15	7.250	8.02	9.59	10.96
6.93	7.28	7.375	8.15	9.75	11.15
7.05	7.40	7.500	8.29	9.92	11.33
7.16	7.52	7.625	8.43	10.09	11.52
7.28	7.65	7.750	8.57	10.25	11.71
7.40	7.77	7.875	8.71	10.42	11.90
7.52	7.89	8.000	8.85	10.58	12.09
7.63	8.02	8.125	8.98	10.75	12.28
7.75	8.14	8.250	9.12	10.91	12.47
7.87	8.26	8.375	9.26	11.08	12.66
7.99	8.39	8.500	9.40	11.24	12.85
8.10	8.51	8.625	9.54	11.41	13.04
8.22	8.63	8.750	9.67	11.57	13.22
8.34	8.76	8.875	9.81	11.74	13.41
8.46	8.88	9.000	9.95	11.90	13.60
8.57	9.00	9.125	10.09	12.07	13.79
8.69	9.13	9.250	10.23	12.23	13.98
8.81	9.25	9.375	10.37	12.40	14.17
8.93	9.37	9.500	10.50	12.57	14.36
9.04	9.50	9.625	10.64	12.73	14.55
9.16	9.62	9.750	10.78	12.90	14.74
9.28	9.74	9.875	10.92	13.06	14.92
9.40	9.87	10.000	11.06	13.23	15.11

Table 5 True Surface Power *(continued)*

Where: $TP = \frac{(MP)(n' - 1)}{0.530}$

True Power n'=1.498	True Power n'=1.523	MARKED POWER n'=1.530	True Power n'=1.586	True Power n'=1.701	True Power n'=1.801
9.51	9.99	10.125	11.19	13.39	15.30
9.63	10.11	10.250	11.33	13.56	15.49
9.75	10.24	10.375	11.47	13.72	15.68
9.87	10.36	10.500	11.61	13.89	15.87
9.98	10.48	10.625	11.75	14.05	16.06
10.10	10.61	10.750	11.89	14.22	16.25
10.22	10.73	10.875	12.02	14.38	16.44
10.34	10.85	11.000	12.16	14.55	16.62
10.45	10.98	11.125	12.30	14.71	16.81
10.57	11.10	11.250	12.44	14.88	17.00
10.69	11.22	11.375	12.58	15.05	17.19
10.81	11.35	11.500	12.72	15.21	17.38
10.92	11.47	11.625	12.85	15.38	17.57
11.04	11.59	11.750	12.99	15.54	17.76
11.16	11.72	11.875	13.13	15.71	17.95
11.28	11.84	12.000	13.27	15.87	18.14
11.39	11.96	12.125	13.41	16.04	18.32
11.51	12.09	12.250	13.54	16.20	18.51
11.63	12.21	12.375	13.68	16.37	18.70
11.75	12.33	12.500	13.82	16.53	18.89
11.86	12.46	12.625	13.96	16.70	19.08
11.98	12.58	12.750	14.10	16.86	19.27
12.10	12.70	12.875	14.24	17.03	19.46
12.22	12.83	13.000	14.37	17.19	19.65
12.33	12.95	13.125	14.51	17.36	19.84
12.45	13.08	13.250	14.65	17.53	20.03
12.57	13.20	13.375	14.79	17.69	20.21
12.68	13.32	13.500	14.93	17.86	20.40
12.80	13.45	13.625	15.06	18.02	20.59
12.92	13.57	13.750	15.20	18.19	20.78
13.04	13.69	13.875	15.34	18.35	20.97
13.15	13.82	14.000	15.48	18.52	21.16
13.27	13.94	14.125	15.62	18.68	21.35
13.39	14.06	14.250	15.76	18.85	21.54
13.51	14.19	14.375	15.89	19.01	21.73
13.62	14.31	14.500	16.03	19.18	21.91
13.74	14.43	14.625	16.17	19.34	22.10
13.86	14.56	14.750	16.31	19.51	22.29
13.98	14.68	14.875	16.45	19.67	22.48
14.09	14.80	15.000	16.58	19.84	22.67

Table 5 *(continued)*

Where: $TP = \frac{(MP)(n' - 1)}{0.530}$

True Power n'=1.498	True Power n'=1.523	MARKED POWER n'=1.530	True Power n'=1.586	True Power n'=1.701	True Power n'=1.801
14.21	14.93	15.125	16.72	20.00	22.86
14.33	15.05	15.250	16.86	20.17	23.05
14.45	15.17	15.375	17.00	20.34	23.24
14.56	15.30	15.500	17.14	20.50	23.43
14.68	15.42	15.625	17.28	20.67	23.61
14.80	15.54	15.750	17.41	20.83	23.80
14.92	15.67	15.875	17.55	21.00	23.99
15.03	15.79	16.000	17.69	21.16	24.18
15.15	15.91	16.125	17.83	21.33	24.37
15.27	16.04	16.250	17.97	21.49	24.56
15.39	16.16	16.375	18.11	21.66	24.75
15.50	16.28	16.500	18.24	21.82	24.94
15.62	16.41	16.625	18.38	21.99	25.13
15.74	16.53	16.750	18.52	22.15	25.31
15.86	16.65	16.875	18.66	22.32	25.50
15.97	16.78	17.000	18.80	22.48	25.69
16.09	16.90	17.125	18.93	22.65	25.88
16.21	17.02	17.250	19.07	22.82	26.07
16.33	17.15	17.375	19.21	22.98	26.26
16.44	17.27	17.500	19.35	23.15	26.45
16.56	17.39	17.625	19.49	23.31	26.64
16.68	17.52	17.750	19.63	23.48	26.83
16.80	17.64	17.875	19.76	23.64	27.01
16.91	17.76	18.000	19.90	23.81	27.20
17.03	17.89	18.125	20.04	23.97	27.39
17.15	18.01	18.250	20.18	24.14	27.58
17.27	18.13	18.375	20.32	24.30	27.77
17.38	18.26	18.500	20.45	24.47	27.96
17.50	18.38	18.625	20.59	24.63	28.15
17.62	18.50	18.750	20.73	24.80	28.34
17.74	18.63	18.875	20.87	24.96	28.53
17.85	18.75	19.000	21.01	25.13	28.72
17.97	18.87	19.125	21.15	25.30	28.90
18.09	19.00	19.250	21.28	25.46	29.09
18.21	19.12	19.375	21.42	25.63	29.28
18.32	19.24	19.500	21.56	25.79	29.47
18.44	19.37	19.625	21.70	25.96	29.66
18.56	19.49	19.750	21.84	26.12	29.85
18.68	19.61	19.875	21.98	26.29	30.04
18.79	19.74	20.000	22.11	26.45	30.23

Table 6

Center- or Edge-Thickness Comparison Chart for Select Powers of Various Index Lenses

Where: ed = effective or finished lens diameter of 56mm

F′ = maximum plus or least minus lens power; and n′ = lens index

For plus lenses, chart values are center thickness (c) with a knife edge thickness (e) of 0mm; for minus lenses, chart values are edge thickness (e) with a center thickness (c) of 0mm; add 2.2mm (e.g. to the knife edge or zero center) to obtain the final lens thickness

based on: $(c) \text{ or } (e) = \frac{[(ed*ed)/4]\,(F')}{2000\,(n'-1)}$

Note: Chart values are for 56mm effective diameter only.

lens power F' +/−	CR−39 n'=1.498 center/edge thickness	Spec Crown n'=1.523 center/edge thickness	Spectralite n'=1.537 center/edge thickness	Polycarbonate n'=1.586 center/edge thickness	High Index n'=1.701 center/edge thickness	High Index n'=1.801 center/edge thickness
0.50	0.4	0.4	0.4	0.3	0.3	0.2
1.00	0.8	0.7	0.7	0.7	0.6	0.5
1.50	1.2	1.1	1.1	1.0	0.8	0.7
2.00	1.6	1.5	1.5	1.3	1.1	1.0
2.50	2.0	1.9	1.8	1.7	1.4	1.2
3.00	2.4	2.2	2.2	2.0	1.7	1.5
3.50	2.8	2.6	2.6	2.3	2.0	1.7
4.00	3.1	3.0	2.9	2.7	2.2	2.0
4.50	3.5	3.4	3.3	3.0	2.5	2.2
5.00	3.9	3.7	3.6	3.3	2.8	2.4
5.50	4.3	4.1	4.0	3.7	3.1	2.7
6.00	4.7	4.5	4.4	4.0	3.4	2.9
6.50	5.1	4.9	4.7	4.3	3.6	3.2
7.00	5.5	5.2	5.1	4.7	3.9	3.4

7.50	5.9	5.6	5.5	5.0	4.2	3.7
8.00	6.3	6.0	5.8	5.4	4.5	3.9
8.50	6.7	6.4	6.2	5.7	4.8	4.2
9.00	7.1	6.7	6.6	6.0	5.0	4.4
9.50	7.5	7.1	6.9	6.4	5.3	4.6
10.00	7.9	7.5	7.3	6.7	5.6	4.9
10.50	8.3	7.9	7.7	7.0	5.9	5.1
11.00	8.7	8.2	8.0	7.4	6.2	5.4
11.50	9.1	8.6	8.4	7.7	6.4	5.6
12.00	9.4	9.0	8.8	8.0	6.7	5.9
12.50	9.8	9.4	9.1	8.4	7.0	6.1
13.00	10.2	9.7	9.5	8.7	7.3	6.4
13.50	10.6	10.1	9.9	9.0	7.5	6.6
14.00	11.0	10.5	10.2	9.4	7.8	6.9
14.50	11.4	10.9	10.6	9.7	8.1	7.1
15.00	11.8	11.2	10.9	10.0	8.4	7.3
15.50	12.2	11.6	11.3	10.4	8.7	7.6
16.00	12.6	12.0	11.7	10.7	8.9	7.8
16.50	13.0	12.4	12.0	11.0	9.2	8.1
17.00	13.4	12.7	12.4	11.4	9.5	8.3
17.50	13.8	13.1	12.8	11.7	9.8	8.6
18.00	14.2	13.5	13.1	12.0	10.1	8.8
18.50	14.6	13.9	13.5	12.4	10.3	9.1
19.00	15.0	14.2	13.9	12.7	10.6	9.3
19.50	15.3	14.6	14.2	13.0	10.9	9.5
20.00	15.7	15.0	14.6	13.4	11.2	9.8
20.50	16.1	15.4	15.0	13.7	11.5	10.0
21.00	16.5	15.7	15.3	14.0	11.7	10.3
21.50	16.9	16.1	15.7	14.4	12.0	10.5
22.00	17.3	16.5	16.1	14.7	12.3	10.8

Table 7

Thickness Difference (t), in Millimeters, of a Sharp-Edged Prism for Various Lenses

Apex angle (A) in degrees	Thin prism diopter power	CR–39 Allyl Diglycol Carbonate Plastic, n=1.498 t = diameter (in mm)* tan(A) (in degrees) at diameters:				
		48mm	52mm	56mm	60mm	64mm
0.29	0.25	0.2	0.3	0.3	0.3	0.3
0.58	0.50	0.5	0.5	0.6	0.6	0.6
0.86	0.75	0.7	0.8	0.8	0.9	1.0
1.15	1.00	1.0	1.0	1.1	1.2	1.3
1.44	1.25	1.2	1.3	1.4	1.5	1.6
1.72	1.50	1.4	1.6	1.7	1.8	1.9
2.01	1.75	1.7	1.8	2.0	2.1	2.2
2.30	2.00	1.9	2.1	2.2	2.4	2.6
2.58	2.25	2.2	2.3	2.5	2.7	2.9
2.87	2.50	2.4	2.6	2.8	3.0	3.2
3.16	2.75	2.6	2.9	3.1	3.3	3.5
3.44	3.00	2.9	3.1	3.4	3.6	3.9
3.73	3.25	3.1	3.4	3.6	3.9	4.2
4.01	3.50	3.4	3.6	3.9	4.2	4.5
4.30	3.75	3.6	3.9	4.2	4.5	4.8
4.58	4.00	3.8	4.2	4.5	4.8	5.1
4.86	4.25	4.1	4.4	4.8	5.1	5.4
5.15	4.50	4.3	4.7	5.0	5.4	5.8
5.43	4.75	4.6	4.9	5.3	5.7	6.1
5.71	5.00	4.8	5.2	5.6	6.0	6.4
5.99	5.25	5.0	5.5	5.9	6.3	6.7
6.27	5.50	5.3	5.7	6.2	6.6	7.0
6.55	5.75	5.5	6.0	6.4	6.9	7.4
6.83	6.00	5.8	6.2	6.7	7.2	7.7

7.11	6.25	6.0	6.5	7.0	7.5	8.0
7.39	6.50	6.2	6.7	7.3	7.8	8.3
7.67	6.75	6.5	7.0	7.5	8.1	8.6
7.94	7.00	6.7	7.3	7.8	8.4	8.9
8.22	7.25	6.9	7.5	8.1	8.7	9.2
8.49	7.50	7.2	7.8	8.4	9.0	9.6
8.77	7.75	7.4	8.0	8.6	9.3	9.9
9.04	8.00	7.6	8.3	8.9	9.5	10.2
9.31	8.25	7.9	8.5	9.2	9.8	10.5
9.58	8.50	8.1	8.8	9.5	10.1	10.8
9.85	8.75	8.3	9.0	9.7	10.4	11.1
10.12	9.00	8.6	9.3	10.0	10.7	11.4
10.39	9.25	8.8	9.5	10.3	11.0	11.7
10.66	9.50	9.0	9.8	10.5	11.3	12.0
10.93	9.75	9.3	10.0	10.8	11.6	12.4
11.19	10.00	9.5	10.3	11.1	11.9	12.7
11.45	10.25	9.7	10.5	11.3	12.2	13.0
11.72	10.50	10.0	10.8	11.6	12.4	13.3
11.98	10.75	10.2	11.0	11.9	12.7	13.6
12.24	11.00	10.4	11.3	12.1	13.0	13.9
12.50	11.25	10.6	11.5	12.4	13.3	14.2
12.76	11.50	10.9	11.8	12.7	13.6	14.5
13.02	11.75	11.1	12.0	12.9	13.9	14.8
13.27	12.00	11.3	12.3	13.2	14.2	15.1
13.53	12.25	11.5	12.5	13.5	14.4	15.4
13.78	12.50	11.8	12.8	13.7	14.7	15.7
14.03	12.75	12.0	13.0	14.0	15.0	16.0
14.28	13.00	12.2	13.2	14.3	15.3	16.3
14.53	13.25	12.4	13.5	14.5	15.6	16.6
14.78	13.50	12.7	13.7	14.8	15.8	16.9
15.03	13.75	12.9	14.0	15.0	16.1	17.2
15.28	14.00	13.1	14.2	15.3	16.4	17.5
15.52	14.25	13.3	14.4	15.6	16.7	17.8
15.76	14.50	13.5	14.7	15.8	16.9	18.1
16.01	14.75	13.8	14.9	16.1	17.2	18.4
16.25	15.00	14.0	15.2	16.3	17.5	18.6

Table 7 Thickness Difference *(continued)*

Apex angle (A) in degrees	Thin prism diopter power	Spectacle/ophthalmic crown glass, n=1.523 t = diameter (in mm)* tan(A) (in degrees) at diameters: 48mm	52mm	56mm	60mm	64mm
0.27	0.25	0.2	0.2	0.3	0.3	0.3
0.55	0.50	0.5	0.5	0.5	0.6	0.6
0.82	0.75	0.7	0.7	0.8	0.9	0.9
1.10	1.00	0.9	1.0	1.1	1.1	1.2
1.37	1.25	1.1	1.2	1.3	1.4	1.5
1.64	1.50	1.4	1.5	1.6	1.7	1.8
1.92	1.75	1.6	1.7	1.9	2.0	2.1
2.19	2.00	1.8	2.0	2.1	2.3	2.4
2.46	2.25	2.1	2.2	2.4	2.6	2.8
2.73	2.50	2.3	2.5	2.7	2.9	3.1
3.01	2.75	2.5	2.7	2.9	3.2	3.4
3.28	3.00	2.7	3.0	3.2	3.4	3.7
3.55	3.25	3.0	3.2	3.5	3.7	4.0
3.82	3.50	3.2	3.5	3.7	4.0	4.3
4.09	3.75	3.4	3.7	4.0	4.3	4.6
4.36	4.00	3.7	4.0	4.3	4.6	4.9
4.63	4.25	3.9	4.2	4.5	4.9	5.2
4.90	4.50	4.1	4.5	4.8	5.1	5.5
5.17	4.75	4.3	4.7	5.1	5.4	5.8
5.44	5.00	4.6	5.0	5.3	5.7	6.1
5.71	5.25	4.8	5.2	5.6	6.0	6.4
5.98	5.50	5.0	5.4	5.9	6.3	6.7
6.24	5.75	5.3	5.7	6.1	6.6	7.0
6.51	6.00	5.5	5.9	6.4	6.8	7.3
6.78	6.25	5.7	6.2	6.7	7.1	7.6
7.04	6.50	5.9	6.4	6.9	7.4	7.9

7.31	6.75	6.2	6.7	7.2	7.7	8.2
7.57	7.00	6.4	6.9	7.4	8.0	8.5
7.83	7.25	6.6	7.2	7.7	8.3	8.8
8.10	7.50	6.8	7.4	8.0	8.5	9.1
8.36	7.75	7.1	7.6	8.2	8.8	9.4
8.62	8.00	7.3	7.9	8.5	9.1	9.7
8.88	8.25	7.5	8.1	8.7	9.4	10.0
9.14	8.50	7.7	8.4	9.0	9.7	10.3
9.40	8.75	7.9	8.6	9.3	9.9	10.6
9.65	9.00	8.2	8.8	9.5	10.2	10.9
9.91	9.25	8.4	9.1	9.8	10.5	11.2
10.16	9.50	8.6	9.3	10.0	10.8	11.5
10.42	9.75	8.8	9.6	10.3	11.0	11.8
10.67	10.00	9.0	9.8	10.6	11.3	12.1
10.93	10.25	9.3	10.0	10.8	11.6	12.4
11.18	10.50	9.5	10.3	11.1	11.9	12.6
11.43	10.75	9.7	10.5	11.3	12.1	12.9
11.68	11.00	9.9	10.7	11.6	12.4	13.2
11.93	11.25	10.1	11.0	11.8	12.7	13.5
12.17	11.50	10.4	11.2	12.1	12.9	13.8
12.42	11.75	10.6	11.5	12.3	13.2	14.1
12.67	12.00	10.8	11.7	12.6	13.5	14.4
12.91	12.25	11.0	11.9	12.8	13.8	14.7
13.15	12.50	11.2	12.2	13.1	14.0	15.0
13.40	12.75	11.4	12.4	13.3	14.3	15.2
13.64	13.00	11.6	12.6	13.6	14.6	15.5
13.88	13.25	11.9	12.8	13.8	14.8	15.8
14.12	13.50	12.1	13.1	14.1	15.1	16.1
14.35	13.75	12.3	13.3	14.3	15.4	16.4
14.59	14.00	12.5	13.5	14.6	15.6	16.7
14.83	14.25	12.7	13.8	14.8	15.9	16.9
15.06	14.50	12.9	14.0	15.1	16.1	17.2
15.29	14.75	13.1	14.2	15.3	16.4	17.5
15.52	15.00	13.3	14.4	15.6	16.7	17.8

Table 7 Thickness Difference *(continued)*

Apex angle (A) in degrees	Thin prism diopter power	Sola Spectralite, n=1.537 t = diameter (in mm)* tan(A) (in degrees) at diameters:				
		48mm	52mm	56mm	60mm	64mm
0.27	0.25	0.2	0.2	0.3	0.3	0.3
0.53	0.50	0.4	0.5	0.5	0.6	0.6
0.80	0.75	0.7	0.7	0.8	0.8	0.9
1.07	1.00	0.9	1.0	1.0	1.1	1.2
1.33	1.25	1.1	1.2	1.3	1.4	1.5
1.60	1.50	1.3	1.5	1.6	1.7	1.8
1.87	1.75	1.6	1.7	1.8	2.0	2.1
2.13	2.00	1.8	1.9	2.1	2.2	2.4
2.40	2.25	2.0	2.2	2.3	2.5	2.7
2.66	2.50	2.2	2.4	2.6	2.8	3.0
2.93	2.75	2.5	2.7	2.9	3.1	3.3
3.19	3.00	2.7	2.9	3.1	3.3	3.6
3.46	3.25	2.9	3.1	3.4	3.6	3.9
3.72	3.50	3.1	3.4	3.6	3.9	4.2
3.99	3.75	3.3	3.6	3.9	4.2	4.5
4.25	4.00	3.6	3.9	4.2	4.5	4.8
4.51	4.25	3.8	4.1	4.4	4.7	5.1
4.78	4.50	4.0	4.3	4.7	5.0	5.3
5.04	4.75	4.2	4.6	4.9	5.3	5.6
5.30	5.00	4.5	4.8	5.2	5.6	5.9
5.56	5.25	4.7	5.1	5.5	5.8	6.2
5.82	5.50	4.9	5.3	5.7	6.1	6.5
6.08	5.75	5.1	5.5	6.0	6.4	6.8
6.34	6.00	5.3	5.8	6.2	6.7	7.1
6.60	6.25	5.6	6.0	6.5	6.9	7.4
6.86	6.50	5.8	6.3	6.7	7.2	7.7

7.12	6.75	6.0	6.5	7.0	7.5	8.0
7.38	7.00	6.2	6.7	7.2	7.8	8.3
7.63	7.25	6.4	7.0	7.5	8.0	8.6
7.89	7.50	6.7	7.2	7.8	8.3	8.9
8.14	7.75	6.9	7.4	8.0	8.6	9.2
8.40	8.00	7.1	7.7	8.3	8.9	9.4
8.65	8.25	7.3	7.9	8.5	9.1	9.7
8.90	8.50	7.5	8.1	8.8	9.4	10.0
9.16	8.75	7.7	8.4	9.0	9.7	10.3
9.41	9.00	8.0	8.6	9.3	9.9	10.6
9.66	9.25	8.2	8.8	9.5	10.2	10.9
9.91	9.50	8.4	9.1	9.8	10.5	11.2
10.16	9.75	8.6	9.3	10.0	10.7	11.5
10.40	10.00	8.8	9.5	10.3	11.0	11.8
10.65	10.25	9.0	9.8	10.5	11.3	12.0
10.90	10.50	9.2	10.0	10.8	11.6	12.3
11.14	10.75	9.5	10.2	11.0	11.8	12.6
11.39	11.00	9.7	10.5	11.3	12.1	12.9
11.63	11.25	9.9	10.7	11.5	12.3	13.2
11.87	11.50	10.1	10.9	11.8	12.6	13.5
12.11	11.75	10.3	11.2	12.0	12.9	13.7
12.35	12.00	10.5	11.4	12.3	13.1	14.0
12.59	12.25	10.7	11.6	12.5	13.4	14.3
12.83	12.50	10.9	11.8	12.8	13.7	14.6
13.06	12.75	11.1	12.1	13.0	13.9	14.9
13.30	13.00	11.3	12.3	13.2	14.2	15.1
13.53	13.25	11.6	12.5	13.5	14.4	15.4
13.77	13.50	11.8	12.7	13.7	14.7	15.7
14.00	13.75	12.0	13.0	14.0	15.0	16.0
14.23	14.00	12.2	13.2	14.2	15.2	16.2
14.46	14.25	12.4	13.4	14.4	15.5	16.5
14.69	14.50	12.6	13.6	14.7	15.7	16.8
14.92	14.75	12.8	13.9	14.9	16.0	17.1
15.14	15.00	13.0	14.1	15.2	16.2	17.3

Table 7 Thickness Difference *(continued)*

Apex angle (A) in degrees	Thin prism diopter power	Polycarbonate, n=1.586 t = diameter (in mm)* tan(A) (in degrees) at diameters: 48mm	52mm	56mm	60mm	64mm
0.24	0.25	0.2	0.2	0.2	0.3	0.3
0.49	0.50	0.4	0.4	0.5	0.5	0.5
0.73	0.75	0.6	0.7	0.7	0.8	0.8
0.98	1.00	0.8	0.9	1.0	1.0	1.1
1.22	1.25	1.0	1.1	1.2	1.3	1.4
1.47	1.50	1.2	1.3	1.4	1.5	1.6
1.71	1.75	1.4	1.6	1.7	1.8	1.9
1.95	2.00	1.6	1.8	1.9	2.0	2.2
2.20	2.25	1.8	2.0	2.1	2.3	2.5
2.44	2.50	2.0	2.2	2.4	2.6	2.7
2.68	2.75	2.3	2.4	2.6	2.8	3.0
2.93	3.00	2.5	2.7	2.9	3.1	3.3
3.17	3.25	2.7	2.9	3.1	3.3	3.5
3.41	3.50	2.9	3.1	3.3	3.6	3.8
3.65	3.75	3.1	3.3	3.6	3.8	4.1
3.90	4.00	3.3	3.5	3.8	4.1	4.4
4.14	4.25	3.5	3.8	4.1	4.3	4.6
4.38	4.50	3.7	4.0	4.3	4.6	4.9
4.62	4.75	3.9	4.2	4.5	4.8	5.2
4.86	5.00	4.1	4.4	4.8	5.1	5.4
5.10	5.25	4.3	4.6	5.0	5.4	5.7
5.34	5.50	4.5	4.9	5.2	5.6	6.0
5.58	5.75	4.7	5.1	5.5	5.9	6.3
5.82	6.00	4.9	5.3	5.7	6.1	6.5
6.06	6.25	5.1	5.5	5.9	6.4	6.8
6.29	6.50	5.3	5.7	6.2	6.6	7.1

6.53	6.75	5.5	6.0	6.4	6.9	7.3
6.77	7.00	5.7	6.2	6.6	7.1	7.6
7.00	7.25	5.9	6.4	6.9	7.4	7.9
7.24	7.50	6.1	6.6	7.1	7.6	8.1
7.47	7.75	6.3	6.8	7.3	7.9	8.4
7.71	8.00	6.5	7.0	7.6	8.1	8.7
7.94	8.25	6.7	7.3	7.8	8.4	8.9
8.17	8.50	6.9	7.5	8.0	8.6	9.2
8.41	8.75	7.1	7.7	8.3	8.9	9.5
8.64	9.00	7.3	7.9	8.5	9.1	9.7
8.87	9.25	7.5	8.1	8.7	9.4	10.0
9.10	9.50	7.7	8.3	9.0	9.6	10.3
9.33	9.75	7.9	8.5	9.2	9.9	10.5
9.56	10.00	8.1	8.8	9.4	10.1	10.8
9.79	10.25	8.3	9.0	9.7	10.3	11.0
10.01	10.50	8.5	9.2	9.9	10.6	11.3
10.24	10.75	8.7	9.4	10.1	10.8	11.6
10.46	11.00	8.9	9.6	10.3	11.1	11.8
10.69	11.25	9.1	9.8	10.6	11.3	12.1
10.91	11.50	9.3	10.0	10.8	11.6	12.3
11.14	11.75	9.4	10.2	11.0	11.8	12.6
11.36	12.00	9.6	10.4	11.2	12.1	12.9
11.58	12.25	9.8	10.7	11.5	12.3	13.1
11.80	12.50	10.0	10.9	11.7	12.5	13.4
12.02	12.75	10.2	11.1	11.9	12.8	13.6
12.24	13.00	10.4	11.3	12.1	13.0	13.9
12.46	13.25	10.6	11.5	12.4	13.3	14.1
12.67	13.50	10.8	11.7	12.6	13.5	14.4
12.89	13.75	11.0	11.9	12.8	13.7	14.6
13.10	14.00	11.2	12.1	13.0	14.0	14.9
13.32	14.25	11.4	12.3	13.3	14.2	15.1
13.53	14.50	11.6	12.5	13.5	14.4	15.4
13.74	14.75	11.7	12.7	13.7	14.7	15.7
13.95	15.00	11.9	12.9	13.9	14.9	15.9

Table 7 Thickness Difference *(continued)*

Apex angle (A) in degrees	Thin prism diopter power	High Index Glass, n=1.701; t = diameter (in mm)* tan(A) (in degrees) at diameters: 48mm	52mm	56mm	60mm	64mm
0.20	0.25	0.2	0.2	0.2	0.2	0.2
0.41	0.50	0.3	0.4	0.4	0.4	0.5
0.61	0.75	0.5	0.6	0.6	0.6	0.7
0.82	1.00	0.7	0.7	0.8	0.9	0.9
1.02	1.25	0.9	0.9	1.0	1.1	1.1
1.23	1.50	1.0	1.1	1.2	1.3	1.4
1.43	1.75	1.2	1.3	1.4	1.5	1.6
1.63	2.00	1.4	1.5	1.6	1.7	1.8
1.84	2.25	1.5	1.7	1.8	1.9	2.1
2.04	2.50	1.7	1.9	2.0	2.1	2.3
2.24	2.75	1.9	2.0	2.2	2.4	2.5
2.45	3.00	2.1	2.2	2.4	2.6	2.7
2.65	3.25	2.2	2.4	2.6	2.8	3.0
2.85	3.50	2.4	2.6	2.8	3.0	3.2
3.06	3.75	2.6	2.8	3.0	3.2	3.4
3.26	4.00	2.7	3.0	3.2	3.4	3.6
3.46	4.25	2.9	3.1	3.4	3.6	3.9
3.66	4.50	3.1	3.3	3.6	3.8	4.1
3.87	4.75	3.2	3.5	3.8	4.1	4.3
4.07	5.00	3.4	3.7	4.0	4.3	4.6
4.27	5.25	3.6	3.9	4.2	4.5	4.8
4.47	5.50	3.8	4.1	4.4	4.7	5.0
4.67	5.75	3.9	4.2	4.6	4.9	5.2
4.87	6.00	4.1	4.4	4.8	5.1	5.5
5.07	6.25	4.3	4.6	5.0	5.3	5.7
5.27	6.50	4.4	4.8	5.2	5.5	5.9

5.47	6.75	4.6	5.0	5.4	5.7	6.1
5.67	7.00	4.8	5.2	5.6	6.0	6.4
5.87	7.25	4.9	5.3	5.8	6.2	6.6
6.07	7.50	5.1	5.5	6.0	6.4	6.8
6.26	7.75	5.3	5.7	6.1	6.6	7.0
6.46	8.00	5.4	5.9	6.3	6.8	7.2
6.66	8.25	5.6	6.1	6.5	7.0	7.5
6.85	8.50	5.8	6.3	6.7	7.2	7.7
7.05	8.75	5.9	6.4	6.9	7.4	7.9
7.25	9.00	6.1	6.6	7.1	7.6	8.1
7.44	9.25	6.3	6.8	7.3	7.8	8.4
7.64	9.50	6.4	7.0	7.5	8.0	8.6
7.83	9.75	6.6	7.2	7.7	8.3	8.8
8.02	10.00	6.8	7.3	7.9	8.5	9.0
8.22	10.25	6.9	7.5	8.1	8.7	9.2
8.41	10.50	7.1	7.7	8.3	8.9	9.5
8.60	10.75	7.3	7.9	8.5	9.1	9.7
8.79	11.00	7.4	8.0	8.7	9.3	9.9
8.98	11.25	7.6	8.2	8.9	9.5	10.1
9.17	11.50	7.8	8.4	9.0	9.7	10.3
9.36	11.75	7.9	8.6	9.2	9.9	10.6
9.55	12.00	8.1	8.7	9.4	10.1	10.8
9.74	12.25	8.2	8.9	9.6	10.3	11.0
9.93	12.50	8.4	9.1	9.8	10.5	11.2
10.11	12.75	8.6	9.3	10.0	10.7	11.4
10.30	13.00	8.7	9.5	10.2	10.9	11.6
10.49	13.25	8.9	9.6	10.4	11.1	11.8
10.67	13.50	9.0	9.8	10.6	11.3	12.1
10.86	13.75	9.2	10.0	10.7	11.5	12.3
11.04	14.00	9.4	10.1	10.9	11.7	12.5
11.22	14.25	9.5	10.3	11.1	11.9	12.7
11.41	14.50	9.7	10.5	11.3	12.1	12.9
11.59	14.75	9.8	10.7	11.5	12.3	13.1
11.77	15.00	10.0	10.8	11.7	12.5	13.3

Table 7 Thickness Difference *(continued)*

Apex angle (A) in degrees	Thin prism diopter power	High Index Glass, n=1.801 t = Diameter (in mm)* tan(A) (in degrees) at diameters:				
		48mm	52mm	56mm	60mm	64mm
0.18	0.25	0.1	0.2	0.2	0.2	0.2
0.36	0.50	0.3	0.3	0.3	0.4	0.4
0.54	0.75	0.4	0.5	0.5	0.6	0.6
0.72	1.00	0.6	0.6	0.7	0.7	0.8
0.89	1.25	0.7	0.8	0.9	0.9	1.0
1.07	1.50	0.9	1.0	1.0	1.1	1.2
1.25	1.75	1.0	1.1	1.2	1.3	1.4
1.43	2.00	1.2	1.3	1.4	1.5	1.6
1.61	2.25	1.3	1.5	1.6	1.7	1.8
1.79	2.50	1.5	1.6	1.7	1.9	2.0
1.96	2.75	1.6	1.8	1.9	2.1	2.2
2.14	3.00	1.8	1.9	2.1	2.2	2.4
2.32	3.25	1.9	2.1	2.3	2.4	2.6
2.50	3.50	2.1	2.3	2.4	2.6	2.8
2.68	3.75	2.2	2.4	2.6	2.8	3.0
2.85	4.00	2.4	2.6	2.8	3.0	3.2
3.03	4.25	2.5	2.8	3.0	3.2	3.4
3.21	4.50	2.7	2.9	3.1	3.4	3.6
3.39	4.75	2.8	3.1	3.3	3.5	3.8
3.56	5.00	3.0	3.2	3.5	3.7	4.0
3.74	5.25	3.1	3.4	3.7	3.9	4.2
3.91	5.50	3.3	3.6	3.8	4.1	4.4
4.09	5.75	3.4	3.7	4.0	4.3	4.6
4.27	6.00	3.6	3.9	4.2	4.5	4.8
4.44	6.25	3.7	4.0	4.4	4.7	5.0
4.62	6.50	3.9	4.2	4.5	4.8	5.2

4.79	6.75	4.0	4.4	4.7	5.0	5.4
4.97	7.00	4.2	4.5	4.9	5.2	5.6
5.14	7.25	4.3	4.7	5.0	5.4	5.8
5.32	7.50	4.5	4.8	5.2	5.6	6.0
5.49	7.75	4.6	5.0	5.4	5.8	6.2
5.66	8.00	4.8	5.2	5.6	5.9	6.3
5.84	8.25	4.9	5.3	5.7	6.1	6.5
6.01	8.50	5.1	5.5	5.9	6.3	6.7
6.18	8.75	5.2	5.6	6.1	6.5	6.9
6.35	9.00	5.3	5.8	6.2	6.7	7.1
6.53	9.25	5.5	5.9	6.4	6.9	7.3
6.70	9.50	5.6	6.1	6.6	7.0	7.5
6.87	9.75	5.8	6.3	6.7	7.2	7.7
7.04	10.00	5.9	6.4	6.9	7.4	7.9
7.21	10.25	6.1	6.6	7.1	7.6	8.1
7.38	10.50	6.2	6.7	7.3	7.8	8.3
7.55	10.75	6.4	6.9	7.4	7.9	8.5
7.72	11.00	6.5	7.0	7.6	8.1	8.7
7.88	11.25	6.6	7.2	7.8	8.3	8.9
8.05	11.50	6.8	7.4	7.9	8.5	9.1
8.22	11.75	6.9	7.5	8.1	8.7	9.2
8.39	12.00	7.1	7.7	8.3	8.8	9.4
8.55	12.25	7.2	7.8	8.4	9.0	9.6
8.72	12.50	7.4	8.0	8.6	9.2	9.8
8.89	12.75	7.5	8.1	8.8	9.4	10.0
9.05	13.00	7.6	8.3	8.9	9.6	10.2
9.21	13.25	7.8	8.4	9.1	9.7	10.4
9.38	13.50	7.9	8.6	9.2	9.9	10.6
9.54	13.75	8.1	8.7	9.4	10.1	10.8
9.71	14.00	8.2	8.9	9.6	10.3	10.9
9.87	14.25	8.3	9.0	9.7	10.4	11.1
10.03	14.50	8.5	9.2	9.9	10.6	11.3
10.19	14.75	8.6	9.3	10.1	10.8	11.5
10.35	15.00	8.8	9.5	10.2	11.0	11.7